GLUTEN
TOXICITY

The Mysterious Symptoms of
Celiac Disease, Dermatitis Herpetiformis,
and Non-Celiac Gluten Intolerance

SHELLY L. STUART, B.SC.N.
REGISTERED NURSE

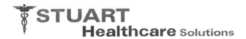

STUART
Healthcare Solutions

Gluten Toxicity

Published by:
Stuart Healthcare Solutions
British Columbia, Canada
www.stuarthealthcare.com

ISBN 13: 978-1453864111
ISBN 10: 1-453864113

Library and Archives Canada Cataloguing in Publication

Stuart, Shelly, 1966-
    Gluten toxicity : the mysterious symptoms of celiac disease, dermatitis
herpetiformis and non-celiac gluten intolerance / Shelly Stuart.

Includes bibliographical references and index.
ISBN 978-1-4538-6411-1

    1. Celiac disease--Diagnosis.   2. Dermatitis herpetiformis--Diagnosis.
3. Gluten-free diet.   I. Title.

RC862.C44S78 2010   616.3'99   C2010-907862-4

Cover & Book Design by:
Randal W. Stuart, P.Eng.

Cover Photo by:
Shelly L. Stuart, R.N., B.Sc.N.

Table of Contents

Chapter 18
Thirty Lifestyle Tips To Help Ease The Transition

Chapter 19
Celiac Disease: Helping The Villi Heal

Chapter 20
What If The Gluten-Free Diet Doesn't Work?

Chapter 21
Could A Grain-Free, Specific Carbohydrate, Paleolithic, Or Elimination
Diet Be Helpful?

Chapter 22
Charts To Track Progress

Chapter 23
Two Alternative Approaches To Relieve Allergies

Chapter 24
Food Can Heal Or Make You Ill: Could Other Autoimmune Diseases Be Triggered By Immune Reactions To Food?

Chapter 25
Food For Thought: Would A Healthy Gluten-Free Diet During Childhood Along with Probiotics Decrease The High Prevalence Of Other Food Allergies?

Bibliography

Acknowledgments

First, I would like to thank my husband, Randal, and my 3 wonderful daughters, Sydney, Madeline, and Nicole for their endless support and encouragement. They are my pillars of inspiration and strength. My mission to increase awareness and to help people who are suffering would not be possible without their understanding and support.

Secondly, I would like to thank my parents for teaching me how to maintain a good work ethic, a positive view and for teaching me that the possibilities in this world are endless. Other family acknowledgments include my four brothers, my brother's spouses, and other relatives who have contributed. Their encouragement and ongoing support is greatly appreciated.

Thirdly, I would like to thank the professors, at Ryerson University in Toronto, for teaching me to think outside of the box, to continually strive for self improvement, and to always question and pursue a better way. Respect for others, perseverance, and pursuit of excellence were continuously promoted. Thank you, I will always benefit from your teachings.

In finishing my acknowledgments, I would like to extend my warmest gratitude to the researchers, doctors (naturopathic, chiropractic, and medical), nurses, dietitians, and support groups who recognize the three forms of gluten intolerance. Their collaborative efforts have significantly improved the health of people, globally, who have been suffering from undiagnosed celiac disease, dermatitis herpetiformis, and non-celiac gluten intolerance. They are truly the heroes and heroines in this race to end the suffering and to save lives.

Disclaimer

The information contained in this book is merely intended to communicate material which is helpful and educational to the reader. It is not intended to replace a medical diagnosis or treatment by a doctor, but rather to provide information which may help increase the rate of diagnosis with celiac disease, dermatitis herpetiformis and non-celiac gluten intolerance. The tips and information provided in this book should be reviewed with your doctor. This book should never be used as medical advice or in place of a visit to a physician. You should always seek the advice of a qualified health care professional with any questions you may have and have all of your symptoms assessed by a medical doctor. If you have or suspect you have a medical problem, promptly contact a doctor.

Information about my gluten-free diet is shared, but this information shouldn't replace a doctor or registered dietitian's advice. As well, toxicities can occur with vitamin or mineral supplements, please consult a doctor and registered dietitian before supplementing. Always seek the advice of your physician and a registered dietitian prior to starting any new diet, treatments, supplements, before making any health related changes, or with any questions you may have regarding a medical condition.

There are no warranties. In no event will the author of this book be liable, based on any legal theory, for any damages of any kind, howsoever caused, resulting from the use of this information including, without limitation, for any error or misstatement that may exist within this book. Review everything in this book with a physician (preferably one who is knowledgeable about gluten intolerance) before making any changes.

Websites, blogs, books, or health professionals mentioned in this book are to be used at your own risk, there are no guarantees or endorsements. Their knowledge, credentials, skills and services that they offer will have to be individually assessed by each consumer. Any consultations are at your own risk.

Some of the studies I used for this book are case studies. The case studies do not conclusively mean that a link between gluten intolerance and the symptoms (mentioned in each case study) exist. Case studies are not conclusive because the association may be a coincidence, they just demonstrate that a link may exist. Large controlled studies can clarify if a link is present. I still mentioned these symptoms in this book because I think everyone should be aware of the possibilities.

Introduction

Wheat was a staple food in our house. During my childhood, I loved how the lovely smell of fresh pies, bread, cookies, buns, or other treats baking in the oven filled the entire house. Waking up to the smell of pancakes or my grandmother's Chelsea buns was always a special treat. I grew to love and appreciate the value of making baked products from scratch, using primarily wheat flour, but also rye, barley and oats. In my own kitchen, I frequently made French loaves, cinnamon bread, Chelsea buns, pie crusts, cakes, apple strudel, tarts, homemade pasta, and many other tasty treats from scratch. I never suspected these foods that I lovingly made for myself and my family, could have toxic effects on every physiological system in our bodies. The realization of that reality was quite a shock!

The path of ill health that led to my diagnosis was long, twisted, full of potholes (symptoms), and broken bridges (misdiagnoses). Only after diagnosis, did the path begin to straighten, the potholes filled, and the bridges mended. With this new path, I finally was able to heal myself and truly nourish my body with the gluten-free foods that I was genetically designed to eat.

Even though this journey was a struggle, I know I am very lucky. Currently, only 3% (approximately) of the people with celiac disease are diagnosed. Unfortunately, the other 97% are unaware that their symptoms are related to the ingestion of gluten (wheat, rye, barley, and for some people oats), and are living a decreased quality of life with the risk of multiple complications [7].

As well, many are living with a non-celiac gluten intolerance, which is both very under recognized and under diagnosed. Combined, all the forms of undiagnosed gluten intolerance can lead to unnecessary suffering, increased doctor's visits, increased hospital visits, and possible death due to all the associated complications. This can drastically reduce an individual's quality of life and adds an additional strain to an already overstressed healthcare system.

This book will discuss the many elusive ways gluten can affect all the systems of the body in gluten intolerant individuals. I reviewed large and small quantitative studies, case studies, and multiple articles while compiling this book. Also included, are my personal stories, patient's stories and many other stories from people internationally. These stories help to demonstrate how the symptoms can range from vague to very pronounced and obvious.

While reviewing the literature and conversing with doctors, I noticed that many physicians have different views related to the diagnosis and management of celiac disease, dermatitis herpetiformis, and non-celiac gluten intolerance. Therefore, patients who are consulting their doctor about gluten intolerance may only hear one point of view. My goal is to present all approaches in a collective and objective style. My hope is that this information will empower people so that they can have a knowledgeable discussion with their doctor and co-actively create a plan for diagnosis and a plan of care that is individualized to their needs. My belief is that more patient involvement equals better patient outcomes.

Lack Of Awareness Put Me At Risk

I was misdiagnosed and given a variety of explanations for my vague symptoms for most of my life. Unfortunately, even when the symptoms were obvious, misdiagnosis still occurred. For example, I was misdiagnosed with irritable bowel syndrome when I had classic celiac disease symptoms for 5 years prior to my diagnosis.

Eventually, I diagnosed myself by doing my own research and initiating a gluten-free diet to see if it provided symptom relief. Successful, I approached a gastroenterologist and confirmed my diagnosis.

This lack of awareness put me at risk for complications and at risk for a false negative test result since consuming a gluten-free diet prior to diagnosis can lead to false negatives. Unfortunately, delayed diagnosis is very common in many countries. This often leads to an increased risk of developing other autoimmune diseases, lymphomas, cancers, allergies, complications from malabsorption issues, possible decreased immune response to other illnesses, and many other health complications that will be discussed in this book.

What Inspired Me To Create This Book?

Inspiration #1: My love for my family has been a powerful motivator for the creation of this book. Gluten intolerance is very prevalent in my family. Therefore, this book is my gift to my current and future family members (grandchildren, great grandchildren, etc). I feel that this guide provides the information they will need to get diagnosed and to help improve their health once diagnosed. For many years to come, my infinite love and guidance can be passed on through this book.

Inspiration #2: Many are suffering and quite likely many are dying globally due to undiagnosed celiac disease, dermatitis herpetiformis and non-celiac gluten intolerance. This breaks my heart when I think of grandparents being lost due to dementia or illness, couples dealing with infertility or pregnancy issues (potentially leading to loss of a baby), mothers and fathers struggling with illness, children with cognitive disabilities affecting their ability to achieve their potential in life, and many others who are suffering with a variety of misdiagnoses.

This is what I visualized while I wrote this book. I shed tears a number of times just thinking of all the people who are afflicted by gluten intolerance. I am hoping that this book will help others to recognize that a link may exist between their symptoms and the ingestion of gluten. Recognition, diagnosis, and a gluten-free diet may be all that is needed to increase their quality of life and end the suffering.

CHAPTER 1
The Three Types Of Gluten Intolerance

This chapter describes gluten and the three types of gluten intolerance, celiac disease (CD), dermatitis herpetiformis (DH), and non-celiac gluten intolerance. As well, gender differences and the need for increased diagnosis is discussed.

Gluten: Gluten is a protein found in wheat, rye, and barley. Some people may react to oats as well. My gluten-free diet, including more information about oats, is discussed in Chapter 17.

Celiac Disease: The ingestion of gluten causes bowel damage in individuals with CD. The associated inflammation, nutrient deficiencies, and auto-immune activity can lead to a variety of symptoms throughout the body.

Dermatitis Herpetiformis: The ingestion of gluten can lead to immune related damage that can cause an itchy skin rash. Bowel damage can occur in this population, but isn't always present. Other symptoms can occur throughout the body.

Non-Celiac Gluten Intolerance: With non-celiac gluten intolerance, the tests for CD and DH are negative, but symptoms occur with the ingestion of gluten. Damage, inflammation, and related symptoms can occur throughout the body.

Gluten Intolerance Or Gluten Sensitivity: General names used for the three types of gluten intolerance including celiac disease, dermatitis herpetiformis, and non-celiac gluten intolerance.

Treatment: The treatment for all three types of gluten intolerance is a strict gluten-free diet. After a period of time, symptoms usually disappear with this diet. Although, some symptoms may not resolve if the damage is permanent or if there are other contributing factors (see Chapter 20, "What If The Gluten-Free Diet Doesn't Work").

Other treatments, such as digestive enzyme therapy, probiotics, medications to treat damaged or inflamed areas and vitamins may also be recommended by your doctor.

The previous definitions provide a very simple description for people that don't want the extra detail. For others, continue reading this chapter for more information.

What Is Gluten?

Gluten is made of two types of peptides, glutenin and prolamins. In gluten intolerant individuals, the prolamins are the specific antigens within gluten that can trigger a cascade of immune reactions. The toxic prolamins include gliadin (in wheat), secalin (in rye), and hordein (in barley). Some people react to the prolamin in oats (avenin) as well. Chapter 17 discusses concerns with oat consumption in more detail.

There are other prolamins, found in rice (orzenin) and corn (zein). However, these two prolamins do not appear to trigger a reaction in people with a gluten intolerance, unless the person has developed a separate rice and/or corn allergy. For example, I have a gluten intolerance (CD) and an allergy to rice and corn.

In dough, gluten is valued for its elasticity and its ability to give baked products structure and form with a pleasant texture. It is also valued for its ability to trap air and make products rise while baking. For these reasons, gluten is in most processed or baked foods, not just breads, cakes and pasta.

Since gluten has been valued traditionally for these amazing culinary properties, grains have been genetically modified to contain a higher content of gluten. Once ingested, our digestive system is ill equipped to deal with this gluten overload, since we are deficient in the digestive enzymes that are needed to deal with the large protein chains in gluten. The result, undigested gluten remaining in the bowel begins to cause a cascade of events that can lead to many symptoms. Chapter 2, "Pathophysiology: The Chain Of Reactions That Lead to Symptoms" discusses this further.

What Is Celiac Disease And Dermatitis Herpetiformis?

Celiac Disease

Celiac disease (CD) is a permanent autoimmune disease that can cause inflammation and damage to the small intestine. Alternate names for celiac disease include coeliac disease, c(o)eliac sprue, gluten sensitive enteropathy, Gee-Herter-Heubner disease, endemic sprue, gluten intolerance and non-tropical sprue.

In individuals with undiagnosed CD, the immune system reacts when gluten is ingested. The small intestinal (bowel) villi, responsible for absorbing nutrients, become damaged, creating a flattened mucosal surface (villus flattening) that is less able to absorb nutrients. Autoimmune reactions to ingested gluten, cross-react with intestinal villi and this leads to the villi damage. Various nutrient deficiencies can occur, and this can affect every physiological system, resulting in many symptoms. Furthermore, autoimmune reactions can cause damage to other areas of the body which can lead to inflammation, tissue destruction and more symptoms. Without treatment, permanent damage can occur.

Villi are finger-like projections in the small intestine and are discussed more in Chapter 19, "Celiac Disease: Helping The Villi Heal".

Dermatitis Herpetiformis

Autoimmune reactions can lead to dermatitis herpetiformis (DH), a form of celiac disease (CD) that affects the skin with an itchy blistering rash. In many with DH, bowel damage can occur as well. The additional presence of nutrient deficiencies, resulting from bowel damage, can add to the severity of the skin lesions, impair the healing process, and affect other parts of the body. With DH, autoimmune activity may cause damage and symptoms in other areas of the body as well.

Other individuals with DH don't appear to have any bowel damage. However, these people may have bowel changes occurring, but the tests used may not be detecting the damage yet. As a result, this group only shows positive results with the DH skin biopsy and can have negative celiac tests results. A positive skin biopsy for DH means that the person should maintain a gluten-free diet (even if the CD tests results are negative).

See Chapter 7 about skin rashes for more detail.

What Is Non-Celiac Gluten Intolerance?

Like CD, individuals with non-celiac gluten intolerance experience symptoms when they eat gluten. However, it is different from CD in that these individuals don't appear to have any villi damage in the small intestine.

Unfortunately, this diagnosis could be due to false negative blood tests and false negative intestinal biopsy results for CD, which can occur, and is discussed more in the diagnosis chapter. In this situation, the limitations of the CD tests may miss the true CD diagnosis and lead to a non-celiac gluten intolerance diagnosis. This misdiagnosis can put patients at risk, since related nutrient deficiencies may not be recognized, and this could lead to many ongoing symptoms and permanent damage [7].

With a true non-celiac gluten intolerance, immune related damage is present in other areas of the body (with no intestinal villi damage). However, bowel symptoms can still develop. The removal of gluten from the diet makes the symptoms disappear, unless the person has other additional food allergies, an intolerance, or other factors (diseases, infections, etc) contributing to the symptoms (see more in Chapter 20, "What If The Gluten-Free Diet Doesn't Work").

To summarize, CD and non-celiac gluten intolerance have similarities. Both are triggered by the ingestion of gluten, both can affect almost every physiological system in the body with many possible symptoms, and gastrointestinal (bowel) symptoms can occur with both. The only difference is that intestinal villi damage along with related nutrient deficiencies appear to only occur with CD (and in some with DH).

It is important to recognize that nutrient deficiencies may also occur in non-celiac gluten intolerance for a variety of other reasons, such as poor diet, poor appetite, lack of digestive enzymes, the presence of diarrhea and vomiting, or other malabsorption issues.

Why Are So Few Diagnosed?

Only 3% of individuals with CD are diagnosed [27]. This is mainly due to lack of awareness amongst doctors and nurses in the health care system and in the general public. The percentage of people diagnosed with non-celiac gluten intolerance is likely greater, since it is even less recognized than CD.

Only people who are very ill tend to get diagnosed (if they are lucky), while others are diagnosed only through association with a celiac relative. Some individuals may also get diagnosed if there is a screening program in place or if a study requires screening for a designated number of people. Unfortunately, the screening programs are not plentiful enough and there are not enough studies to effectively diagnose everyone.

The medical profession needs to increase their awareness so that people can be diagnosed before they become critically ill, sometimes with permanent psychological, cognitive and/or physiological damage. Gluten intolerance is a worldwide global issue. Every ethnic community and age group can potentially be affected. Millions are suffering unnecessarily.

Are There Gender Differences?

The prevalence of CD is fairly equal between men and women [27,28]. Historically, doctors believed that CD was more prevalent in females because it was diagnosed more in women. The higher rate of diagnosis in females may have occurred because women are conditioned to see the doctor regularly for gynecological and obstetrical issues. Regular contact with the doctor may increase the chance that women may share their symptoms on a frequent basis. This could increase the chances of being diagnosed.

As well, the symptoms of CD may become more pronounced during a woman's child-bearing years due to malabsorption issues. There are more nutritional demands on the body while pregnant and a compromised bowel may not be able to meet the demands. Anemia, infertility, miscarriages, intrauterine growth restriction of the fetus, or other obstetrical symptoms may have led to a higher rate of diagnosis in the past.

The prevalence of DH is also fairly equal between men and women [27,34]. Historically, research showed a higher prevalence in men. The reason for this is unclear. Perhaps, men generally had more obvious skin symptoms than woman. This could have increased their chance of diagnosis and led to a higher prevalence in the past.

Future research will help to reveal if there are any gender differences in non-celiac gluten intolerance.

CHAPTER 2

Pathophysiology: The Chain Of Reactions That Lead to Symptoms

This chapter contains information about the chain of reactions that can lead to the symptoms in celiac disease (CD), dermatitis herpetiformis (DH), and non-celiac gluten intolerance. With CD and DH, the ingestion of gluten triggers an immune response that leads to damage, inflammation and symptoms in many different parts of the body. The presence of bowel damage can lead to nutrient deficiencies and this can lead to many additional symptoms [1].

With non-celiac gluten intolerance, the ingestion of gluten can lead to a variety of symptoms throughout the body, but the chain of reactions that lead to these symptoms is less clear. There are a few theories that are outlined in the following pages.

Three Contributing Factors

A combination of three contributing factors can trigger the development of CD and DH. These factors include a genetic predisposition, an environmental influence (i.e. gluten, lectins, stress, infection, pregnancy, etc), and a leaky gut leading to an immune response and physiological damage (i.e. damaged villi in small intestine and/or damaged skin) [61-63].

The triggers for non-celiac gluten intolerance are less clear, but may follow the same path. The ingestion of gluten and increased bowel permeability is certainly a factor. Research has demonstrated immune involvement with gluten ataxia so it is reasonable to suspect there is immune activity with other forms of non-celiac gluten intolerance [29,31,32]. As well, the presence of antigliadin antibodies (antibodies against gliadin) in patients with non-celiac gluten intolerance helps to confirm that there is immune activity [73-75]. More research is needed to look at genetic susceptibilities, to clarify the types of immune activity involved and to investigate other environmental influences.

For me, a genetic component is obvious since my mother, my daughter, and I all have
CD. I believe my environmental triggers included the ingestion of gluten, perhaps a

virus, the physiological stress of my pregnancies and the hormonal shifts that occurred at the 3 week postpartum period.

I had vague symptoms for most of my life. However, my pronounced symptoms seemed to be triggered and re-triggered at the 3 week postpartum period with all 3 of my pregnancies.

Antigliadin antibodies are discussed further in the diagnosis chapter.

Is Gluten Difficult For Everyone To Digest And How Does This Lead To A Leaky Gut?

Unfortunately, gluten appears to be a difficult protein for everyone to digest. Humans don't have all of the gastric (stomach), brush border (intestinal), and pancreatic (pancreas) enzymes necessary to break it into individual micromolecules so that it can be digested easily [52,53,60]. As a result, these large protein chains remain more or less intact and its presence in the small intestine tends to relax the tight intercellular junctions (like gates) between the intestinal cells [51,54,65,88].

The relaxed gates stimulate the increased expression of zonulin, a human protein, in the intestinal tissues. Zonulin stimulates the gates to open further, breaking the body's first line of defense against invaders (i.e. undigested gluten). These open gates allow the undigested gluten to enter into the body where it can interact with the immune system and trigger a reaction [60,64,88]. This demonstrates that gluten can potentially promote a leaky gut in everyone and this increases the risk of an immune response. Once an immune response is triggered, the immune-related damage, inflammation, and nutrient deficiencies can further impair bowel integrity.

One study highlights the possibility that all individuals may have an immune reaction to gluten [29]. In this study, researchers found that an immune factor in all of the biopsied intestinal tissue, from patients with CD and without CD, reacted to crude gliadin. All of the cultures reacted with an immune response (interleukin-15).

The immune response, mentioned above, supports the theory that everyone could have an immune system response to gluten. This reaction could lead to cellular damage, inflammation and increased intestinal permeability (leaky gut). This leaky gut effect would potentiate the effect of undigested gluten on gut permeability. With these two influencing factors combined, there would be an increased risk of developing CD, DH, or a non-celiac gluten intolerance.

Other factors can also increase the leaky gut effect. These factors can include certain medications, viruses, bacterial infections, stress, nutrient deficiencies (from a poor diet), caffeine, alcohol, lectins, refined carbohydrates, and the presence of other diseases or parasites.

Like a ticking time bomb, perhaps, everyone who is ingesting gluten has the potential for an unfavorable outcome (i.e. cancer, autoimmune damage, other immune reactions, nutrient deficiencies and possibly permanent damage). For some, gluten may be the only trigger needed to cause a cascade of immune reactions. For others, additional triggers (virus, stress, pregnancy, etc), may also be needed before the immune system reacts and the onset of symptoms is noticed.

The Pathophysiology Of Celiac Disease

As described previously, undigested gluten relaxes the gates between the intestinal cells, zonulin is released and this further impairs the body's first line of defense (the mucosal barrier). With CD, the undigested gluten enters the body and then it triggers a cascade of immunological events in people that are genetically predisposed [56,60,64,88].

Tissue transglutaminase, an enzyme responsible for tissue repair, has an affinity for undigested gluten peptides, it chemically alters (deamidates) it into a more toxic form. Then, antigen presenting cells (APC) in the innate immune system act as a second line of defense. These cells are continuously policing our bodies looking for invaders that shouldn't be there (i.e. viruses, bacteria, undigested deamidated gluten). In CD, the antigen presenting cells can include macrophages, dendritic cells , and also B-cells [1,2,44,48,55,56,72].

The APC, in the submucosa of the bowel, with the expressed genes HLA-DQ2 and HLA-DQ8 (may be other genes too), has an affinity for this toxic deamidated gluten (also called negatively charged glutamic acid residues) and engulfs it. This leads to another type of molecular complex that stimulates the activated APC to release cytokines and interferon (chemical messengers) that alert the adaptive immune system (third line of defense) [1,2,44, 48,55,56,72].

The adaptive immune system has two parts, the humoral immune system (makes antibodies) and the cell-mediated immune system (makes T-cells). The humoral part of the adaptive immune system produces B cells which create antibodies that can tag invader cells (i.e. gluten) for destruction. Unfortunately, in celiac disease, the immune system doesn't just make antibodies against the gliadin in gluten (antigliadin antibodies) or the deamidated gluten, it cross reacts and produces antibodies against tissue transglutaminase (this can further hinder tissue repair) and against the endomysial tissue lining the intestinal tract. The presence of these auto-antibodies is destructive because they can tag our own tissue in our bowel for destruction [1,2,44].

Antibodies can also cause their own destructive damage by attacking the antigens (i.e. gliadin, deamidated gluten or our tissue) with chemicals called complement, neutralizing the antigens, or by recruiting other immune cells (i.e. T-cells, phagocytes) to help destroy the perceived invader. The development of additional auto-antibodies can tag tissue in other areas of our body as well leading to a variety of symptoms [2,49].

Once the T-cells are activated, the destructive damage intensifies. Helper T cells produce cytokines that help to direct immune responses and cytotoxic T cells (killer T cells) produce granules that are toxic to the perceived invader cells. In CD, this attack is launched on the invaders that have been tagged in the small intestinal mucosa (i.e. gluten, deamidated gluten, tissue transglutaminase, endomysial tissue) and elsewhere in the body. An immunological war ensues with an intense inflammatory reaction and tissue damage [2, 49].

In the small intestinal villi, intraepithelial lymphocytes (natural killer cells, B-cells, T-cells) infiltrate, intestinal cell production decreases, circulation can be affected, the crypts (area at base of and between villi) thicken and the structural support for the villi is threatened. The villi flatten in a patchy nature typically starting in the duodenum (area below the stomach) and this damage works its way distally in the small intestine [49].

Prior to the intestinal damage, the small intestinal villi release digestive enzymes while mixing with the ingested food. Once digested, the food is absorbed into the body through the villi. Due to immune reactions, the flattened dysfunctional villi can no longer do this and deficiencies develop. The deficiencies and other autoimmune reactions combined can lead to many symptoms that can potentially affect every part of the body.

The Pathophysiology Of Dermatitis Herpetiformis

With dermatitis herpetiformis (DH), the immune reactions lead to a skin rash. Approximately 80% of these patients have all of the immunological reactions that lead to intestinal villi damage as well. In the other 20 %, there is no evidence of small intestinal villi damage, but there may be intraepithelial lymphocytes evident in the small intestinal villi. Since so many do have intestinal involvement, this disease is considered a form of celiac disease [4-6].

As discussed under CD, IgA anti-tissue transglutaminase antibodies can develop against tissue transglutaminase 2 in the intestinal mucosa. Scientists theorize that these auto-antibodies can also cross react to epidermal (in the skin) transglutaminase 3 (eTG) which is an enzyme that contributes to skin cell health. For me, this makes sense, if antibodies can react to one type of transglutaminase in the body (i.e. in the bowel), then these antibodies will quite likely react to other transglutaminases (i.e. eTG) since the various types are homologous in nature. The associated cell destruction and inflammation could lead to the skin rash associated with DH [4-6].

Scientists also suspect that the IgA/eTG complex could circulate in the bloodstream and deposit in different skin regions. The immune system would react to the IgA/eTG deposits in the skin since they would be viewed as foreign. This type of reaction could add to the inflammation and skin damage characteristic of DH. Anti-eTG IgA auto-antibodies (antibodies against transglutaminase in the skin) have been found in the blood of DH patients and granular IgA deposits with eTG has also been found in skin biopsies of affected individuals which helps to strengthen this theory [4-6].

Other immune factors may also contribute, the pathophysiology isn't completely clear. There are still some mysteries that future research will help to clarify.

The fact that dermatitis herpetiformis can just affect the skin with no intestinal damage demonstrates that gluten intolerance (complete with auto-immune reactions) can affect other areas of the body without damaging the intestine. Therefore, gluten intolerance is not just an intestinal condition.

The Pathophysiology Of Non-Celiac Gluten Intolerance

In people with a non-celiac gluten intolerance, the chain of reactions that lead to symptoms is less clear. As previously discussed, undigested gluten in the small intestine can lead to increased bowel permeability (leaky gut) and this can increase the likelihood of an immune reaction. Antibodies to gliadin have been found in patients with a non-celiac gluten intolerance which helps to demonstrate that an immune reaction is involved. With gluten ataxia, antibodies to transglutaminase 6 have also been found which demonstrates that an autoimmune reaction is possible [29,50,74,76-81]. I suspect that autoimmune reactions are involved with other forms of non-celiac gluten intolerance as well.

Gluten ataxia is a form of non-celiac gluten intolerance that affects the nervous system.

In a study, IgA deposits on transglutaminase 2 were found in jejunal biopsies taken from the small intestine of patients with gluten ataxia [74]. With this in mind, perhaps, all patients with non-celiac gluten intolerance have these deposits in their jejunal tissue demonstrating that there is some intestinal involvement. I wouldn't be surprised, it seems plausible that there would be immune reactions in the bowel since the gluten would first encounter the immune system in that location. Perhaps, CD, DH, and non-celiac gluten intolerance are more similar than we realize.

More research is needed to thoroughly examine the pathophysiology behind non-celiac gluten intolerance. For now, some research and emerging theories have attempted to shed light on this type of intolerance. Some of the following theories are currently being considered by researchers, others are just hypothetical possibilities.

Theory 1: Reactions Against Transglutaminases

Like celiac disease, dermatitis herpetiformis and gluten ataxia [4-6,59], perhaps, immune responses to gluten and transglutaminase in the gut leads to autoimmune activity against various forms of transglutaminases throughout the body. The result, IgA and IgG antibodies against tissue transglutaminase reactions could lead to inflammation and autoimmune damage in organs and tissues with transglutaminase. For example, transglutaminase can be found in the bowel, skin, bone, nervous system, lungs, heart, bladder, liver, pancreas, factor XIII (involved in clotting), prostate, uterus, etc. Theoretically, auto-antibodies against tranglutaminases could cause inflammation and damage in these areas. This could lead to a variety of symptoms.

Hypothetically, immune reactions to gluten and cross reactions against tissue transglutaminase could be the underlying culprit in the varying forms of non-celiac gluten intolerance. Inflammation and damage could result in symptoms throughout the body. This type of reaction could be responsible for many diseases, syndromes, and autoimmune diseases not yet linked to gluten intolerance. I believe researchers need to take a close look at tissue transglutaminase's role in various areas of the body, how it is affected with different illnesses, and how the ingestion of gluten may be promoting a cross reaction against tissue transglutaminase in those illnesses.

Tissue transglutaminase is a very important enzyme. Without it, tissue repair is hindered, possibly leading to inflammation and damage in the area of the body where the enzyme is not available. With CD, tissue transglutaminase 2 is damaged by antibodies in the bowel, antibodies against tissue transglutaminase 3 occur in DH and antibodies attack tissue transglutaminase 6 in gluten ataxia [1,4,50]. It seems reasonable to suspect that cross reactions to tissue transglutaminase could occur throughout the body in gluten intolerant individuals.

Theory 2: Undigested Gluten, Deamidated Gluten, And Immune Complexes

Possibly, the undigested gluten, toxic deamidated gluten, or other immune complexes could circulate and cause many problems in various organs and tissues in the body. It could become lodged and affect the function of the organ or tissue. This would likely elicit an immune response since the complex would be perceived as an invader.

As well, undigested gluten in the bowel may provide food for the bad bacteria, fungi, and other microorganisms leading to many intestinal symptoms (i.e. vomiting, diarrhea, gas, abdominal distension and nausea). Ongoing growth of the fungi (i.e. candidiasis) or bacteria could lead to other symptoms in the body as well.

Theory 3: Exomorphins

Gluten may have pharmacological effects on our bodies. Exomorphins are opiate type proteins found in casein (a milk protein) and gluten. These proteins may have a sedating, analgesic type of effect, on individuals who are sensitive (morphine-like effect) [82,83].

This may contribute to neurological and cognitive symptoms. People who feel they have a non-celiac gluten and dairy intolerance may have a sensitivity to the exomorphins in these foods.

Of interest, some people may experience withdrawal when these foods are removed from their diet.

The diagnosis chapter discusses exomorphins further under "Urinary Peptide Tests".

Theory 4: Lectins

Lectins are glycoproteins that are present in grains (even gluten-free grains) and some other foods such as legumes, seeds, nightshades (i.e. potatoes, tomatoes, etc) and dairy. Like gluten, lectins are difficult to digest. However, due to their small size and possible effect on bowel permeability, they are easily absorbed [8-28,30-47,66-70].

Lectins can be toxic to humans. Research (animal and human) suggests that lectins may increase inflammation, can increase bowel permeability, and may stimulate immune responses, possibly increasing the risk for autoimmune diseases. According to studies,

13

lectins may also affect the nervous system, the joints, hormonal levels, the cell cycle, the health of platelets, our renal system and may be disruptive to our endocrine system (affecting insulin levels) [8-28,30-47,66-70].

IgA and IgG antibodies against wheat germ agglutinin (WGA), a type of lectin, have been found in patients with celiac disease demonstrating that our immune system can react to these glycoproteins. The fact that these antibodies don't react to gluten, only WGA, further demonstrates that they are specifically reacting to lectins [8,9,32].

Theoretically, lectins may increase the risk for a gluten intolerance due to the effects on bowel permeability [15,27,28,34,46,77]. As well, the antibodies against lectins along with other immune responses may add to the damage associated with non-celiac gluten intolerance. The presence of a lectin intolerance could also add to CD and DH symptoms. With this in mind, people who think they have a non-celiac gluten intolerance may actually have a sensitivity to lectins or they may have both a gluten and lectin intolerance. An individual with a lectin sensitivity would benefit from a paleolithic diet (see Chapter 21, "Could A Grain-Free, Specific Carbohydrate, Paleolithic, Or Elimination Diet Be Helpful?).

Unfortunately, testing for lectins doesn't seem to be widely available. Hopefully, testing for IgA and IgG antibodies against wheat germ agglutinin (WGA) and antibodies against other forms of lectins will be widely available in the future. Identifying a lectin intolerance early could prevent many complications.

Note: Lectins are a problem if increased bowel permeability occurs and the lectins encounter the immune system or the circulation. Due to gluten and lectin's combined effect on bowel permeability, this seems likely.

Theory 5: Glutamic Acid And Aspartic Acid

According to John B. Symes, D.V.M., wheat, dairy, and soy contain high levels of glutamic acid and aspartic acid. These two non-essential amino acids can over activate the receptors of the nerve cells and lead to excitotoxicity in animals. His research suggests that this can lead to nerve and brain impairments which are evident in many neurodegenerative diseases. Possibly, his findings could be applicable to humans.

With his theory in mind, people who think they have a non-celiac gluten intolerance may have a sensitivity to glutamic acid and aspartic acid.

Website: dogtorj.com

Theory 6: Allergies To Wheat, Rye, Barley, Or Oats

People who think they have a non-celiac gluten intolerance may find that IgE mediated allergies to wheat, rye, barley or oats are responsible for their symptoms. This isn't really a theory since it is well known that this type of allergy can result in a variety of symptoms [86].

People with CD, DH, or non-celiac gluten intolerance typically have negative results with IgE allergy tests for grains that contain gluten (unless they have IgE allergies as well). These conditions are usually IgA and IgG antibody mediated. However, it is possible to have a gluten intolerance and an IgE mediated allergy to these grains. For example, I have celiac disease and an IgE mediated allergy to wheat.

Theory 7: Allergies To Other Foods

An allergy to foods (other than gluten) may also be responsible for a variety of symptoms [86]. This isn't really a theory since it is well known that allergies to foods can cause a variety of symptoms. An allergist and a naturopathic doctor can help to identify the offending foods. An allergist typically just tests for IgE reactions and a naturopathic doctor usually offers blood tests for IgE, IgA, and IgG mediated reactions. Both may offer an elimination diet to help figure out your allergies or to confirm the blood test results (discussed more in Chapters 16 and 21).

People who think they have a non-celiac gluten intolerance may find that other foods are responsible for their symptoms. It is also possible to have a gluten intolerance along with allergies to other foods.

Theory 8: A Food Intolerance

It is possible to have an intolerance to a food due to a lack of enzymes. If a digestive enzyme is diminished or absent, then the food (or part of the food) may sit undigested in the bowel. As the food ferments, it can cause a variety of symptoms. For example, lactose intolerance can lead to a variety of gastrointestinal symptoms.

With this in mind, people who think they have a non-celiac gluten intolerance may really have a different food intolerance. It is also possible to have both a gluten intolerance along with an additional food intolerance. Ask your doctor for testing to investigate this possibility. Enzyme supplementation may be necessary.

Note: The immunological responses in the three types of gluten intolerance are very complex. Many mysteries remain and new information is continuously being released. Therefore, the previous information is a summary of my current under-standing of the pathophysiology related to celiac disease, dermatitis herpetiformis, and non-celiac gluten intolerance.

More Research Needed

More research is needed to help solve the mysteries and to clarify the similarities and differences in pathophysiology between celiac disease, dermatitis herpetiformis and non-celiac gluten intolerance.

With ongoing research, likely many more theories will emerge and more immunogenic proteins may be identified in grains and other foods that we may not be genetically designed to eat.

CHAPTER 3
The Symptoms

Under Recognized And Under Diagnosed

Celiac Disease (CD), dermatitis herpetiformis (DH), and non-celiac gluten intolerance are all very under recognized and under diagnosed by the medical community.

With CD, the current estimated prevalence is on average around 1 out of every 100 people (1%). Although, in some countries, studies have suggested that the prevalence is higher (i.e. 5.6% in the Sahara people) [14,15,17]. The prevalence in each country is based on population studies that have randomly tested people for CD. Unfortunately, the studies often only include 2-3 tests from the celiac panel of tests (see diagnosis chapter) and an endoscope is only offered if the blood test is positive. Therefore, many people could be missed with this approach.

As discussed in the diagnosis chapter, false negatives can occur with all the celiac tests. Therefore, false negatives could occur with the blood tests or the endoscope in these studies. In particular, I noticed that many studies don't mention testing to check for IgA and IgG deficiencies. These tests are important to include because deficiencies can cause false negative blood test results. The risk of an IgA deficiency is high since there are more Celiacs with an IgA deficiency than in the average population [16]. Due to all the possible shortfalls associated with testing, I believe the prevalence of CD is much, much higher than is reported through population sampling.

With DH, the estimated prevalence has been shown to be as high as 1 in 400, to as low as 1 in 100,000 [5,11,18-20]. I suspect that the prevalence is higher than these estimates due to the fact that DH can present with a variety of skin symptoms (most are very under recognized) and false negatives can occur with testing, just like CD.

With non-celiac gluten intolerance, the prevalence is likely a staggering number due to the fact that it is even more under recognized than CD and DH. I wouldn't be surprised if most individuals suffered from varying degrees of non-celiac gluten intolerance. Future research will help to reveal the true prevalence. However, identifying a specific number for prevalence will be a challenge due to the pitfalls associated with the diagnostic tests.

Typical vs Atypical Symptoms

Gastrointestinal (GI) symptoms, such as diarrhea, bloating, and weight loss, are generally recognized as typical CD symptoms. Other extra-intestinal symptoms, such as epilepsy, learning problems, migraines, osteoporosis, dementia, and infertility are not as widely recognized and often referred to as atypical [3-5,8,9,11].

An itchy blistering skin rash is thought of as typical for DH, although, DH can present with various types of atypical skin rashes. With non-celiac gluten intolerance, more research is needed to define atypical vs typical symptoms [3-5,8,9,11].

Personally, I think all of the symptoms discussed in this book are likely typical in individuals with a gluten intolerance, just not recognized yet as being typical. Once the other 97% of Celiacs and others with a gluten intolerance are diagnosed, we will have a better picture of what typical is for celiac disease (CD), dermatitis herpetiformis (DH), and non-celiac gluten intolerance.

Silent And Latent Forms Of Gluten Intolerance

Some people develop a latent form of CD and DH, only developing symptoms, associated intestinal and skin damage later in life. This appears to occur with non-celiac gluten intolerance as well.

Other people have a silent form of gluten intolerance with vague or no symptoms. However, immune reactions to gluten are still occurring placing them at risk for complications.

With the latent forms of gluten intolerance, it is possible that the intolerance, as a silent form of CD, DH, or non-celiac gluten intolerance, existed for many years prior to the presentation of symptoms. Due to the late onset of symptoms, diagnosis may only occur once the symptoms and damage become significant enough to be recognized and diagnosed [3-5,8,9, 11].

Incomplete Diagnoses And Misdiagnoses Are Common

Due to lack of awareness, the elusive nature of gluten intolerance may lead some doctors to provide an incomplete diagnosis by only diagnosing the symptoms, such as anemia, gastric reflux (heartburn), lactose intolerance, infertility, ataxia, failure to thrive, lactose intolerance, arthritis, miscarriage, infertility, osteoporosis, aphthous stomatitis (canker sores), dermatitis, epilepsy, myopathies or migraines to mention a few. As well, gluten intolerance can be misdiagnosed as irritable bowel syndrome, lupus erythematosus, fibromyalgia and many other conditions mentioned in the following chapters [3-5,8,9,11].

Unfortunately, delayed diagnosis can place individuals at risk for many complications and sometimes permanent damage. Therefore, early recognition and diagnosis is important for primary prevention.

I was partially diagnosed and misdiagnosed with vague symptoms for 32 years and my mom had vague symptoms for 60 years. From age 32-37yrs, I experienced obvious symptoms.

We both experienced anemia for decades, this should have alerted the doctors to consider a malabsorption issue, but this was never investigated. Only a band-aid (iron pills) was offered as a solution. Eventually, I had obvious gastrointestinal symptoms that were misdiagnosed as irritable bowel syndrome for 5 years. I finally figured out that it was related to gluten and testing confirmed a CD diagnosis.

What If Bowel Symptoms, Stunted Growth, And Weight Loss Are Absent?

While reviewing the symptoms, be aware that gluten intolerance can be present in children that are growing normally so normal growth rate should not be a factor that excludes this possibility [7].

Many individuals with the various forms of gluten intolerance will have no bowel symptoms. As well, weight loss may or may not occur in CD and DH and is dependent on the amount of the intestine that is damaged [5]. It is possible to be overweight with a gluten intolerance. Overall, many of the symptoms discussed in this book could occur in the absence of stunted growth, weight loss, or bowel symptoms.

Presentation Of Symptoms Is Unique With Each Person

Another consideration: Some individuals will only have one or two symptoms (for example, anemia and a rash) and others may have many symptoms. Individuals with silent or latent gluten intolerance may have no symptoms.

Any Gender, Ethnic Group, Or Age Group can Be Affected

One final consideration: Gluten toxicity does not spare any gender, ethnic group, or age group, anyone can be affected.

Could Your Symptoms Be Caused By A Gluten Intolerance?

Ready? Let's proceed and see if you think any of your symptoms could be related to the ingestion of gluten. Chapters 4-13 discuss the symptoms. Chapter 14 discusses some of the associated diseases and there is a symptom checklist in Chapter 15.

Note: Quite likely, there are many other symptoms not mentioned in this book. The science behind all of the various forms of gluten intolerance is still young. The most extensively researched form of gluten intolerance is CD. However, even the knowledge around this disease has many gaps.

Overall, there are several unsolved mysteries and more research may link other symptoms and diseases to gluten intolerance, to lectin intolerance, or may reveal an intolerance to additional proteins present in grains. For now, many people experiencing symptom relief with a gluten-free diet or other therapeutic diets such as a grain free (see Chapter 21), specific carbohydrate (Chapter 21), or paleolithic diet (Chapter 21) are thrilled to finally have a better quality of life.

CHAPTER 4
Gastrointestinal (Digestive) Symptoms

The gastrointestinal (GI) system is essentially a long muscular tube that extends from the mouth to the rectum. It digests and absorbs nutrients, excretes dead intestinal cells, food residues, water, liver and intestinal secretions, and symbiotic bacteria. The salivary glands, stomach, pancreas, liver, and gallbladder aid the process of digestion and absorption. The enteric nervous system located within the intestinal wall controls bowel motility which propels nutrients through the intestinal tube. The enteric nervous system also stimulates the intestine and associated organs to secrete substances necessary for digestion and absorption [1].

The GI system is host to the majority of lymphocytes (players in the immune system) in the body, which means it plays a significant role in immune mediated responses to viruses, bacteria, and parasites. Unfortunately, this also means that GI epithelium, mucosa, villi, and associated organs are particularly susceptible to damage from autoimmune reactions [2]. In celiac disease (CD) and in many patients with dermatitis herpetiformis (DH), this can lead to gastrointestinal damage and a variety of symptoms. With non-celiac gluten intolerance, many of the following digestive symptoms may occur without the bowel damage that defines celiac disease.

Unfortunately, many are misdiagnosed with irritable bowel syndrome.

I was misdiagnosed for 5 years when I had Celiac symptoms that would flare up with diarrhea, bloating, and flatulence. The symptoms would last for awhile, then the symptoms would lessen or disappear for a few months. I saw a Gastroenterologist, was checked for parasites and bacterial infections, had a scope of my colon, and had some blood tests completed. All of the results were normal and I was told I had Irritable Bowel Syndrome. An upper endoscopy of the small intestine with biopsies would have revealed the true source of my symptoms. I wouldn't have had to suffer for an additional 5 years.

21

Diarrhea

Many individuals with an undiagnosed gluten intolerance will have no or very vague bowel symptoms [3,4]. In others, the gastrointestinal tract's transit time is altered, resulting in diarrhea. Loose watery stool can be continuous with many stools per day, or episodic with periods of normal stool occurring in between the episodes of diarrhea, lasting for a few hours, days, or months. Weight loss may or may not occur, is dependent on the amount of the intestine that is damaged (it can be very patchy) and whether diarrhea and vomiting are present [1,4,11].

I didn't have any diarrhea until after I gave birth to my first child, then it was episodic in nature and was usually worse at night and in the morning. My daughter and mother, both with CD, didn't have any loose stools.

There are many influencing factors that promote the development of diarrhea. In CD (and many with DH), an autoimmune reaction to gluten in the proximal small intestine (near the stomach) ignites a cross reaction with the intestinal mucosa, resulting in a damaged flattened mucosal surface (villous flattening). Since the intestinal villi are responsible for absorbing nutrients, malabsorption issues occur, and this contributes to the production of diarrhea. The intestinal nutrient and fluid load exceeds the absorptive capacity of the affected small intestine [9-11].

In addition to issues with the damaged villi, absorption can also be compromised by impaired intestinal endocrine cell secretion of secretin and cholecystokinin (CCK). Since S cells in the duodenum (area in bowel near the stomach) release secretin and I cells in the duodenum release CCK, secretion can be impaired with the CD damage that occurs in this region. These hormones are secreted in response to food, and stimulate the pancreas and gallbladder to release substances to aid digestion. Therefore, impaired secretion of these hormones decreases pancreatic (enzymes and bicarbonate) and gallbladder (bile) secretions into the lumen of the intestine. This hinders the digestive process since pancreatic enzymes and bile help to digest carbohydrates, protein, and fat [1,5,6,20,21,39,45].

Fat malabsorption, evident in steatorrhea (fatty stool), can increase the osmotic load, and the fat along with unabsorbed carbohydrates, electrolytes, protein, and other nutrients can increase stool volume in the colon (large intestine) [8,9,10]. The unabsorbed fat can also contribute to the proliferation of bacteria that feeds on fatty acids, and if damage occurs in the ileum (lower small bowel), then malabsorbed bile salt may also have a cathartic effect [7]. As well, with damaged villi, the secretion of intestinal peptides (digestive enzymes) may be hindered and this can also contribute to the undigested foods in the bowel (i.e. lactose intolerance) [44].

There is one other factor that may contribute to diarrhea as well [1]. As previously mentioned in Chapter 2, no one appears to digest gluten very well. It is possible that undigested gluten in the bowel ferments, producing excess gas and some loose stool. The undigested gluten may also contribute to the proliferation of bacteria and gastrointestinal infections. This could lead to vomiting, diarrhea, gas, abdominal distension and nausea.

Overall, the maladaptive state of the bowel can lead to malabsorption with resulting infections that add to the bulk of diarrhea seen in people with an undiagnosed gluten intolerance.

Steatorrhea

Fatty stool with a foul odor, called steatorrhea, may be seen if the bowel damage in CD (and many with DH) progresses past the proximal small intestine. The color of this stool is greyish or a light tan with a greasy appearance. Stools floating in the toilet bowl can result from the high content of malabsorbed fat in the stool. [11]

I didn't notice any steatorrhea until I was quite ill with extensive weight loss. My mother and daughter didn't have this symptom.

Constipation

Some people experience periods of constipation, either in isolation or alternating with periods of diarrhea. Periods of constipation can follow periods of diarrhea due to the resulting dehydration.

I had constipation that would occur after severe episodes of diarrhea. My daughter and mother didn't have any problems with constipation.

In CD (and many with DH), constipation can occur from compensatory ileal hypertrophy which occurs when the ileum compensates for a chronically inflamed jejunum (area below duodenum) due to longstanding undiagnosed CD. An autoregulatory mechanism (biological adjustments by body) or neurogenic influence (affected by the nervous system) in this adaptive response may be responsible for the bowel's ability to compensate. This functional change may alter the motility of the bowel, resulting in constipation [12].

With all forms of gluten intolerance, reduced intestinal motility (sluggish bowel) might also occur due to immune related damage to intestinal neurocrine (intestinal nervous system), hormonal endocrine (glands that secrete hormones) or the paracrine (endocrine hormone secretion into cells or tissue) tissues [1,9,10].

Abdominal Discomfort, Bloating, And Flatulence

Undigested nutrients, resulting from poor digestion, can ferment in the bowel, resulting in proliferation of bacteria and excess gas production. Copious malodorous flatus can make the abdomen distended, and uncomfortable. Increased stomach grumbling, can result from excess gas in the bowels [8,11].

I intermittently experienced all of these symptoms and often looked like I was 5-6 months pregnant after a meal. My mother had some bloating and my daughter didn't have any of these symptoms.

Nausea and Vomiting

Some, with an undiagnosed gluten intolerance, experience nausea and vomiting [13]. The precise reason for this type of response is unclear, but it may be that chemoreceptor trigger zone stimulation, in the postrema of the medulla area of the brain, stimulation of the nucleus tractus solitarius (also in the brain), and stimulation of the brain stem vomiting center may occur in response to gluten consumption [1].

As well, gastritis (inflamed stomach) is associated with gluten intolerance. The presence of gastritis can lead to nausea and vomiting [46,47].

My daughter and I often experienced nausea.

Heartburn, Burping, And Feelings Of Fullness

Indigestion, burping, belching, and feelings of fullness (dyspepsia) can result from the impaired stomach contractions, poor stomach emptying, and immunological effects associated with an undiagnosed gluten intolerance [4,23].

During flare ups, I would burp after meals, feel uncomfortably full after a meal with a high gluten content, such as pasta or bread, and would experience indigestion with acid reflux post meals. I lived fully stocked with Tums and Maalox. My daughter would comment frequently after meals that she ate too much and felt very full (uncomfortable heavy feeling in her stomach) even though she hadn't eaten very much. My mom didn't have these symptoms.

Oral (Mouth) Changes

Oral ulcers can result from vitamin deficiency or immune activity. Aphthous stomatitis (canker sores) affects many people and may be the only symptom [8,11,14].

My mother and I both had difficulties with oral ulcers for most of our lives. My daughter didn't have this problem.

Decreased tongue papillation with glossitis (tongue inflammation), angular cheilosis (scales and fissures on lips and in mouth), and dental enamel defects are also commonly seen [15]. Dental enamel defects can result from demineralization that can occur during the development of tooth buds in children and can lead to frequent dental caries [11].

My mother, daughter, and I didn't have these problems.

A link has been found between Sjögren's Syndrome and CD. Orally, Sjögren's Syndrome can cause a dry mouth, resulting from inflammation in the salivary glands leading to decreased saliva production (other symptoms can occur as well). A study found that the incidence of CD in Sjögren's disease was higher than in the healthy control group and recommends screening of all Sjögren's patients for CD [2,4].

Recurrent Intestinal Bacterial And Candidiasis (Yeast) Infections

As previously mentioned, the unabsorbed fat in the large intestine can be one contributing factor to the proliferation of bacteria and yeast in the intestines [11]. As well, the overstressed intestinal immune system, maladaptive intestinal environment, a diet high in sugars, damaged intestinal mucosa and use of some medications (such as antibiotics) may increase the risk for bacterial bowel infections or the overgrowth of candidiasis.

Symptoms of bacterial infections and candidiasis (yeast) can include bloating, flatulence, abdominal cramps, and diarrhea. Candida infection of the tongue and oral areas can occur. This usually presents with white patches and raw areas in the mouth.

I didn't have any difficulties with bowel infections or candidiasis when I was undiagnosed. Perhaps that was due to the fact that I was taking digestive enzymes and probiotics during the 5 years when my digestive symptoms were most prevalent.

Lactose Intolerance

Lactose is natural sugar found in dairy products. It requires lactase, an enzyme produced within the intestines, to digest it. Usually, this enzyme is produced by the small intestinal villi. In CD (and some with DH), the intestinal villi damage impairs the production of lactase. Loss of this brush border enzyme results in a condition called lactose intolerance [1,2,4].

Once the lactose passes undigested into the colon, it is broken down by commensal bacteria. This process produces CO_2 and hydrogen which can cause abdominal discomfort, bloating, flatulence, and possibly diarrhea. This may be temporary, since lactase production may resume once the bowel has healed [1,2,4].

Liver Disease

The liver is an extremely important organ. Metabolism of endogenous hormones, synthesis of proteins, storing and releasing glucose as needed, acting as a glucose buffer, and metabolism of carbohydrates and fats are some of its functions. It also helps to detoxify the blood of colonic bacteria, other particulates, drugs, xenbiotics, and ammonia.

Liver disease can be an associated symptom of gluten intolerance. Elevated transaminase levels (of unknown cause), autoimmune hepatitis, primary biliary cirrhosis, fatty liver disease, primary sclerosing cholangitis, and autoimmune cholangitis have been associated with CD [11,16,17].

It is reasonable to suspect that immune mediated reactions in non-celiac gluten intolerance could negatively impact the liver as well. Immune complexes could circulate and become lodged in the liver causing inflammation and damage. As well, transglutaminase is present in the liver. Perhaps, auto-antibodies are reacting against this type of transglutaminase, just as the antibodies in the bowel react against transglutaminase 2. This is likely since we know this can occur in DH (antibodies react against transglutaminase 3), and with gluten ataxia (antibodies react against transglutaminase 6) [11,33,34,37]. Future research will help to reveal the under lying mechanisms behind this possible association.

My liver enzymes were elevated when I was very ill with symptoms, but returned to normal with a gluten-free diet.

Gallbladder Problems

Bile is made in the liver, and the gallbladder is like a storage unit, where bile is stored in between meals. Bile digests fat. In patients with suspected typical gallbladder disease, a biliary scintigraphy (HIDA scan) with injected cholecystokinin (hormone) is used to check for blockages, disease, or problems emptying bile contents. The amount the gallbladder empties with this hormonal stimulation is called the ejection fraction. Typically, a low ejection fraction and return of gallbladder discomfort during the procedure are criteria used to diagnose gallbladder disease. Individuals with CD may have an unusual elevated ejection fraction, which could lead medical staff to mistakenly rule out a diseased gallbladder. This is important for doctors to know because an elevated ejection fraction could be one of the first symptoms to be noticed during a hospital admission or during an assessment [18-21,38,39, 44]. As well, this knowledge can be considered while assessing celiac patients for gallbladder problems.

With all forms of gluten intolerance, perhaps the altered intestinal microbiota (flora) could affect the gallbladder in an adverse way. In mice, a study suggested that altered gut microbiota may contribute to a fatty liver [17]. Due to the liver's close proximately to the gallbladder, it is reasonable to suspect altered microbiota may affect the gallbladder as well. With bowel involvement, often the intestinal flora is affected so this possibility is likely.

Chapter 27 under "Imbalance Intestinal Flora Theory" discusses the intestinal microbiota and how it is affected in more detail.

Pancreatic Problems

The pancreas has exocrine and endocrine functions that may be affected by undiagnosed gluten intolerance.

Endocrine Pancreas

The endocrine pancreas manufactures hormones that help keep the body in a state of homeostasis (stable condition). The islets of Langerhans located throughout the pancreas have four types of islet cells that produce 4 types of secretory granules called insulin, glucagon, somatostatin, and pancreatic polypeptide. Type 1 diabetes develops when the pancreas fails to produce insulin and type 2 diabetes occurs when the body is unable to effectively utilize the insulin that is produced. There is an association of type 1 diabetes with CD. This group of people would benefit from CD screening shortly after diagnosis and periodically after [4,22].

It is possible that a gluten intolerance may influence the onset of type 2 diabetes as well. In one study, Dr. Jay Woortman found that a low carbohydrate, low sugar diet beneficially lowered blood sugar, blood pressure, and cholesterol in himself and a group of Namgis First Nation people in Alert Bay, British Columbia Canada. Some of the diabetic patients were actually able to reduce their diabetic medications (with the doctor's supervision). I noticed that this diet appears to have eliminated grains from the diet of the study subjects. Were the beneficial effects from the low carbohydrate diet, from the lack of grain (eliminates gluten) in their diet, or both? Dr. Woortman's blog can be found at

www.drjaywortman.com/blog/wordpress/

In another study, there is some evidence that impairment of transglutaminase 2 (TG2) may impair insulin secretion in mice and make them glucose intolerant. This implies that there is a role for transglutaminase 2 activity in the pancreas. With gluten intolerance, it is reasonable to suspect that auto-antibodies could impair this enzyme and lead to various pancreatic symptoms including the endocrine symptoms that the mice had [36].

With bowel damage in CD and DH, transglutaminase 2 (in the bowel) is one of the targets for auto-antibodies. In a study, IgA deposits on transglutaminase 2 were found in jejunal biopsies taken from the small intestine of patients with gluten ataxia [41]. This demonstrates that antibodies against transglutaminase 2 can occur in various types of gluten intolerance, not just with CD. Theoretically, the presence of transglutaminase 2 in the pancreas could increase the risk for damage in this organ as well.

Exocrine Pancreas

The exocrine pancreas releases 4 types of digestive enzymes called proteases, amylolytic enzymes, lipases, and nucleases. A "monitor peptide" is produced, which monitors the digestive needs of the intestine and increases the secretory capacity of the pancreas as needed. Colipase and trypsin inhibitors are also produced and function to modulate the pancreatic secretions.

Digestive enzymes are required to help us digest our meals. If the production of digestive enzymes is affected, an individual can suffer from pancreatic insufficiency and have many bowel symptoms.

Some people with undiagnosed CD can suffer from pancreatic insufficiency. This can be an issue after diagnosis as well [11,22,28]. More research is needed to examine how non-celiac gluten intolerance may be associated with pancreatic insufficiency. Theoretically, the presence of auto-antibodies against pancreatic transglutaminase or lodged immune complexes in the pancreas may lead to inflammation and damage. This could result in pancreatic insufficiency.

When I was undiagnosed, I found that consuming digestive enzymes appeared to moderately improve my bowel symptoms. Likely, I was suffering from a lack of digestive enzymes in my intestine and may have had pancreatic insufficiency.

Pancreatitis

Pancreatitis can be a problem as well. In a recent case study, a young boy presented with the symptoms of pancreatitis (along with positive blood tests) from the ages of 1-3 years old [31]. At age 3 he was finally diagnosed with CD. Another study mentioned that celiac disease should be ruled out when a patient presents with papillary stenosis or idiopathic recurrent pancreatitis [32].

Pancreatic symptoms might occur with a non-celiac gluten intolerance. We know that auto antibodies can attack a variety of physiological areas in gluten ataxia, CD, and DH. It is reasonable to suspect that immune mediated reactions in non-celiac gluten intolerance could negatively impact the pancreas as well.

Other People's Experiences

Case 1: Prior to my diagnosis, I experienced canker sores in my mouth, anemia, bloating, nausea, burping, indigestion, and I felt a feeling of fullness after eating. I had recurrent vaginal yeast infections, elevated liver enzymes, and recurrent pneumonia. It took 6 years to get a diagnosis. Once I started eating gluten-free, the symptoms went away. I finally feel like I can start living life again.

Case 2: My spouse didn't seem to have any symptoms except an elevated blood sugar. The dietitian put him on a low carbohydrate diet for the blood sugar issues. At this time, I noticed that he was gluten-free due to his food choices.

When he introduced anything with gluten, the bowel symptoms would return. He requested celiac tests from his doctor and they were all negative following a 3 month gluten challenge. He has always been very thin and pale. He did stool tests with

Enterolab and they found antigliadin antibodies in his stool. Now he is gluten-free and symptom-free. His mouth sores and heartburn went away too.

Case 3: *My 7 year old son was diagnosed with type 1 diabetes. He was pale, tall, and thin. I read about Type 1 diabetes and celiac disease on a blog and requested testing. The result was positive. He now has gained weight, is not pale, and his diabetes is controlled. Could an earlier diagnosis have prevented the diabetes?*

Case 4: *My daughter was having stomach aches, constipation, and dark circles under her eyes. Her aunt has celiac disease so I tested her with the celiac home test and the result was positive. A gastroenterologist confirmed the diagnosis and her symptoms are gone with a gluten-free diet.*

Case 5: *I was diagnosed with irritable bowel syndrome for 8 years and really suffered with this. It was an embarrassing condition. Then, I read an article about CD and requested a test. My doctor said I couldn't have CD because I was overweight. I went to another doctor and insisted on the test. It came back positive. Eight years of suffering and all I needed to do was eat gluten-free. Why didn't my doctor recognize the symptoms? Now, I feel great.*

Case 6: *I was diagnosed with lactose intolerance when I was a teenager. I also had anemia and some indigestion. Through a blog, I realized that these symptoms can be a symptom of celiac disease. I requested testing and the result was positive. The symptoms are gone with a gluten-free diet.*

Case 7: *Even though my celiac test was negative, a gluten-free diet took away my diarrhea, bloating, heartburn and snoring. Through a blog, I discovered that this was possible.*

CHAPTER 5

Fatigue, Anemia, And Abnormal Bleeding

In this chapter, factors that contribute to fatigue (tiredness), anemia, abnormal bleeding and bruising will be discussed.

Nutrient Losses May Contribute

With undiagnosed celiac disease (CD) and in many with dermatitis herpetiformis (DH), the intestinal villi, responsible for absorbing nutrients, becomes damaged, creating a flattened mucosal surface (villus flattening) that is less able to absorb nutrients. Autoimmune reactions to ingested gluten cross-react with intestinal villi and create this damage. Food allergies can also contribute to villi damage as well. Various nutrient deficiencies can occur and this, along with inflammation and other factors, can lead to fatigue, anemia, and abnormal bleeding [6-8,15].

With a non-celiac gluten intolerance, the presence of nausea, vomiting, a poor appetite, food allergies and certain medications may lead to deficiencies as well. If a lectin intolerance is occurring, anti-nutritive effects may also cause nutrient deficiencies [47].

Malabsorption of each nutrient listed in this chapter may or may not occur with CD. Severity of nutrient loss and related symptoms are dependent on the location, length and severity of intestinal villi damage, which can be patchy in nature, and the availability of digestive enzymes and transport proteins/carriers that take nutrients to the cells, organs, tissues, and other systems of the body. Nutrient losses may impair production of these enzymes and transport proteins/carriers, which can hinder absorption and mobilization of nutrients [1,3,7, 8,13,16,23].

Malabsorption is compounded by the fact that many nutrients are dependent on other nutrients for successful absorption to occur. A deficiency in one nutrient may affect the absorption of other nutrients since many are co-dependent. The impaired villi is also reliant on nutrients, so nutrient deficiencies may add to the intestinal autoimmune damage further hindering the villi's ability to absorb fat and water soluble vitamins, minerals, trace elements, electrolytes, proteins, fats, and carbohydrates [1,3,7,8,13,16,23].

With all three forms of gluten intolerance, bacterial overgrowth, viral infections, or diarrhea and/or vomiting may result in greater nutrient losses. Presence of a fish tape worm or parasites may also contribute to a deficiency, since they are nutrient dependent.

A poor diet, medications that affect nutrient absorption, past stomach and intestinal surgery, and/or the presence of other associated autoimmune diseases, such as Crohn's Disease, Graves Disease (hyperthyroidism-diarrhea, weight loss), Sjögren's Syndrome, Microscopic Colitis, or Addison's Disease can also add to the severity of nutrient losses [1,3,7,8,23].

Fatigue

Fatigue (feelings of being tired) can be a symptom of gluten intolerance and can result from a variety of factors. These factors can include inflammation, malabsorption of nutrients, hypoglycemia (low blood sugar), anemia (low hemoglobin), adrenal gland hypofunction, muscle weakness, nervous system problems, cognitive (brain) changes, an overstressed immune system (leading to more infections), heart and lung problems, or psychological issues such as depression.

Feelings of helplessness can add to the fatigue. A reduced quality of life and lack of an accurate diagnosis for symptoms can increase this risk. The presence of additional auto-immune diseases (more common with delayed CD diagnosis), associated cancers, or parasites can compound this symptom. Collectively, all of these factors can contribute to feelings of fatigue.

Hypotension (low blood pressure) can result from protein/amino acid deficiencies (i.e. low albumin), dehydration (due to fluid losses and electrolyte depletion with vomiting and/or diarrhea), blood loss, impaired cardiac function, or as a side effect from a medication. Low blood pressure can cause dizziness, edema (if from protein losses), fatigue, weakness, cardiac symptoms and possibly fainting.

Since electrolytes are also necessary for nerve and muscle function, a deficiency can lead to muscle weakness and possibly arrhythmias (abnormal heart rhythm and rate) that can add to the fatigue.

Presence of allergies or sensitivities to other foods, possibly due to increased intestinal permeability (leaky gut), may also add to the fatigue. Medications used to treat allergic symptoms and other health problems may increase feelings of fatigue due to possible side effects.

As you can see, the causes of fatigue can be complex, since many factors with a gluten intolerance may be contributing. Thorough investigations can help uncover the causes and assist an individual to regain their stamina and quality of life.

I had intermittent fatigue for years. This was likely due to anemia, the inflammatory effects of CD, low blood pressure (sometimes as low as 80/40), low albumin level, and likely many other nutrient deficiencies.

I had periods of foggy thinking, palpitations, and frequent lung infections. Once diagnosed and consuming a gluten-free diet, my fatigue, anemia, and low blood pressure resolved.

Anemia

Various nutrient deficiencies, combined with inflammation, can lead to anemia. With anemia, the quantity of red blood cells (RBC) and hemoglobin (Hgb) is less than normal. Since RBCs and specifically Hgb carry oxygen to all the bodily cells and tissues for cell respiration, a deficiency can lead to cell hypoxia (lack of oxygen). This can cause clinically mild to severe symptoms that are dependent on the severity of the anemia, underlying medical problems such as heart or lung conditions, and other contributing factors such as low vitamin K levels leading to blood loss. Anemia is common in CD (also in many with DH) and can occur in non-celiac gluten intolerance for a variety of reasons mentioned previously.

Menstruation, poor dietary habits, medications that affect nutrient absorption, past stomach and intestinal surgery, age (decreased absorption in elderly), smoking, kidney problems, pregnancy, breast feeding, growth spurts, or the presence of other auto-immune diseases may may also add to the severity of anemia and presenting symptoms.

Symptoms

Anemia symptoms can include pallor (pale skin, nail beds, and mucosa), shortness of breath, chest pain/heart attack, palpitations (arrhythmias), and tachycardia (rapid heart rate). Other symptoms can include muscular weakness, dizziness/fainting from low blood pressure (due to heart symptoms or blood loss) hypoxia, fatigue, enlarged spleen, poor concentration, poor appetite, hair loss, dry skin, and feeling cold or having cold hands and feet.

As well, anemia symptoms can include an inflamed and sore tongue, increased susceptibility to infections, cravings for non-nutritive substances (pica-low iron), dark half circles under the eyes, intermittent claudication in the legs, koilonychia (flat or concave nails from low iron), brittle nails, headaches, murmurs, clubbing of finger tips (if chronic iron deficiency), restless leg syndrome (crawling or tingling feeling-low iron), difficulty learning, behavioral problems, or jaundice with yellow eyes or skin (from hemolysis).

Nutrient Deficiencies Contributing To Anemia

When many nutrient deficiencies co-exist, as often seen in active CD, it can be difficult to identify which deficiency is specifically responsible for the resulting anemia. Iron, B-12, and folate (folic acid) deficiencies are well recognized as causes of anemia in undiagnosed CD [7,8,23].

Additional nutrients that may contribute to anemia are vitamins A, C, E, B-2, B-6, niacin, the mineral copper, and protein. These nutrients can also be malabsorbed due to intestinal villi damage [1,2,7,9,17-20]. Although each of the additional nutrients appear to contribute anemia, more conclusive research is needed to clarify the precise role each nutrient executes.

Anemia Is Common With Celiac Disease

Anemia can be the only presenting symptom in undiagnosed CD and can occur without gastrointestinal symptoms or weight loss. The Canadian Celiac Association Health Survey (2007) found that 40% of children and 66% of adults with active CD have anemia [12].

Women who are menstruating should not be denied testing for CD due to an assumption that the anemia is caused by menstruation. As well, heavy menstruation could be due to a vitamin K deficiency.

> *My mother and I, both with CD, had anemia without bowel symptoms for most of our lives. We had pallor, palpitations, muscular weakness, occasional dizziness, low blood pressure, fatigue, hair loss, cold hands and feet, brittle nails, increased susceptibility to infections, and restless leg syndrome.*

> *Doctors told me that my anemia was likely due to ongoing normal menstruation and that perhaps I wasn't eating enough iron. I ate red meat regularly plus I supplemented with iron tablets and a daily multivitamin. A celiac screen and an upper endoscopy with biopsies would have revealed the cause of my anemia.*

Abnormal Bleeding Or Bruising

With intestinal damage, fat malabsorption can occur and this can lead to impaired absorption of fat soluble vitamin K. Bacteria in the intestine can synthesize some vitamin K (menaquinones). However, the maladaptive state of the intestine, in some individuals, may lead to decreased production and absorption of this vitamin resulting in a deficiency. If a vitamin K deficiency occurred, it could impair clotting and lead to abnormal bleeding. An additional issue, blood loss can make the anemia and related symptoms worse.

Vitamin K contributes to the production of prothrombin and other clotting system proteins in the blood. Calcium and protein also contribute to normal coagulation, a deficiency might add to abnormal bleeding or bruising. As well, fragile capillaries may result from a vitamin C deficiency and this may lead to blood loss through damaged capillary walls.

Auto-antibodies can attack various transglutaminases in CD, DH, and with gluten ataxia. It seems reasonable to suspect that auto-antibodies could attack plasma transglutaminase involved in clotting (i.e. Factor XIII). This might also contribute to bleeding problems in CD, DH, or with non-celiac gluten intolerance.

Symptoms

If bleeding occurs, it may be seen in the nose (epitaxis), eyes (red eyes), ears, gums when brushing teeth, in emesis (if vomiting), in the urine (hematuria), in the stool (black, tarry or bloody stool), with abnormal vaginal bleeding, petechia (red spots on skin), ecchymoses (bruising), or increased bleeding with injuries.

With an injury, internal bleeding or a large blood loss externally may lead to shock-like symptoms and/or pain that may be dependent on the cause and type of bleeding. Shock symptoms may include tachycardia, hypotension, restlessness, anxiety, weakness, lethargy, cool, moist skin, pallor, low body temperature, rapid and shallow respiration, dizziness, unconsciousness, confusion, and reduced urinary output.

Bleeding in the brain (intracerebral hemorrhage) is life threatening and may lead a variety of neurological symptoms including headache, a change in level of consciousness, difficulty swallowing, difficulty communicating or comprehending speech, weakness or loss of function, loss of balance or coordination, tremors, nausea, vomiting, changes in behavior, changes in sensation, visual or taste changes, pupil changes, and confusion. As you can see, an undiagnosed gluten intolerance can lead to serious medical conditions that are medical emergencies.

I know the above symptoms can sound intimidating. Keep in mind that many people don't experience any of the above symptoms, even with CD. Everyone's presentation of symptoms is very unique. With those that are affected, the good news is that a strict gluten-free diet along with good medical care should alleviate the above symptoms and lead to a better quality of life.

Other People's Experiences

Case 1: I had anemia my whole life and was only treated with iron pills. No one tested me for celiac disease or did tests to examine why I wasn't absorbing iron. Last year I started to have bowel symptoms so the Doc tested me and I have celiac disease. Finally on a gluten-free diet, I am absorbing iron and no longer have to take pills.

Case 2: I had anemia and thyroid problems for years. My daughter was diagnosed with celiac disease so I was tested and the result was positive. I now know that thyroid problems and anemia are associated with celiac disease. I wonder if an earlier diagnosis could have prevented the thyroid problems. The anemia is gone.

Case 3: For years, bruising happened very easily to me. I would barely bump against something and I would have a big bruise. I also had problems with nose bleeds and anemia for years. Then I had a bout of diarrhea with vomiting that lasted 3 months. I even got bruising around my eyes. My doctor tested me for everything and celiac came back positive. No bruising now and no anemia or vomiting while on a gluten-free diet.

Case 4: After the birth of my 3 children, I had very heavy and frequent unexpected periods. It was awful. I would be in the grocery store or at a dance and gush! Exhausted, I started staying at home and not going out very much. It was depressing. The doctor had to remove my uterus so I could live normally. Eventually, I started to have gas, bloating, and diarrhea which led to my celiac diagnosis.

CHAPTER 6
Sensory Symptoms (Vision, Hearing, Taste, Smell, and Touch)

In this chapter, five sensory symptoms (vision, hearing, taste, smell, and touch) will be discussed. In many with undiagnosed celiac disease (CD) and dermatitis herpetiformis (DH), the intestinal villi, responsible for absorbing nutrients, becomes damaged. Various nutrient deficiencies can occur and this, along with inflammation and other autoimmune factors, can lead to various sensory symptoms [8,70,71,73]. Some of the following symptoms have been reported by patients with a non-celiac gluten intolerance as well. However, the underlying reasons for their symptoms is less clear.

Vision Symptoms

Functional vision is reliant on a healthy nervous system, vascular system, muscular system and structural eye integrity. Immune reactions to gluten can affect all 3 systems comprom-ising visual health. As well, these systems are dependent on nutrients, it is thought that vision loss may result from nutrient deficiencies that cause pathological changes in these systems. Vitamin A deficiency is well known for causing vision problems and can be common with bowel damage. Many other nutrient deficiencies can occur as well [1-4,8,71,74].

Nutrient deficiencies can be primarily responsible for many of the pathological changes that can occur to the conjunctiva, cornea, and retina. Some of the symptoms may only occur if the deficiency is chronic, this is probable since misdiagnosis can occur for years.

Visual symptoms may include difficulty seeing in a dimly lit room, night blindness, conjunctival xerosis (dryness of the eye), corneal xerosis (cornea rough, dry, and hazy), keratoconjunctivitis sicca (dry cornea and conjunctiva), Bitot's spots (pearly foamy patch on conjunctiva and cornea), keratomalacia (corneal necrosis, corneal ulceration), corneal scar, and formation of corneal opacity (cornea white or clouded over) [1,3,4,75,77,86].

Other symptoms include xerophthalmia (dry and inflamed eye), xerophthalmic fundus (white or gray linear or oval opacities in the retina), blindness, conjunctivitis with corneal vascularization and lens opacity, blepharitis (inflammation of the eyelids), styes, and eye

37

infections. As well, red (bloodshot) eyes or central retinal vein occlusion may occur if coagulation problems exist [1,3,4,75,77,86].

Optic neuropathy is another complication that could arise from nutritional deficiencies or, theoretically, from autoimmune damage. Symptoms usually present symmetrically and simultaneously, and are not painful. One eye may have visual symptoms prior to the other, but symptoms in the other generally follow. Dyschromatopsia (defect in color vision) may be the first symptom. Colors (one or more) may not seem as bright and vivid as they were previously. Foggy, cloudy, or blurred vision may occur and may be more prevalent at the point of fixation. Vision may deteriorate rapidly. Centrocecal or central scrotomas (blind spots) may also occur [2].

Vision symptoms resulting from muscular problems could happen. Ocular myopathy in a 12 year old girl with CD has been documented. The ocular myopathy corrected itself with a gluten-free diet and vitamin supplementation [85]. In theory, extraocular palsy and nystagmus could also occur due to a thiamine deficiency causing a central nervous system lesion [2].

There may also be a correlation between CD, macular degeneration and cataracts since these conditions tend to improve with supplementation of nutrients, such as vitamins A, C, E, zinc, lutein, zeaxanthin, and omega #3 (when they are given collectively) [6,76]. Perhaps individuals who show improvement with supplementation suffer from malab-sorption issues due to an undiagnosed gluten intolerance. More research is needed.

Nutrient deficiencies contributing to the above symptoms can include vitamin A, B complex, C, E, K, zinc, copper, iron, taurine, and essential amino and fatty acids [1-4,5,7]. More research is needed to specifically identify which nutrients are directly involved in each visual symptom and to investigate how common each symptom is in the three forms of gluten intolerance.

My visual symptoms included night blindness, blurred vision, Bitot's spots, flashes of light, occasional partial loss of vision (I was told this was likely due to ocular migraines), and periodically it appeared as if a cloud of fog was in the room. I also suffered occasionally from styes, and dry eyelids.

I used prescription glasses in university to see the blackboard and to drive. After my diagnosis, my vision corrected itself. My mother, also with CD, has some visual impairment and wears glasses.

I wonder whether everyone with unexplained visual symptoms could benefit from testing, especially children who get prescription glasses so early in life. Is the prescription a band aide approach? Could the underlying reason really be a gluten intolerance? Could a gluten-free diet improve sight for many who are affected with visual symptoms? Future research is needed.

Auditory (Hearing) Symptoms

Functional hearing is reliant on a healthy nervous system, vascular system, and skeletal system. Since these systems are dependent on nutrients, it is theorized that hearing loss may result from nutrient deficiencies that cause pathological changes in these systems [9-13]. Multiple nutrient deficiencies can occur with bowel involvement and, theoretically, this may cause a variety of symptoms.

With non-celiac gluten intolerance, immune reactions might compromise hearing by affecting the nervous or vascular system. The nervous system can be affected in gluten ataxia, it seems reasonable to suspect that auto-antibodies could affect the nervous system or vascular system that supports hearing. More research is needed to examine this possible connection.

In humans and animals with nutritional deficiencies, many types of auditory dysfunction has occurred [13-16]. Symptoms could include tinnitus or ringing in the ears, auditory hallucinations, middle ear infections, loss of hearing, dizziness, and other hearing impairments [13-15, 22].

In human studies, vitamin A [3,4], B-12 [13,17-20,59], folate [13,21-25,59], vitamin D [13,26-32], calcium [33,34], and iron deficiency [7,35,36] is associated with an alteration in hearing [13]. In animal studies, vitamin B-12 [38], thiamine [39], riboflavin [39], vitamin B-6 [39-43], vitamin A [39], vitamin C [39,44], vitamin D [39,45-47], vitamin E [39,48], copper [49], iron [37,50-53], magnesium [54-57], and zinc [58] deficiencies have had various effects on hearing.

I had intermittent tinnitus.

Olfactory (Smell) And Gustatory (Taste) Symptoms

It is thought that nutrients are important for gustatory and olfactory function since the epithelial cells in these areas have high metabolic needs. More research is needed to identify specific nutrient requirements. Vitamin A, thiamine, riboflavin, pantothenic acid, pyridoxine, niacin, cobalamin, folic acid, vitamin E, copper, iodine, iron, zinc, and nickel deficiencies have been identified as possible contributing factors to smell and taste impairments [3,4,13,61-66,78]. Since all of these nutrients can be deficient with a gluten intolerance, taste and smell impairments may be possible.

Theoretically, olfactory (smell) symptoms could include anosmia (unable to smell), hyposmia (decreased detection of odors), dysosmia (incorrect identification of odors), parosmia (perception of smell is altered), phantosmia (false odor detected), agnosia (can smell, but difficulty in identifying odor) [62,65].

Taste symptoms affecting the 5 tastes (salty, sweet, bitter, sour, and umami) could include ageusia (unable to taste), hypogeusia (decreased taste function), or dysgeusia (taste function is distorted/altered) [65].

If gustatory and olfactory senses are impaired, then appetite may be decreased leading to further malnutrition. Other symptoms affecting appetite include lesions in the oral mucosa (esp. dorsal tongue), dry nose and mouth, papillary atrophy and degeneration of the tongue, atrophic glossitis, or pica cravings [62,65].

I found that I couldn't smell as well as others and I often had a strange taste in my mouth (like metallic tin). Once eating gluten-free, these symptoms disappeared.

Touch Symptoms

Peripheral neuropathy can be the only presenting symptom with a gluten intolerance and can occur without bowel symptoms or weight loss [70]. Symptoms can include burning, tingling, numbness, or a loss of feeling in the hands and feet. These sensations can spread to the arms, legs, face, and body [69,79,80].

Pain may also occur and may feel like an electric shock. Some feel an increased sensitivity to touch. Many other symptoms can occur as well [69,79,80]. These additional symptoms will be discussed in Chapter 11, about neurological symptoms.

Nutrient deficiencies contributing to peripheral neuropathy can include vitamins E, B complex, amino and fatty acids, calcium, magnesium, phosphorus, copper, electrolytes, and inositol. Malabsorption of these nutrients along with immune reactions in CD, DH, and non-celiac gluten intolerance may lead to touch symptoms [3,4,79,81,82].

I had intermittent tingling, numbness, vibrations, cold and burning feelings, and pain in my head, face, arms, and legs. I also had carpal tunnel for awhile in my wrist and had to wear a brace. My daughter had tingling and numbness in her feet. These symptoms have disappeared now.

Other Influencing Factors

Other factors that may contribute to sensory symptoms are diabetes (diabetic retinopathy and neuropathy), certain medications, occupational exposures, smoking, diet, past eye surgery, age, low or high blood pressure, increased homocysteine levels, upper respiratory infections, trauma, infections, alcoholism, certain medications, candidiasis, gingivitis, genetic differences, and brain surgery. [1,2,8,9,13,60-62,79,80]

The presence of other autoimmune diseases or conditions, such as scleroderma, downs syndrome, Alzheimer's disease, Huntington's disease, multiple sclerosis, Parkinson's dementias, idiopathic Parkinson's disease, complex of Guam, epilepsy, age, multi-infarct dementia, schizophrenia, tumors, lupus, Crohn's disease, kidney disease, liver disease, or hypothyroidism can add to the symptoms [1,2,8,10,13,60-62,79,80].

Other People's Experiences

Case 1: Along with my other celiac symptoms, I had night blindness, a tin taste in my mouth, and tingling in my fingertips. After diagnosis, the symptoms resolved. It took about 3 months.

Case 2: I had ringing in my ears, irritable bowel syndrome, and burning type of pain on my legs before diagnosis. Now no symptoms.

Case 3: I had tingling in my feet, headaches, and anemia before I was diagnosed. A gluten-free diet worked to remove symptoms.

Case 4: *I heard voices (when no one was there) prior to my diagnosis. I ignored the voices because they didn't make sense. I had other symptoms too which led to a diagnosis of celiac disease. Once I was eating gluten-free for 4 months, the voices went away for the first time in years and have never returned.*

CHAPTER 7
Skin Rashes, Hair, and Nail Symptoms

In this chapter, skin rashes, hair, and nail symptoms will be discussed. In many with undiagnosed celiac disease (CD) and dermatitis herpetiformis (DH), the intestinal villi, responsible for absorbing nutrients, becomes damaged. Various nutrient deficiencies can occur and this, along with inflammation and other immune factors in the three forms of gluten intolerance, can lead to various skin rashes, hair, and nail symptoms.

Skin Rashes And Other Skin Symptoms

Dermatitis Herpetiformis (Duhring's Disease)

Dermatitis herpetiformis (DH) occurs when autoimmune reactions lead to a skin rash. Unfortunately, this form of CD is often misdiagnosed as other skin disorders such as psoriasis, shingles, hives, poison ivy, dermatitis, eczema, and a variety of other skin conditions [1,3,4].

Typically, symptoms include a blistering (papulovesicular eruptions) or scabbed rash that is very itchy. As well, the rash can have pimple type lesions, look like little bumps, or look similar to psoriasis with raised red patches of skin. Often, the rash occurs bilaterally on the body and is commonly found on the buttocks, back, elbows, forearms, back of knees, scalp and on the face. In children, the rash may only present as purpura on the palms of their hands (in isolation or in addition to other symptoms). Clinically, the rash can present anywhere on the body [1-4].

I have met patients who have encountered dermatologists who continue to prescribe medication for dermatitis herpetiformis, without prescribing a strict gluten-free diet. Unfortunately, these patients may continue to have a high risk of associated cancers, other autoimmune damage or malabsorption issues (even without bowel symptoms) with this approach. If you have DH, you have a gluten intolerance and should follow a strict gluten-free diet. This is well researched and proven [1,4,77,80].

One Recreational Therapist that I worked with was diagnosed with DH and put on Dapsone without being told about a gluten-free diet. The dermatologist did ask her if she had any bowel symptoms. She said no. Further tests were not completed and a gluten-free diet was not mentioned.

Unfortunately, she suffered with side effects from the medication for 2 years with this approach. Following a discussion with me on a lunch break, she saw her MD, a gastroenterologist, and her dermatologist. She started a gluten-free diet and was able to discontinue the Dapsone following a discussion with her doctor. Now, she is the picture of health, living rash and drug free.

List Of Other Skin Rashes/Conditions Associated With A Gluten Intolerance

- Cutaneous vasculitis
- Hereditary Angioneurotic Edema
- Urticaria
- Linear IgA bullous dermatosis
- Erythema nodosum
- Necrolytic migratory erythema
- Erythema elevatum diutinum
- Psoriasis
- Eczema
- Vitiligo
- Behçet's disease
- Dermatomyositis
- Porphyria
- Ichthyosiform dermatoses
- Pellagra
- Generalized acquired cutis laxa
- Atypical mole syndrome and cogenital giant naevus
- Prurigo nodularis (Hyde's prurigo)
- Pityriasis rubra pilaris
- Erythroderma
- Acne
- Acquired hypertrichosis lanuginosa
- Ichthyosis
- Transverse Leukonychia
- Follicular Hyperkeratosis
- Scleroderma
- Sarcoidosis

- Oral Lichen Planus
- Bullous pemphigoid
- Angular cheilitis, glossitis, ulcerative stomatitis, and aphthous ulcers
- Pale skin (from anemia)
- Melanoma
- Dermatitis or acrodermatitis
- IgA Linear dermatosis
- Lupus erythematosus
- Lichen sclerosus
- Cutaneous amyloidosis
- Annular erythema
- Partial lipodystrophy
- Atopic dermatitis
- Palmoplantar pustulosis
- seborrheic dermatitis-from riboflavin deficiency
- Facial butterfly Rash-from niacin deficiency
- Increased skin pigmentation
- Spontaneous ecchymoses
- Bruised skin
- Purpura
- Petechia
- Bleeding under the skin
- Dry and/or cracked skin from dehydration and malabsorption of nutrients
- Delayed wound healing (malabsorption of nutrients)
- Edema (swollen skin)
- Any itchy skin rashes

I experienced generalized dry skin and cracked peeling skin on the heels of my feet. My lips would crack at the corners and I had canker sores in my mouth. Occasionally, intensely itchy red raised areas would occur on various parts of my body.

As well, a rash would develop over my nose about once a week for awhile, then it would disappear for a month or two (lupus tests were negative). I was always pale, and I did tend to bruise easily.

My mother, also with CD, bruised easily, was pale, had dry skin (especially on her feet), and would develop an unusual blotchy rash around her neck area. My daughter, at age 4 (also with CD), had red itchy patches that would last a few hours, then disappear. My mother and daughter did not have bowel symptoms. My bowel symptoms started after the birth of my first child.

My middle child tested negative for CD. She had eczema of moderate severity, hyperactivity, occasional diarrhea, and abdominal discomfort. All medical tests ordered by the pediatric allergist (including the IgE mediated allergy test) were negative. An elimination diet revealed that she was sensitive to corn and corn derivatives (which are in most grocery store products). All symptoms resolved when I removed corn from her diet. All symptoms return with accidental ingestion of corn.

Nutrient Deficiencies

Nutrient deficiencies partially or fully contributing to the above skin symptoms may include vitamin A, B complex, C, K, essential fatty and amino acids, iron, zinc, biotin, copper, and manganese [73,74].

Hair Symptoms

Alopecia Areata (patches of hair loss) has been associated with CD. In CD, it may be the result of an immunological attack and/or nutrient deficiencies. Alopecia can be the only presenting symptom in CD [1,8,73-77]. It seems reasonable to suspect that immune reactions in non-celiac gluten intolerance may also lead to alopecia areata.

An individual with a gluten intolerance may have dry, thin, brittle, slow growing hair due to nutrient deficiencies. Hair might change color due to malabsorption issues with pantothenic acid or manganese deficiencies [73,74].

My mother and I had hair that grew slowly, was fine, and brittle.

Nail Symptoms

Individuals with CD and DH may have nails that are dry, brittle, thin, malformed, and that break easily. This can be due to nutrient deficiencies or associated conditions. Nails may grow slowly and can also have white bands, longitudinal striations, horizontal or vertical ridges, color changes, white spots, splinter hemorrhages, a deformed nail shape that is curved up or down (ex. spoon shaped with anemia), hang nails, or be clubbed [78,79].

Muehrcke's lines (white lines) may indicate albumin levels are low. Beau's lines (deep grooved lines) can result from nutrient deficiencies disrupting nail growth, onycholysis (nail starts detaching from nail bed) can be associated with psoriasis or sarcoidosis, and the nails might be pitted (associated with psoriasis and alopecia). Telangiectasia (small dilated blood vessels under nail) may develop with underlying lupus, dermatomyositis, or scleroderma [78,79].

Nutrient Deficiencies

Nutrients Deficiencies that can contribute to nail abnormalities can include, vitamin A, B complex, C, K, protein, calcium, iron, and zinc [73,74].

I had dry, brittle, nails that broke easily. Hang nails were continuously present and my nails frequently had white spots. My mother had horizontal ridges on her dry, brittle nails.

Other People's Experiences

Case 1: I was diagnosed with psoriasis for years. It was better in the summer and always worse in the winter. I also was diagnosed with type 1 diabetes as a child. Later in life I started to have bowel symptoms and I was tested for CD. The result was positive. All my symptoms except the diabetes went away. The rash took longer to resolve than the other symptoms.

I wonder if an early diagnosis and a gluten-free diet could have prevented my diabetes and my years of dealing with needles and blood sugar monitoring.

Case 2: I had a weird rash on my legs and arms for years. My sister has celiac disease so I was tested. My test and scope was negative. I had a skin biopsy and it was negative. I decided to try a gluten-free diet and my rash that I had for years went away.

Case 3: My child had eczema with diarrhea and weight loss. The celiac test was positive and all disappeared with a gluten-free diet.

Case 4: I had an itchy rash that would come and go for years. It looked like little bumps (like bug bites). My doctor just prescribed a steroid ointment. I now know that I have dermatitis herpetiformis and a gluten-free diet took the symptoms away. I didn't have any bowel symptoms.

CHAPTER 8
Musculoskeletal (Muscle And Bone) Symptoms

In this chapter, musculoskeletal symptoms will be discussed. With a gluten intolerance, various nutrient deficiencies can occur and this, along with inflammation and other autoimmune factors, can lead to various musculoskeletal symptoms [1-4].

Rickets And Osteomalacia

Autoimmune factors, associated inflammation and malabsorption of nutrients can start demineralizing skeletal bones in infancy or childhood (rickets) and this can continue into adulthood (osteomalacia). In some, the pathological demineralizing effects of CD may not be triggered until adulthood [1-3,5,6,8-12,70].

The bone structure becomes soft, weak, and bendable loosing it's rigidity. This can lead to disfiguring disabilities such as bow legs, pigeon chest, pelvic deformities, deformed skull, and spine deformities (ex. lordosis, scoliosis, and kyphosis) possibly decreasing mobility. Osteomalacia can coexist with arthritis and osteoporosis [1-3,5,6,8-12,70].

Over the past 6 years, I have met many people who have scoliosis and CD. Is this a coincidence or is there a connection? With malabsorption issues and autoimmune involvement, a connection is very likely.

The damaging life long effects can be permanent. A gluten intolerance diagnosis and a gluten-free diet could be the perfect primary prevention. Unfortunately, the symptoms can be so elusive that diagnosis is often delayed for years.

Symptoms of rickets in infancy and childhood may include bone pain or tenderness, muscle weakness, seizures, failure to thrive, dental deformities and cavities, delayed or impaired growth, short stature, bone fractures, skeletal deformities (ex. bowed legs, pigeon chest, pelvic deformities, deformed skull, and/or curvature of the spine that is abnormal) muscle cramps/spasms, tetany, numbness, tingling, abnormal heart rhythms, difficulty crawling and sitting, and delayed walking [3,6,64].

Early symptoms of osteomalacia in adulthood may initially be absent. During this initial phase, it may be diagnosed if apparent on a x-ray or other tests. As osteomalacia becomes chronic, symptoms may include muscle weakness, muscle cramps/spasms, tetany, seizures, numbness, tingling, abnormal heart rhythms, bone pain or tenderness, spine deformities, skeletal deformities, fractures, rachitic rosary, dental caries, reduced mobility, a change in gait, and a waddling gait [4,64,70].

Osteopenia And Osteoporosis

A number of studies and articles have identified an association between osteoporosis and CD [1,2,4,5,9-15]. Demineralization of the bones in CD may result from an immunological process that is destructive to bones combined with malabsorption of important nutrients, primarily vitamin D, calcium, magnesium, and phosphorus. Decreased mineral content of the bone is evident in osteopenia and chronic osteopenia can lead to weak, brittle bones (fragile and porous) evident in osteoporosis. This increases the risk for fractures [1,2,4,5,9-17].

Symptoms may be absent initially. As the disease progresses, symptoms may include tetany, muscle weakness, muscle cramps/spasms, numbness, tingling, palpitations (irregular heart rhythms), convulsions, loss of height, low back or neck pain, stooped posture, bone pain or tenderness, collapsed vertebrae or other fractures [1,5,17-21,70].

Testing for CD is recommended for all individuals with osteoporosis, even in the absence of bowel symptoms [4,5,45]. Since autoimmune activity is involved with non-celiac gluten intolerance (i.e. gluten ataxia), it is reasonable to suspect that antibodies could react against bones in non-celiac gluten intolerance as well. Therefore, testing for a non-celiac gluten intolerance is likely beneficial for this population.

When I was diagnosed with CD, I was told I had osteopenia (borderline osteoporosis) and the bone density of my spine was comparable to a 76 year old (I was 37).

I did some research, and then decided to choose the medication-free approach. My bone density returned to normal within 2 years on a strict gluten-free, nutrient dense diet. I also did bone building exercises and consumed vitamin plus mineral supplements. I met with a registered dietitian and my MD monitored me closely (with the gastroenterologist's guidance) during this time.

While undiagnosed, I also experienced muscle weakness, muscle cramps/spasms in my calves and feet, numbness, tingling, palpitations, and tenderness in my lower back and my neck. I was informed about 10 years ago that I had a healed fracture on one of my ribs. I skydived, rock climbed, and white water kayaked frequently prior to having children and assumed the fracture may have happened during this time.

I'm surprised I didn't have more fractures given that my bone density was likely poor for many years prior to diagnosis. My mother was diagnosed with osteoporosis and has CD. My daughter, also with CD, had occasional leg cramps. My mother and daughter did not have bowel symptoms prior to diagnosis.

Nutrient Deficiencies Contributing To Rickets, Osteomalacia, Osteopenia, And Osteoporosis

Nutrient deficiencies (common in CD and can be in DH) that may contribute to skeletal symptoms include vitamins A, D, E, K, and calcium, magnesium, phosphorus, protein, fatty acids, manganese, molybdenum, copper, boron, fluoride, and zinc. Allergies to certain foods can also affect the intestinal villi and this can lead to flattened villi and possibly deficiencies [1,4,5,62-65].

It is possible for nutrient deficiencies to be present in a non-celiac gluten intolerance with the presence of vomiting, diarrhea, a poor diet (possibly due to a poor appetite), and/or the presence of other autoimmune diseases that affect digestion.

Arthritis And Joint Pain

Various types of arthritis, such as rheumatoid arthritis, osteoarthritis, polyarthritis, monoarthritis, sacroiliitis, ankylosing spondylitis and psoriatric arthritis, have been associated with gluten intolerance. In arthritis, joint inflammation can lead to destructive tissue damage within and around the joints. In addition to this, some types of arthritis can also damage other areas of the body (ex. skin and organs) [1,2,22-29,43,44,48].

Arthritis symptoms can include swelling, pain, stiffness, redness, tenderness, and warmth in the affected areas, loss of function in affected area, and disfigured joint areas.

More research needs to be done to look at the effect gluten and other food sensitivities have on various types of arthritis. The effects of chronic arthritis symptoms can be debilitating affecting an individual's psychological (decreased quality of life) and physical health. The risks associated with changing one's diet is minimal (need to ensure foods are nutrient dense and that you consume all essential nutrients) compared with the possible risks associated with the side effects of medication. Many have found relief from arthritis

51

symptoms by identifying a gluten intolerance or allergies, then avoiding those foods [2,22-27,29-31,46,47,50,51,74,75].

Nutrient deficiencies that may contribute to arthritis symptoms include vitamins A, D, C, E, K, niacin, pantothenic acid, pyridoxine, and protein, fatty acids, calcium, magnesium, iron, selenium, manganese, boron, copper, and zinc [62,64,65].

As mentioned previously, nutrient deficiencies can be present in non-celiac gluten intolerance as well.

Prior to diagnosis, I experienced pain and stiffness in both knees, my shoulder, my wrist, and my hip. Once diagnosed and gluten-free, the pain and stiffness disappeared only to return occasionally. I removed dairy from my diet and the pain and stiffness went away. A consultation with an allergist confirmed that I have a diary allergy.

Muscular Symptoms

Muscle symptoms may result from immunological reactions affecting the nerves or muscle tissue, a compromised blood supply to the muscles, intramuscular bleeding, and/or nutrient deficiencies.

Muscular symptoms can include cramps, stiffness, spasms, weakness, aching, pain, fatigue, swallowing difficulties (dysphagia), droopy eyelids, difficulty moving eyes, eye paralysis, limb weakness, weakness after exertion, tetany, decreased mobility, difficulty climbing stairs, difficulty breathing, myocarditis, decreased muscle mass, difficulty lifting objects or doing activities of daily living [1,2,8,9,30-39,52-55,57-61].

If gluten intolerance tests are negative, keep in mind that muscular symptoms can occur with food allergies as well. An allergist or naturopathic doctor may be helpful to identify the offending foods. A naturopathic doctor tends to do a wider variety of tests for food allergies.

Myopathy involves a disease process that leads to dysfunctional muscle fibers. Various myopathies have been associated with gluten intolerance including dermatomyositis, polymyositis, inclusion body myositis, rhabdomyolysis, ocular myopathy, muscular dystrophy, neutrophilic myositis, muscular hypotonia (muscle weakness) of the infant or child, proximal myopathy and generalized myopathy [8,9,31-35,37-39,51,52,54-56,58-60, 67]. Intramuscular hemorrhage was also identified in one case study and this symptom was due to a vitamin K deficiency [66].

Nutrient deficiencies that may contribute to muscular symptoms include vitamins A, D, E, K, niacin, thiamine, pantothenic acid, pyridoxine, cobalamin, protein, fat, carbohydrates, calcium, magnesium, phosphorus, potassium, iodine, iron, and copper [62-65].

> *I experienced muscle cramps, stiffness, weakness, aching, and fatigue. There were times I felt so weak that I had to sit or lie down for awhile. My daughter and mother both had muscle cramps.*

Other Influencing Factors

Other factors that may contribute to musculoskeletal symptoms include a poor diet, past stomach or intestinal surgery, decreased sun exposure, gender, age, obesity, type of work, pregnancy, lactation, exclusively breast feeding without infant vitamin D supplements (inquire with MD), certain medications, low body weight, smoking, family history, early menopause, alcoholism, increased homocysteine levels, chronic bed rest, lack of exercise, and the presence of diarrhea and vomiting [1,5,43,71].

The presence of other conditions such as renal failure, renal tubular acidosis, tumor-induced osteomalacia, cancer, acquired disorders of vitamin D metabolism, liver disease, Crohn's disease, hypoparathyroidism, hyperthyroidism, compensatory secondary hyperparathyroidism, Cushing's Syndrome, Paget's disease, scleroderma, lupus, and Sjögren's Syndrome may contribute to the symptoms as well [1,5,43,71].

Other People's Experiences

Case 1: I was misdiagnosed with fibromyalgia for years. After my dad was diagnosed with celiac disease, I was tested and my result was positive. Now, my symptoms are gone.

Case 2: I was diagnosed with osteoporosis at age 55. I had problems with constipation and bloating. I thought I wasn't eating enough fiber. At age 60, I started having some diarrhea and I was diagnosed with celiac disease. Early diagnosis may have prevented my osteoporosis.

Case 3: I had low back pain and leg cramps prior to diagnosis. It was difficult to sit for long periods. I also had fatigue and muscle weakness. I would break out in a sweat and have to sit or lie down. It began to affect my work.

After I was diagnosed with celiac, I found out that I had severe osteopenia. The gluten-free diet has worked to remove my symptoms and my osteopenia is almost gone now after 2 years.

Case 4: *Prior to my celiac diagnosis, I was diagnosed with scoliosis. Could an earlier celiac diagnosis have prevented this?*

Case 5: *I had anemia, scoliosis, and migraines. I had surgery to help correct my scoliosis. Then, I came across a blog describing how undiagnosed celiac disease might lead to soft bendable bones. I bought a celiac home test and it was positive. My doctor confirmed a Celiac diagnosis. I keep wondering if a gluten-free diet could have prevented all of my suffering and the surgery I needed to have for my scoliosis.*

Case 6: *I was very short as a child and my 3 daughters were short as well. Never once was celiac disease investigated. I am sure that celiac disease caused our short stature since my 3 children have been diagnosed with CD and 1 with dermatitis herpetiformis. An earlier diagnosis may have helped my kids reach a taller height. It is too late now for that.*

CHAPTER 9
Reproductive Symptoms

In this chapter, reproductive symptoms associated with celiac disease (CD), dermatitis herpetiformis (DH), or a non-celiac gluten intolerance will be discussed. There are many studies, books and articles that identify an association between gluten intolerance and reproductive symptoms [1-49]. The presence of nutrient deficiencies provides a possible explanation since the reproductive organs and a developing fetus are dependent on a steady supply of nutrients. However, the pathogenesis of these symptoms due autoimmune damage to the reproductive organs or the fetus is unclear.

Hypothetically, reproductive symptoms may result from auto-antibodies directed at hormones, organs necessary for development in puberty, reproductive organs, or fetal tissue. This is plausible since we know that auto-antibodies (resulting from autoimmune reactions to ingested gluten) can cause damage to a variety of bodily tissues such as the intestinal mucosa (villous flattening), muscles, nerves, skin, pancreas, and liver [50,51,57-59,61].

If intestinal damage occurs, the intestinal villi are less able to absorb nutrients leading to various nutrient deficiencies that may affect sex hormones, health of the reproductive organs, threaten the viability of a fetus, or decrease success with breast feeding. With a non-celiac gluten intolerance, the presence of diarrhea or vomiting, a poor diet, certain medications or the presence of other autoimmune diseases that could affect digestion may lead to nutrient deficiencies as well [39,40,62].

Collectively, the above influencing factors are likely responsible for the reproductive symptoms evident with gluten intolerance. Reproductive symptoms may be the first to develop and can occur without bowel or other extra-intestinal symptoms [8,19,32,47,48].

Symptoms

Reproductive symptoms may include hypogonadism (decreased function of the ovaries or testes), pubertal delay (failure to develop secondary sex characteristics), delayed or retarded menarche (delayed period) or amenorrhea (no period). Other symptoms may include secondary amenorrhea (no period for 6 or more months), chronic pelvic pain, dysmenorrhea (severe uterine menstrual pain), dyspareunia (intercourse is painful), vaginal infections, and vaginitis (inflamed vagina) [1-49].

As well, people may experience a decreased sex drive (decreased libido), impotence (inability to sustain an erection), sperm abnormalities, infertility (in men or women), preeclampsia (high blood pressure in pregnancy), miscarriages (loss of fetus) and zygote (first stage in fetal development) abnormalities. Fetal complications (birth defects, intrauterine fetal growth restriction, decreased growth of baby in uterus), lower birth weight, premature birth, abnormal bleeding or infections post birth in mother, poor breast milk quality and production, and early menopause may also be a problem [1-49].

The sense of loss experienced by individuals with these symptoms can be overwhelming and psychologically scarring. Imagine the loss of reproductive years due to infertility, the loss of a baby, or dealing with birth defects (stress, worry), only to find out later that it was due to the ingestion of gluten. Diagnosis and the implementation of a gluten-free diet is key to the primary prevention of reproductive symptoms in those with a gluten intolerance. Unfortunately, diagnosis can be delayed for years due to the elusive presentation of symptoms.

I was diagnosed at age 37. I didn't suffer from infertility and had 3 children. I did have delayed menarche and also had some problems with my pregnancies.

My first child was born 3 weeks early due to my water breaking. I had anemia and palpitations during the pregnancy. I did not have any intestinal symptoms (classic CD symptoms) until after the birth of my first child.

With my second pregnancy, I was hospitalized and put on bed rest due to premature inter-uterine contractions and pain. I also had anemia with this pregnancy and delivered 2 weeks early.

With my third pregnancy, I had inter-uterine fetal growth restriction and had to decrease my activity. I remember adding lots of pasta and bread into my diet to help increase weight (exactly the opposite of what I needed since the pasta and bread had a high gluten content). My third child was born 1 1/2 weeks early at 6 pounds, 6 ounces.

My mother (diagnosed with CD at age 60) almost lost her second child during her child bearing years due to pregnancy complications.

I breast fed all 3 babies. However, I had to stop breast feeding the third after six weeks due to poor breast milk quality and production. I was ill with bowel symptoms at that time and likely had multiple nutrient deficiencies.

Note: Delivery of a baby 2-3 weeks early is still considered full-term. However, I thought that the fact that all 3 children were born before their due date is worth mentioning.

Nutrient Deficiencies

Nutrient deficiencies that may contribute to reproductive symptoms include vitamins A, D, E K, B complex, C, essential amino and fatty acids, carbohydrates, iodine, electrolytes, calcium, magnesium, phosphorus, iron, copper, manganese, zinc and molybdenum [37-46].

Severity of nutrient loss and related symptoms are dependent on the location, length and severity of intestinal villi damage, which can be patchy in nature, and the presence of other factors such as diarrhea, vomiting, medications that affect nutrient absorption, other associated diseases, intestinal parasites, a poor diet, past stomach and intestinal surgery, smoking, or alcoholism [1-3,32,39,40,47,48].

Other People's Experiences

Case 1: Along with diarrhea, bloating, and anemia, I had frequent ovarian cysts. All symptoms are gone with a GF diet. My grandmother died from ovarian cancer. Could it have been related to a gluten intolerance?

Case 2: I had 2 miscarriages and 1 very difficult pregnancy. I was diagnosed with IBS as a teenager. Now I'm diagnosed with celiac disease and gluten-free. Could an earlier diagnosis and a GF diet have prevented the miscarriages? I will always wonder about that.

Case 3: While undiagnosed, I had a very difficult pregnancy and my baby died before it was born. Would I have my baby today if I was diagnosed earlier? That is a question that will always haunt me. Doctors need to be more aware.

CHAPTER 10
Urological (Kidney And Bladder) Symptoms

This chapter discusses the variety of ways adverse reactions to food may affect the kidneys, ureters (tube between kidney and bladder), bladder and/or urethra (tube from bladder to outside of body). All of these bodily parts are needed to produce and pass urine.

The Cause: A Gluten Intolerance?

There are studies and articles identifying an association between gluten intolerance and urological symptoms [5,34,35,42,48]. However, the pathogenesis of urological symptoms due to gluten consumption and the resulting autoimmune damage is unclear.

Hypothetically, these symptoms may result from auto-antibodies directed at the kidneys, ureters, bladder, or the urethra. This is plausible since we know that auto-antibodies in the three forms of gluten intolerance can cause damage to a variety of other bodily tissues such as the intestinal mucosa (villous flattening), muscles, nerves, skin, and liver [36,38-41].

Additionally, if intestinal damage occurs, the flattened villi are less able to absorb nutrients leading to various nutrient deficiencies that may affect the urological system [1,2]. We know that nutrient deficiencies can adversely affect muscle, nerve, and mucosal tissue so it is reasonable to expect that the urological system would be affected since it is dependent on these systems.

Another Culprit: Food Allergies?

If urological symptoms persist once diagnosed and gluten-free, then a food allergy may exist. In the absence of a gluten intolerance, food allergies may be the sole or part of the underlying reason for your symptoms [42,43].

Various food allergies have been linked either through research, case studies, or personal experiences to urological symptoms [23-29,31-35,42,43]. This may be due to immune reactions causing damage and inflammation to the kidneys, bladder, ureters or the urethra. This seems plausible since mast cells (release histamine) and histamine (produces inflammation) are involved in immune reactions to food. Histamine has also been detected in bladder washings and mucosal mast cells have been located in the detrusor muscle, lamina propria, and epithelium of the bladder in patients with interstitial cystitis [42,43].

Another theory, the kidneys may be vulnerable to damage if exposed to immune complexes (resulting from reactions with food allergens) that are circulating in the blood since the kidney filters all the blood. An immune complex could become lodged in the kidney and this could lead to inflammation and further immune activity, resulting in kidney damage. Overall, it is reasonable to suspect that a reaction to food antigens could be an underlying contributing factor for the development of urological conditions.

A few studies have examined the effects that reactions to food can have on the urological system. Various food allergens such as milk proteins, soy bean protein, rice protein, gliadin, oat flour extracts, ovalbumin, and bovine serum albumin have been associated with urological symptoms [13,14,18,23,24,26,29-33]. As well, increased intestinal permeability (leaky gut) has been identified in IgA nephropathy [26,27]. As previously discussed, gluten intolerance along with other factors can lead to a leaky gut. Increased intestinal permeability allows food molecules to interact with the immune system and this interaction could theoretically lead to inflammation and damage in the kidney or elsewhere in the urological system.

Almost any food, pesticide, or food additive could potentially cause an immune mediated reaction in the form of an allergy.

Wendy Cohen (RN) [www.wellbladder.com] has identified many possible bladder irritants [28]. Visit her site for tips. Wendy has many comments on her urology articles describing personal experiences with food allergies. She has also just released a new book, "The Better Bladder Book".

More research is needed. Research results demonstrating an association between food allergens and urological symptoms could lead to dietary intervention as the key to primary prevention and treatment of many urological symptoms. Personal and healthcare benefits include decreased hospitalization, decreased physician visits, decreased use of medications, and increased quality of life for individuals suffering with urological symptoms.

Symptoms

Urological symptoms may include chronic prostatitis (inflammation of prostate gland), interstitial cystitis (bladder pain and altered urination), bed-wetting in children, stress incontinence, frequency and urgency to urinate, bladder spasms, chronic or recurrent bladder infections, urethritis (inflamed urethra), IgA nephropathy (inflamed small blood vessels - glomeruli in kidney), and nephrotic syndrome (damaged kidney) [2,5-35].

Other symptoms can include kidney stones (renal calculus), active albuminuria (albumin in urine), proteinuria (protein in urine), haematuria (blood in urine), glomerulonephritis (inflamed small blood vessels in kidney), mesangial nephritis (kidney), glomerulitis (kidney), membranoproliferative glomerulonephritis (kidney), IgA mesangial glomerulonephritis (kidney), immunoglobulin A mesangial nephropathy (kidney), and midaortic syndrome affecting infrarenal aorta or renal arteries. Many of these conditions can lead to renal failure [2,5-35].

Further research may reveal other symptoms or urological conditions such as renal rickets, neurogenic bladder, or polycystic kidney disease.

I experienced frequent ovarian cysts prior to my diagnosis so it seems reasonable to suspect that cysts could occur elsewhere in the body (i.e. the kidneys). I do not have problems with ovarian cysts now.

As well, while undiagnosed, I experienced occasional urine frequency and bladder cramping. The urine dipsticks and urine culture and sensitivity would surprisingly be negative. Perhaps, my symptoms were related to bladder irritants, nutrient deficiencies (affecting the muscles, nerves, or mucosa) or other immune factors such as mast cells and histamine.

Nutrient Deficiencies

Nutrient deficiencies may affect the nervous system, muscular system, and mucosal health in the urological system. Nutrient deficiencies that may contribute to nerve related urological symptoms in the bladder may include vitamins E, B complex, amino and fatty acids, calcium, magnesium, phosphorus, copper, electrolytes, and inositol [45-49].

Nutrient deficiencies that may contribute to muscular related urological symptoms in the bladder may include vitamins A, D, E, K, niacin, thiamine, pantothenic acid, pyridoxine, cobalamin, amino and fatty acids, carbohydrates, calcium, magnesium, phosphorus, potassium, iodine, iron, and copper [44-46].

Nutrients deficiencies that may affect urological mucosal health include vitamin A, B complex, C, D,E, K, amino and fatty acids, carbohydrates, iron, zinc, copper, manganese, and molybdenum [45,46].

Other Factors Affecting Kidney Or Bladder Function

Other factors that may contribute to kidney and bladder symptoms include diabetes, hypotension, hypertension, poor diet, alcoholism, street drugs, past surgery, poor heart function, infections, protein toxicity, tumors, congenital defects, trauma, toxicity from chemicals, certain medications, or vitamin toxicity.

Other People's Experiences

Case 1: I was diagnosed with interstitial cystitis for 5 years prior to my dermatitis herpetiformis diagnosis. Four months after starting the GF diet, the cystitis was gone. I suffered for 4 years with constant pain and all I had to do is remove gluten.

Case 2: I have had interstitial cystitis for 32 years. 6 months ago I was tested for CD and it was negative. Recently, I read a blog and decided to try a GF diet anyway. Well, I am feeling much better now and the IC symptoms are almost gone.

Case 3: Prior to my celiac diagnosis, I was diagnosed with IgA Nephropathy and I had kidney stones. I have diabetes too. I wonder if a gluten-free diet would have prevented all of this from occurring.

CHAPTER 11
Neurological (Brain And Nerve) Symptoms

This chapter discusses a variety of neurological symptoms that can be caused by undiagnosed gluten intolerance. The link between neurological symptoms and gluten intolerance is very under recognized by the medical community, this is sad since ongoing immune reactions and nutrient deficiencies can lead to permanent damage.

There are studies and articles that identify an association between gluten intolerance and neurological symptoms [1-3,5-8,11-90,94,96,98,99,109-117,120,123-123]. The pathogenesis is thought to be due to autoimmune reactions (to ingested gluten) causing inflammation and damage in the central and peripheral nervous systems in gluten sensitive individuals.

Nutrient Deficiencies

The presence of nutrient deficiencies may also lead to neurological symptoms. This can be common in CD or DH, but can also be present with non-celiac gluten intolerance if diarrhea, vomiting, and other diseases or conditions (affecting nutrient absorption) are present. Certain medications and a nutrient poor diet can contribute to deficiencies.

Nutrient deficiencies contributing to neurological symptoms can include vitamins E, B complex, K, amino and fatty acids, calcium, magnesium, phosphorus, copper, electrolytes, l-carnitine, and inositol [8-10,51,80].

Abnormal Findings

With gluten intolerance, some abnormal findings on tests can include abnormal brain waves on electroencephalography (EEG), unusual cerebellar (part of brain) physiology, hypoperfused brain regions (decreased blood flow), brain atrophy (decreased size), inflammation, patchy Purkinje cell (out-put neurons) loss in the cerebellum, and progressive multifocal leukoencephalopathy leading to destruction of myelin sheaths that support neuronal impulses [1,7,11,14,22,33,50,59,65-67,80,81,85,87,91-95,97,123,150].

Other findings include lymphocytic (immune system players) infiltration of the cerebellum and peripheral nerves, damage to the posterior columns of the spinal cord, and widespread IgA deposition around vessels in the brain (showing immune activity). As well, brain white-matter lesions or calcifications, likely resulting from autoimmune reactions, calcium deposits, ischemia (inadequate blood supply), vasculitis (inflammation of blood vessels), or inflammatory demyelination, can occur.

Symptoms

Collectively, immunological reactions, various neurological abnormalities, and nutrient deficiencies can lead to a wide variety of neurological symptoms.

Gluten Ataxia

Gluten ataxia may result from immunological damage to the cerebellum, posterior columns of the spinal cord, and peripheral nerves [16,19,20,22,25,26]. Ataxia symptoms can include staggering gait, lack of balance, poor coordination, unsteadiness with standing or walking, increased falls, and dysarthric speech (may be slurred, slow, and difficult to produce and also the pitch, rhythm, loudness, and other voice qualities may change).

Other symptoms include dysphagia (difficulty swallowing), clumsy exaggerated imprecise limb (arms and legs) movements, difficulty with fine-motor skills (ex. writing, buttoning a shirt, or eating), oculomotor (abnormal eye movements) problems, sensorimotor axonal neuropathy and other peripheral neuropathies.

As well, dysmetria (inability to judge distance or scale), decreased processing of sensory information, sometimes declining cognitive function, and decreased cerebellar processing of afferent information (information from muscles, joints, movement, visual, auditory, somatosensory, cerebral cortex and midbrain) can occur. The progression of symptoms is generally slow. However, in some cases the progression is quick with cerebellar atrophy that can occur within 1 year of the initial symptom.

A gluten-free diet may take a year or more to eliminate antibodies and this along with correction of nutrient deficiencies will hopefully decrease or stop further progression of symptoms. If permanent damage has already occurred, symptoms may not resolve. Children and infants can have ataxia symptoms as well [12,16-19,25,27,43,63,104,122,126].

Neuropathies (Neuritis)

Autoimmune damage to the nerves, inflammation, and nutrient deficiencies may lead to a variety of neuropathies. Symptoms can include burning, tingling, numbness, vibrations, pinching, stabbing, buzzing, pressure, muscle twitches, or a loss of feeling [21,22,25,62,71, 99].

These sensations can spread from an initial localized area to other parts of the body. Pain may also occur and may feel like an electric shock, legs may feel heavy, an increased sensitivity to touch may occur and paresthesias resulting in sensory loss and muscle weakness can occur.

Other symptoms can include carpal tunnel syndrome, vestibular dysfunction (dizziness, lack of balance), myelitis, reduced reflexes, deep sensory loss, proprioceptive (sense of position in space) loss, dysesthesias (abnormal sensations), feeling like you are wearing gloves or stockings, difficulty moving limbs, frequently dropping items, walking with a wide stance (to compensate), and increased falls.

As well, a change in bowel habits, sexual dysfunction, skin problems, organ dysfunction, internuclear ophthalmoplegia, myelopathies, paralysis, and acute paraplegia might occur. Autonomic nerve damage can also cause low blood pressure and dizziness. Onset can be sudden or gradual and neuropathies can affect any age.

I had intermittent tingling, numbness, vibrations, cold and burning feelings, and pain in my head, face, arms, and legs. I also had carpel tunnel for awhile and had to wear a brace. My daughter had tingling and numbness in her feet. Occasionally, I also experienced pressure on top of my head or on an extremity, and transient head and mouth numbness would occur. There were occasions where I actually felt like I was slurring my speech.

Epilepsy (Seizures)

There is mystery regarding the pathogenesis of gluten-sensitive epilepsy, however, a connection between CD, bilateral occipital cerebral calcification (calcification may or may not be present), and seizures has been noted. It is reasonable to suspect that autoimmune reactions, possibly associated vasculitis, inflammation, and nutrient deficiencies may be responsible. The prognosis is influenced by how soon in the disease a gluten free diet is started [32-39,58].

Theoretically, a non-celiac gluten intolerance might lead to epileptic symptoms as well. This could be due to inflammation related to autoimmune activity, immune reactions to lectins, nutrient deficiencies (with vomiting, diarrhea, poor diet), or a sensitivity to glutamic acid or aspartic acid over activating the nerve cells in the brain (see Chapter 2 for more).

Seizure symptoms can include auras (perceptual disturbance prior to seizure), prodromes (ex. early symptom such as disorientation, photosensitivity, euphoria, or aphagia), loss of consciousness, automatisms (involuntary movements), versive (forced and involuntary head movements) or nonversive (mild, seemingly voluntary head movements).

Other symptoms include confusion, vomiting, convulsions, difficulty talking, drooling, incontinence, temporary paralysis, sweating, and tachycardia (increased pulse). Involuntary movements during the seizure may include chewing movements, lip smacking, eyelid fluttering, eyes rolling up, falling, hand waving, stomping feet, may bit tongue, vocal sounds, shaking, stiffening, staring, swallowing, grinding and clenching teeth, tremors, and tensing muscles, altered breathing pattern, and twitching movements. Seizures types may be grand mal, petit mal or focal. Immediate assessment by an MD can help prevent complications and rule out a stroke.

Migraines/Headaches

Episodic, mild to severe headaches, often with some form of transient neurological deficit, is associated with gluten intolerance. Immunological reactions, inflammation, associated vasculitis, brain white matter, hypoperfused brain regions, altered brain waves, and nutrient deficiencies may contribute to this symptom [21,25,28-31,75,123].

A pre-migraine/headache aura can occur and symptoms may include seeing spots, wavy lines, flashing lights, visual distortion of objects, weakness, numbness, confusion, difficulty with words, and/or a feeling of pins and needles. The migraine/headache symptoms may include pain in part or all of the head that is throbbing, pulsating, or stabbing, possibly with temporary visual loss or change (ocular migraine), nausea or vomiting, and sensitivity to light noise and smell.

A complicated headache may involve extra symptoms, such as difficulty understanding speech, difficulty speaking, numbness, tingling, paralysis of a limb, or include another nervous system deficit. Be careful about assuming these symptoms are related to a headache since a stroke may cause similar symptoms.

I experienced ocular migraines. I would have partial vision loss, usually unilaterally, that would last 1-2 hours, then resolve. Occasionally, I would see flashes of light out of the corner of my eye, the room would seem cloudy, and I would see dots blocking my view.

I had a full-check up with an optometrist and an ophthalmologist, but all tests were negative.

Food allergies can cause neurological symptoms as well. Ten to twenty minutes after eating a banana, the roof of my mouth becomes very itchy, and my vision becomes blurred (usually without head discomfort) for 2-3 hours. A consultation with an allergist confirmed that I have a banana allergy.

Cerebral Infarction (Strokes) And Thrombosis (Clots) Formation

Antiphospholipid Syndrome is associated with CD and this can increase the risk for arterial and venous thrombus (clot) formation [53,107,108]. In a case study, three patients with CD had antiphospholipid syndrome. One experienced fetal death, the second case presented with thrombosis in her limb and had renal infarction (lack of blood to kidney). The third case had two spontaneous abortions and a transient ischemic cerebral attack (change in blood supply to the brain that is temporary) [53].

You can see how the presence of antiphospholipid syndrome in CD could possibly lead to strokes, renal (kidney) problems, fetal complications, pulmonary emboli (clot in lungs), heart attacks, or ischemic (inadequate blood supply) attacks in other areas of the body. Thrombosis, leading to ischemia could be the first symptom/diagnosis present in a gluten intolerance [16,25,52,78, 103,127-130].

Other factors that may contribute to stroke or clot formation in a gluten intolerance include associated systemic vasculitis (leading to stenosis, occlusions, or aneurysm of the blood vessels) or the activity of auto-antibodies inhibiting angiogenesis (affecting the health of blood vessels).

As well, vitamin K deficiency (due to malabsorption) may increase the risk for an intracerebral bleed or cause a protein S and protein C deficiency possibly leading to thrombosis. Auto-antibodies to plasma transglutaminase (i.e. Factor XIII) could lead to problems with coagulation and this could increase the risk for a stroke. This seems plausible since we know auto-antibodies react to other types of transglutaminase in the body with a gluten intolerance. Collectively or in isolation, these factors could lead to a variety of ischemic (lack of blood supply) symptoms.

In case studies, strokes in children and adults were linked to CD [68-71,133]. With a stroke, brain function is lost, as a result of ischemia, due to a thrombosis, embolism, or a hemorrhage. Stroke symptoms are dependent on the area of the brain that is compromised.

Collectively, the symptoms may include convulsions, apneic attacks, difficulty swallowing, reduced vibratory and sensory sensation, decreased ability to move extremities (arms and legs) on one side of the body (hemiplegia) and paralysis. Weakness, difficulty understanding or formulating speech (aphasia), visual field changes or defects, headache, facial weakness, numbness, and decreased reflexes (swallow, gag, pupil reactions to light are altered) can also occur.

Other symptoms include tongue weakness (may be unable to protrude or move side to side), ptosis (drooping of eyelid), ocular (eye) muscle weakness, sensory changes (hearing, taste, smell, vision touch), difficulty walking, difficulty with coordination, dizziness, incontinence, difficulty with balance, and nystagmus (involuntary eye movement).

As well, abnormal breathing and heart rate, sternocleidomastoid muscle weakness (difficulty turning head to one side), apraxia (voluntary movements are altered), loss of memory, hemineglect, confusion, disorganized thinking, anosognosia (denial of a deficit), loss of consciousness, vomiting, and headache can occur. Permanent damage can occur. Thrombosis symptoms could also include organ failure, deep vein thrombosis (clot), heart attack, or pulmonary emboli (clot in lung).

Myopathies

Muscle symptoms may result from immunological reactions affecting the nerves or muscle tissue, a compromised blood supply to the muscles, intramuscular bleeding, and/or nutrient deficiencies.

Muscular symptoms can include cramps, stiffness, spasms, weakness, aching, pain, fatigue, swallowing difficulties (dysphagia), droopy eyelids, difficulty moving eyes, eye paralysis, limb weakness, weakness after exertion, tetany, decreased mobility, difficulty climbing stairs, difficulty breathing, myocarditis, hypotonia, decreased muscle mass, difficulty lifting objects or doing activities of daily living [3,33-40,42,43,51-55,57-62,150].

Myopathy involves a disease process that leads to dysfunctional muscle fibers. Various myopathies have been associated with CD and gluten sensitivity including dermatomyositis, polymyositis, inclusion body myositis, rhabdomyolysis, ocular (eye) myopathy, muscular dystrophy, neutrophilic myositis, muscular hypotonia (lack of muscle strength) of the infant or child, proximal myopathy and generalized myopathy [33-40,42,43,51-55,57-62]. Intramuscular hemorrhage was also identified in one case study and this symptom was due to a vitamin K deficiency [183].

Muscle symptoms can occur with the presence of food allergies. An allergist or naturopathic doctor may be helpful to identify offending foods. A naturopathic doctor usually does a wider variety of allergy related blood tests.

Nutrient deficiencies that may contribute to muscular symptoms include vitamins A, D, E, K, niacin, thiamine, pantothenic acid, pyridoxine, cobalamin, protein, fat, carbohydrates, calcium, magnesium, phosphorus, potassium, iodine, iron, and copper [9,10].

I experienced muscle cramps, stiffness, weakness, aching, and fatigue. There were times I felt so weak that I had to sit or lie down for awhile. My daughter and mother both had muscle cramps.

Dementia

Immunological reactions leading to brain atrophy, nerve damage, nutrient deficiencies, hypoperfused (low blood flow) brain regions, vasculitis (inflamed blood vessels), and white matter lesions in the brain may contribute to dementia symptoms. Dementia can be very subtle or obvious. Dementia symptoms may include loss of short term memory, difficulty with finding words, memory loss or forgetfulness (ex. forgetting names or appointments), difficulty doing familiar tasks, personality or mood changes, change in behavior, and poor judgment [50,52].

Other symptoms include paranoia, hallucinations, suspicion, confusion, disorientation in new or usual surroundings, difficulty with activities of daily living, altered sleep habits, difficulty learning, increased falls, aggressiveness, and inappropriate sexual behavior. As well, poor concentration, confabulation, anxiety, impaired swallowing, withdrawal from others, malnutrition (forget to eat), dehydration, seizures, injuries, difficulty with communication, poor organization, decreased motor and coordination function, personality changes, and difficulty reasoning can occur.

Prior to diagnosis, I would experience foggy thinking and memory lapses.

Note: Psychological and other cognitive symptoms will be discussed in the next chapter. If you have any of the previous symptoms, seek medical attention for an assessment.

Other Contributing Factors

Other factors that may contribute to neurological symptoms include smoking, hypertension, diabetes, hyperlipidemia, ischemic heart disease, atrial fibrillation (increases risk for clots), hyperhomocysteinemia (associated with CD), renal failure, thyroid disease, calcium metabolism, inborn error of metabolism, trauma, infections, genetics, toxic-metabolic agents, certain medications, poor diet, vitamin deficiency or toxicity, alcoholism, heavy metals, solvents, street drugs, and gastric surgery (leading to deficiencies).

Associated Conditions

In studies, gluten intolerance is associated with other neurological diseases, such as Huntington's Disease/Chorea [25,40,41,106], Ramsay Hunt Syndrome [24,61], Plummer Vinson Syndrome/Patterson Brown Kelly [5,6,72,73], Stiff Person Syndrome [25,84], and Multiple Sclerosis (MS) [76,109-116].

Gluten intolerance can produce a variety of neurological symptoms so it is reasonable to suspect that associated autoimmune damage, inflammation, and possible nutrient deficiencies may play a role in other autoimmune diseases such as Parkinson's Disease, Amyotrophic Lateral Sclerosis (ALS)/Lou Gehrig's Disease, Guillain–Barré Syndrome (GBS), or numerous other neurological conditions.

If gluten sensitivity isn't the culprit, then perhaps other various food antigens or processing agents are prompting an autoimmune response. In individuals with a gluten intolerance, gluten consumption can lead to increased expression of zonulin (a human protein) in the intestinal tissues. This increases intestinal permeability allowing macromolecules (ex. food antigens, bacterial, and viral particles) exposure to the immune system. The immune systems exposure to gluten and the subsequent reaction is thought to be responsible for the intestinal and other systemic damage seen with a gluten intolerance. The increased bowel permeability can also increase the risk of developing food allergies. Dr. Alessio Fasano and his research team feel that the increased intestinal permeability (due to zonulin) is part of the underlying pathogenesis involved in CD and possibly many other autoimmune diseases [89]. Could increased intestinal permeability, leading to immune exposure to many possible food antigens, be responsible for other neurological diseases such as Parkinson's Disease, Amyotrophic Lateral Sclerosis (ALS) and Guillain–Barré Syndrome?

I am curious about a possible link between ALS, gluten intolerance and other food allergens. My grandfather died from ALS. My mother (his daughter), myself, and my daughter have CD. Could my grandfather have been misdiagnosed? Did he really have neurological and muscular symptoms as a result of undiagnosed CD? One article, identified a 44 year old male who was misdiagnosed with ALS. Further investigation 6 months later revealed that he really had CD. He was put on a gluten-free diet and 9 months later his symptoms had improved [120]. The abstract can be viewed at www.ncbi.nlm.nih.gov/pubmed/17914346.

In another study, a young man had progressive neurological symptoms. The doctor ordered diagnostic imaging of his brain and the results showed white matter lesions that were suggestive of ALS. However, part of the diagnostic blood work-up revealed endomysium antibodies and duodenal biopsies confirmed the presence of celiac disease. A strict gluten-free diet was initiated [134].

Another area of interest is the use of Palaeolithic diets to lesson immune responses and control symptoms. This may help many with symptoms related to a lectin intolerance. All grains, dairy, legumes, nightshade foods, and processed sugar (eliminates corn sweeteners too) are removed from the diet. With this diet, individuals eat very primal foods, with the belief that our bodies may have difficulty immunologically with foods that have been introduced fairly recently in our evolutionary history. There are many studies identifying adverse effects from the ingestion of lectins (see more under Chapter 2, "Pathophysiology Of Non-Celiac Gluten Intolerance". In fact, the symptoms seem to be just as varied as the symptoms of gluten intolerance.

A researcher, Dr. Loren Cordain, PhD, (from Colorado State University, USA) discusses the use of a Palaeolithic diet for Multiple Sclerosis in a 2007 video, "Potential Therapeutic Characteristics of Pre-agricultural Diets In The Prevention And Treatment Of Multiple Sclerosis", www.wildhorse.insinc.com/directms03oct2007/

Dr. Cordain discusses how 4 individuals with MS benefited from this diet and believes this diet may benefit others with various autoimmune diseases as well. The video is located on Dr. Ashton Embry's (Ph.D) website at Direct-MS [www.direct-ms.org/]. The results of this study make sense, according to other studies lectin does appear to have neurological effects once it gains access to the systemic circulation. The effects of lectin on bowel permeability certainly could increase the risk of this occurring (151-153).

More research is needed to investigate possible links between food antigens and other neurological diseases. A therapeutic diet would be an attractive alternative to the use of medications (with possible side effects) and other possibly invasive procedures. Further research, better diagnostic tests, and increased awareness can help medical professionals and patients put the pieces of the gluten/food sensitivity puzzle together.

Other People's Experiences

Case 1: My child was diagnosed with celiac disease. Before she was diagnosed, she had autistic like behavior, poor motor development, poor balance, had difficulty with word finding, complained that her hands and feet felt prickly, had stomach aches, and frequent bed wetting. We have been eating GF for almost 1 year and the symptoms are finally gone.

Case 2: I had numbness and tingling in my hands and feet before diagnosis. I had cold and hot spots that would develop on my legs too. On a GF diet, the symptoms are gone. It took 5 months for this to happen.

Case 3: I would get frequent headaches and was very forgetful before diagnosis. I asked my doctor to check me for Alzheimer's and she said I was too young. On some days it was hard to think.

After some bowel symptoms started I got tested for celiac. It was negative, but I tried a GF diet anyway. I can think better and the headaches and diarrhea are gone.

Case 4: I had a stroke, seizures, and ataxia before my diagnosis. I was in a wheel-chair. I had been diagnosed with fibromyalgia and I was being investigated for MS. My daughter became sick and then was diagnosed with Celiac. I was screened and celiac was found. An earlier diagnosis could have prevented all of the pain and rehabilitation I had to endure.

Case 5: I had a stroke last year, just before my celiac diagnosis. I remember that the right side of my body went numb and then I noticed that I couldn't swallow well. I'm only 47. An earlier diagnosis may have prevented this permanent weakness in my right leg that I have to live with.

Case 6: My daughter had a stroke a little of over a year ago at the age of 12. The specialists couldn't figure out why she had a stroke at such a young age. She had occasional stomach aches too. The doctors couldn't find a reason for the stomach aches and thought she was suffering from constipation and needed more fiber.

Luckily, I came across a blog about celiac disease when I was on the Internet looking for information. I went to a doctor and he tested my daughter for celiac disease. Her antibody levels were sky high and her biopsy was positive. I wonder if the undiagnosed celiac disease caused her stroke. If so, much suffering could have been avoided with a gluten-free diet.

CHAPTER 12
Psychological (Affecting Your Thoughts) Symptoms

In this chapter, psychological symptoms will be discussed. Unfortunately, the medical profession often doesn't associate gluten intolerance with psychological symptoms. This is unfortunate because the presence of these symptoms could have long lasting effects on one's life, affecting their confidence, self esteem, and the ability to pursue the career of their choice. Many of the symptoms can lead to poor academic performance and behavioral issues. A gluten-free diet could be the perfect primary prevention.

There are many studies and articles identifying an association between gluten intolerance and psychological symptoms. The pathogenesis is thought to be due to autoimmune reactions causing inflammation and damage in the brain of affected individuals. As well, enhanced production of cytokines (carry signals between cells) due to immune reactions, may stimulate the brain to produce neuroimmune, neuroendocrine, and neurochemical changes that may influence behavior. With gastrointestinal involvement, nutrient deficiencies, can add to the symptoms [1,3,7,8,12,13,15-20,23,26,27,29,30,43-45].

Nutrient Deficiencies

Nutrient deficiencies contributing to psychological symptoms can include vitamins A, B complex (esp. folic acid, B-6, and B12), D, E, K, essential amino and fatty acids (i.e. tryptophan affects serotonin levels and low cholesterol associated with mental disorders), carbohydrates, low glucose (with associated diabetes), calcium, magnesium, phosphorus, copper, electrolytes, l-carnitine, and inositol, and selenium [1,3,5,6,27,43,44].

Symptoms

Gluten Intolerance Can Affect Thoughts

Many studies and articles have identified psychological symptoms that can occur with a gluten intolerance. Symptoms such as schizophrenia spectrum disorders, anxiety problems, learning disabilities, mood disorders, personality changes, irritability, apathy, sitophobia (abnormal aversion to food), irritability, obsessional neurosis, anorexia/bulimia, and delinquent behavior have been mentioned. Other symptoms can include attention deficit disorder (ADD), attention-deficit/hyperactivity disorder (ADHD), cognitive decline, and dementia [1,7,8,10,11,15,16,18,23,26-28,30,43,44,46,48,75,77,82].

Depression

There are also studies and articles that identify an association between gluten intolerance and depression [1,3,12,13,19,20,23,27,29,30-42,76]. It is reasonable to suspect the central nervous system damage and inflammation combined with nutrient deficiencies (i.e. low B vitamins, low serotonin and cholesterol) may be responsible. Other factors such as a sense of helplessness associated with being ill, misdiagnosed, or only having one's symptoms diagnosed can certainly add to these feelings.

Once diagnosed, depression might continue if underlying nutrient deficiencies are left untreated and unrecognized, if accidental ingestion of gluten occurs, if underlying food allergies are not identified, or if the individual has difficulty adjusting to a new lifestyle. As well, personal coping strategies, adequate support and follow-up from healthcare professionals, family and friend supports, availability of gluten-free food and resources can all influence the outcome.

Autism And Asperger's Syndrome

There has been much controversy questioning a link between gluten and Autism and/or Asperger's Syndrome. After reviewing all of the symptoms and abnormal findings in both the neurological chapter and this chapter, you can see how a link could exist. It certainly appears as if many have intestinal involvement, it seems reasonable to suspect that gluten, casein, and other possible food antigens may be involved.

I often felt like it was difficult to think, learn, and analyze. I managed to graduate from University with Honors. However, I was studying constantly to achieve that. I couldn't seem to retain information very well.

Now that I'm eating gluten-free (and paleolithic), my head finally feels clear and I can analyze and retain information with greater ease. I feel like it only takes about 1/3 of the time to study now. It is difficult to learn when you are living with "Brain Fog".

My daughter, with CD, won an academic award last year. It may have been a very different outcome if she was still undiagnosed. She did have evidence of "brain fog" prior to diagnosis.

Other food allergies can cause psychological changes as well. My middle child tested negative for CD. She had eczema of moderate severity, hyperactivity, lack of focus, occasional diarrhea, and abdominal discomfort. I was worried that she was experiencing some symptoms of ADHD. All medical tests ordered by the pediatrician were negative. An elimination diet revealed that she was sensitive to corn derivatives (which are in most grocery store products). All symptoms resolved when I removed corn derivatives from her diet. All symptoms return with accidental ingestion of corn derivatives. The hyperactivity and lack of focus is very pronounced with accidental ingestion of corn derivatives (i.e. corn syrup, dextrose, glucose/fructose and more) which are in most processed foods. Without corn, she is very focused and does well academically.

Influencing Factors

In Chapter 11 (Neurological Symptoms), many test findings are discussed which help to highlight the variety of abnormalities that can be found in the brain of gluten intolerant individuals (while consuming gluten). It is apparent from these findings that psychological behavior could be affected as well.

In Chapter 2, theories about the pathophysiology in non-celiac gluten intolerance were discussed. Some of these theories (primarily theories 3-5) may shed some light on the effects grains and dairy can have on the brain of intolerant individuals (i.e. discusses exorphins, gliadorphins, lectins, aspartic acid and glutamic acid).

Other factors that may add to psychological symptoms include hypothyroidism, adrenal disorders, diabetes, infections, low oxygen levels, hypotension, epilepsy, sleep disorders, genetics, a traumatic event, certain medications, poor diet, vitamin deficiency or toxicity, lack of resources, alcoholism, heavy metals, solvents, street drugs, and gastric (stomach) surgery (leading to deficiencies).

Other People's Experiences

Case 1: My daughter was having many problems learning at school, the doctor diagnosed her with ADHD and wanted to start her on medications. I went to a naturopathic doctor and he tested her for gluten sensitivity and allergies. She reacts to gluten and casein. On a gluten-free and casein-free diet, she is doing well at school, is less moody, and her eczema and stomach aches are gone too. That naturopathic doctor changed my daughter's life.

Case 2: *My daughter was always very tired and seemed to be in a dream world half the time. She was doing okay at school, but needed a lot of help. She also vomited once in a while with stomach aches. Her grandmother has celiac disease so I tested her with the celiac home test and it was positive. She is alert now and doing very well at school (A in math) and her other symptoms are gone.*

Case 3: *I was diagnosed with celiac disease 9 months ago and then my whole family was screened. My mothers test was positive. Prior to my mom's diagnosis, she was very moody and irritable. She also had obsessional tendencies. She would check the stove over and over before leaving the house and she was obsessed with keeping the house clean. Now she is much calmer and after 8 months on the gluten-free diet, she doesn't seem to be obsessed with cleaning the house and checking the stove. She said she feels like she is enjoying life more and can think clearer. She didn't have any other symptoms.*

CHAPTER 13
Cardiopulmonary (Heart And Lung) Symptoms

In this chapter, heart and lung symptoms will be discussed. There are studies identifying an association between gluten intolerance, cardiac (heart), and pulmonary (lung) symptoms. The pathogenesis is likely due to autoimmune reactions (to ingested gluten), causing inflammation and damage to the cardiopulmonary system. The presence of nutrient deficiencies may add to the symptoms [1-38,43,60,61].

Cardiac (Heart) Symptoms

A functional cardiac system is dependent on intact blood vessels, adequate blood supply, intact cardiac nervous system and functional cardiac muscle. Hypothetically, cardiac symptoms may result from auto-antibodies cross-reacting with blood vessels (might inhibit angiogenesis and blood flow), the cardiac nervous system, or the cardiac muscle. Since we know immune reactions to gluten can affect the nervous system (ex. gluten ataxia or neuropathies) and the muscular system (ex. myopathies), it is reasonable to suspect that these two systems, involved in cardiac health, could be affected [70-74].

Findings

The finding of anti-transglutaminase antibodies (commonly found in CD, DH, and gluten ataxia) in end-stage heart failure and cardiomyopathy strengthens the link to gluten [44].The presence of these auto-antibodies suggests that autoimmune activity can lead to cardiac symptoms. With blood vessels, one study demonstrated angiogenesis (growth of blood vessels) was inhibited in the intestine of CD patients and the researchers suspect that impaired angiogenesis could occur in other areas of the body as well. Auto-antibodies have been found around blood vessels in the brain of CD patients, it is plausible to suspect that autoimmune reactions could occur around the vessels of the heart as well. This could affect the blood supply to the heart [1,6-9,11,12,14,21,43,44,53].

Vasculitis

If associated vasculitis is present, it could lead to stenosis, occlusions, or aneurysm of the blood vessels. This could decrease the blood supply and add to impaired cardiovascular health in gluten intolerant individuals [56-58].

Nutrient Deficiencies

If intestinal damage is present, various nutrient deficiencies can occur and this can cause or add to the severity of the cardiac and pulmonary symptoms. Nutrient deficiencies that may affect the cardiac nervous system, cardiac muscle, and the functional structure of the heart and lungs include vitamins A, D, E, K, B complex, amino and fatty acids, calcium, magnesium, phosphorus, copper, electrolytes, iodine, iron, zinc, manganese, selenium, l-carnitine, antioxidants, and inositol [1,2,39,41,42].

Thiamine deficiency is one example of how a nutrient deficiency can lead to heart symptoms. This deficiency can lead to wet beriberi (like heart failure) or acute pernicious beriberi (low blood pressure, high cardiac output). Other examples of deficiencies include low electrolytes (or magnesium, calcium) leading to arrhythmias, low iron and B vitamins leading to anemia (contributes to less oxygen in the blood), or low vitamin K levels affecting protein S or protein C (involved in clotting) possibly leading to a heart attack. The presence of associated antiphospholipid syndrome could increase the risk of clots as well [42,50-52, 54,55].

Hypotension (a cardiac stressor) could result from low protein levels (ex. albumin), low electrolytes, or dehydration especially if diarrhea and vomiting is present. Overall, the few examples above help to demonstrate the variety of ways deficiencies can affect cardiac health. You can see how a delayed diagnosis could potentially be life threatening.

Symptoms

In studies (including case studies), cardiac conditions associated with gluten intolerance include idiopathic dilated cardiomyopathy (fairly well known association), heart failure, angina, myocardial infarction (heart attack), cardiomegally, pericarditis, myocarditis, arrhythmias, and atrioventricular heart block. ECG and tissue Doppler imaging results were mentioned in 2 studies. ECG changes showed prolonged QT-period with ventricular bigeminus in an adult. Doppler imaging of the heart revealed myocardial systolic wave velocity (of the mitral annulus) was low and the left ventricle had subclinical systolic dysfunction (in children) [6-9,11,12,14-21,43,44,60,66]. Further research is needed to examine the possible role of gluten intolerance in other heart conditions.

The good news is that a strict gluten-free diet should effectively eliminate the auto-antibodies leading to better cardiac health in most individuals. However, there is always a risk though of irreversible permanent damage. You can see why early diagnosis is so important.

Prior to my diagnosis, I experienced palpitations and low blood pressure. There were days (likely when my blood pressure was low) when I experienced dizziness. My albumin level was low and I was anemic.

Pulmonary (Lung) Symptoms

A functional pulmonary system is reliant on the structural integrity of the lungs, the autonomic nervous system, a healthy heart, and a healthy vascular supply of blood. Hypothetically, pulmonary symptoms may result from auto-antibodies directed at blood vessels (might inhibit angiogenesis and blood supply), the autonomic nervous system, the cardiac system (as discussed above), or the lung tissue. As mentioned under cardiac symptoms, we know that auto-antibodies can affect nerves, muscle, and vascular tissue, it is reasonable to suspect that the smooth muscle and other lung tissue along with the autonomic nervous system may be affected with gluten intolerance [46-49,53].

Other Influencing Factors

Other factors may affect pulmonary function as well. The presence of vasculitis or antiphospholipid syndrome, along with protein S and C abnormalities could increase the risk of clots (pulmonary embolus). Conversely, low vitamin K levels, due to malabsorption could lead to diffuse pulmonary bleeding [32,50-58].

The presence of anemia (common in CD) may impair the supply of oxygen to the cells causing further distress. If heart failure occurs, pulmonary edema (fluid in the lungs) could also impair oxygen exchange. An additional concern is that chronic tissue damage might increase the risk of lung cancer.

Collectively or individually, these factors along with nutrient deficiencies (such as vitamin A deficiency leading to loss of cilia and mucin in lungs) could lead to a variety of pulmonary symptoms [64].

Symptoms

In studies (including case studies) and articles, pulmonary conditions associated with gluten intolerance may include lung infections, lung abscesses, increased susceptibility to tuberculosis, bronchiectasis, pneumonia, lymphocytic interstitial pneumonia, pulmonary hemosiderosis, fibrosing alveolitis (interstitial pneumonia, desquamative interstitial pneumonia and the Hamman-Rich syndrome define the different stages of fibrosing alveolitis), and possibly pneumococcal septicemia [1-7,13,22-30,44,48,49,59,60,67].

There were a few case studies mentioning an association between cystic fibrosis and CD as well. In one study, cystic fibrosis patients had a higher prevalence of CD than in the general population. The researchers recommended that individuals with cystic fibrosis should be screened for CD if they live in a population where CD exists. As we know, gluten intolerance can exist anywhere where gluten is being consumed in the diet. There is evidence that tissue transglutaminase is altered in cystic fibrosis. Perhaps auto-antibodies (ex. anti-tissue transglutaminase antibodies) react to the transglutaminase and also with lung tissue, similar to the response seen in the bowel, brain, and heart of individuals with gluten intolerance [22-31].

Further research is needed to examine the cystic fibrosis/gluten intolerance connection, and the possible connection between gluten and other lung diseases, such as asthma. My mother and I have asthma. My mother's asthma symptoms appear to be related to gluten. My asthma symptoms are related to food allergies (see discussion under "The Elimination Diet" in Chapter 21). I have talked to many others with CD and asthma as well. Could gluten sensitivity and other food related reactions be responsible for many other lung diseases? More research is needed.

Other Factors Contributing To Heart And Lung Symptoms

Other factors that may contribute to cardiopulmonary symptoms include smoking, hypertension, diabetes, hyperlipidemia, hyperhomocysteinemia (associated with CD), renal failure, bleeding (hemorrhage), thyroid disease, trauma, infections, genetics, toxic-metabolic agents, certain medications, poor diet, vitamin deficiency or toxicity, alcoholism, heavy metals, solvents, street drugs, and past gastric (stomach) or intestinal surgery (leading to deficiencies) [13,14,41,42,45].

Other People's Experiences

Case 1: I was always pale, anemic and sometimes short of breath. Once diagnosed, the anemia resolved, then the shortness of breath went away too.

Case 2: *I frequently had palpitations, swelling in my ankles, diarrhea, bloating, and the doctor said I had an irregular heart beat. I was diagnosed with celiac disease and a gluten-free diet took all of this away.*

Case 3: *Every winter I would get pneumonia and have to go on antibiotics at least twice. I was so sick once that I spent one week in the hospital. I was diagnosed with IBS while all this was happening. Now I know I have celiac disease and guess what? I didn't have to go on antibiotics once last winter. The GF diet has been a blessing.*

Chapter 14
Some Associated Diseases

In this chapter, a list of associated diseases/syndromes is included. According to research, individuals with celiac disease (CD) have a higher risk of developing other autoimmune diseases and conditions, especially when the diagnosis is delayed [2-4,34]. Therefore, early recognition and diagnosis is important for primary prevention.

The presence of a non-celiac gluten intolerance may result in the same outcome since a leaky gut is present, allowing other food antigens to interact with the immune system. This could lead to further immune reactions and the development of other conditions.

List of Associated Diseases And Syndromes

Hashimoto's Disease (Hypothyroidism)
Grave's Disease (Hyperthyroidism)
Hypoparathyroidism
Secondary Hyperparathyroidism (from low calcium)
Autoimmune Hypoparathyroidism
Diabetes
Addison's Disease
Primary Biliary Cirrhosis
Down's Syndrome
Turner Syndrome
William's Syndrome
Primary Adrenal Insufficiency
Fibrosing Alveolitis of the Lung
Macroamylasemia
Splenic Hypofunction (Hyposplenism)
IgA Nephropathy
IgA Deficiency
Alopecia Areata
Sjögren's Syndrome
Cardiomyopathy
Malignancy

Vasculitis

Antiphospholipid Syndrome

Systemic Lupus Erythematosus

Thrombocytopenic Purpura (ITP)

Hypopituitarism

Autoimmune Adrenal Hypofunction

Systemic Sclerosis

Sarcoidosis

Crohn's Disease

Ulcerative Colitis (Diffuse duodenitis associated with ulcerative colitis)

Raynaud's Phenomenon

Scleroderma

Look in Chapters 4-14 for more associated diseases. This may not be a complete list as ongoing research may reveal more associated diseases and conditions.

CHAPTER 15
Celiac Disease, Dermatitis Herpetiformis And Non-Celiac Gluten Intolerance Symptom Checklist

As you review the symptoms, keep in mind that some individuals will only have one or two symptoms (for example, anemia and night blindness) and others may have many symptoms. Gluten intolerance can be quite elusive, which makes it difficult to diagnose. As well, some people with silent or latent gluten intolerance may not have any symptoms.

Gluten intolerance can be present in children that are growing normally so normal growth rate should not be a factor that excludes the possibility of a gluten intolerance [1].

Many individuals will have no bowel symptoms. Weight loss may or may not occur, and is dependent on the amount of the intestine that is damaged. It is possible to be overweight prior to diagnosis. Overall, the symptoms in this checklist can occur in the absence of stunted growth, weight loss, or bowel symptoms.

There may be symptoms that are not in this list due to the fact that they may not be recognized as being associated with gluten intolerance, yet. I believe that further research will reveal many more symptoms and associated diseases.

Gastrointestinal Symptoms

- ☐ Feeling uncomfortably full after a meal with a high gluten content, such as pasta or bread (some people don't get this symptom)
- ☐ Gastric reflux (heartburn)
- ☐ Atrophic Gastritis (inflamed stomach)
- ☐ Lymphocytic Gastritis (inflamed stomach)
- ☐ Increased risk of Helicobacter pylori infection.
- ☐ Esophagitis
- ☐ Diarrhea or Constipation
- ☐ Increased flatus (intestinal gas). Grumbling sounds in abdomen (borborygmus)
- ☐ Abdominal discomfort from bloated distended abdomen
- ☐ Lactose intolerance

- ☐ Bowel Infections
- ☐ Steatorrhea (fatty stool with a foul odor)
- ☐ Nausea
- ☐ Vomiting
- ☐ Aphthous Stomatitis (canker sores)
- ☐ Decreased tongue papillation
- ☐ Glossitis (tongue inflammation)
- ☐ Angular cheilosis (scales and fissures on lips and in mouth)
- ☐ Dental enamel defects
- ☐ Liver disease (i.e. autoimmune hepatitis, primary biliary cirrhosis, fatty liver disease, primary sclerosing cholangitis, autoimmune cholangitis, elevated liver enzymes)
- ☐ Gallbladder disease (can also have an elevated ejection fraction)
- ☐ Pancreas (type 1 diabetes, pancreatic insufficiency, pancreatitis)
- ☐ Lymphomas
- ☐ Oral, esophageal, or gastrointestinal cancers
- ☐ Low vitamin K could lead to gastrointestinal bleeding and bleeding or bruising in other areas of the body (see symptoms of bleeding in Chapter 5)
- ☐ Malabsorption could lead to low vitamins A, D, E, K, B complex vitamins, C, calcium, magnesium, phosphorus, copper, iron, zinc, selenium, manganese, l-carnitine, taurine, inositol, essential and amino fatty acids, and electrolytes.
- ☐ Fatigue, anemia, hypotension (low blood pressure), hypoglycemia (low blood sugar), failure to thrive, and weight loss may result from malabsorbed nutrients. As well, other symptoms can result from malabsorption and will be mentioned under each physiological system in this checklist.
- ☐ See anemia symptoms in Chapter 5.

Skin, Hair, And Nail Symptoms

- ☐ A skin rash called Dermatitis Herpetiformis (Duhring's Disease) can occur. Symptoms include a blistering (papulovesicular eruptions) or scabbed rash that is very itchy. As well, the rash can have pimple type lesions or look similar to psoriasis with raised red patches of skin. In children, the rash may only present as purpura on the palms of their hands (in isolation or in addition to other symptoms). Usually the rash occurs bilaterally on the body and is commonly found on the buttocks, back, elbows, forearms, back of knees, scalp and on the face. Clinically, the rash can present anywhere on the body

- ☐ If vitamin K levels are low, symptoms may include spontaneous ecchymoses, bruised skin, purpura, petechia, and other bleeding under the skin
- ☐ Dermatitis
- ☐ Pale skin
- ☐ Aphthous stomatitis (canker sores)
- ☐ Facial butterfly rash-from niacin deficiency
- ☐ Increased skin pigmentation
- ☐ Angular cheilosis (scales and fissures on lips and in mouth)
- ☐ Melanoma
- ☐ Atypical mole syndrome and cogenital giant naevus
- ☐ Any itchy skin rashes
- ☐ Psoriasis
- ☐ Pellagra
- ☐ Edema (fluid under skin)
- ☐ Delayed wound healing
- ☐ Dry, cracked skin
- ☐ Acne
- ☐ Vitiligo
- ☐ Eczema
- ☐ Urticaria
- ☐ Acne
- ☐ Alopecia Areata (patches of hair loss)
- ☐ Dry, thin, brittle, slow growing hair due to nutrient deficiencies. Hair might change color due to malabsorption issues with pantothenic acid or manganese deficiencies
- ☐ Nails may be dry, brittle, thin, malformed, grow slowly, break easily, and can also have white bands, longitudinal striations, horizontal or vertical ridges, color changes, white spots, splinter hemorrhages, deformed nail shape that is curved up or down (ex. spoon shaped with anemia), hang nails, or be clubbed. Muehrcke's lines may indicate albumin levels are low. Beau's lines can result from nutrient deficiencies disrupting nail growth, onycholysis can be associated with psoriasis or sarcoidosis, and the nails might be pitted (associated with psoriasis and alopecia).

Other Associated Skin Conditions
- ☐ IgA linear dermatosis
- ☐ Lichen sclerosus

- ☐ Annular erythema
- ☐ Partial lipodystrophy
- ☐ Palmoplantar pustulosis
- ☐ Hereditary Angioneurotic Edema
- ☐ Linear IgA bullous dermatosis
- ☐ Erythema nodosum
- ☐ Necrolytic migratory erythema
- ☐ Erythema elevatum diutinum
- ☐ Behçet's disease
- ☐ Dermatomyositis
- ☐ Porphyria
- ☐ Ichthyosiform dermatoses
- ☐ Generalized acquired cutis laxa
- ☐ Prurigo nodularis (Hyde's prurigo)
- ☐ Pityriasis rubra pilaris
- ☐ Erythroderma
- ☐ Acquired hypertrichosis lanuginosa
- ☐ Ichthyosis
- ☐ Transverse Leukonychia
- ☐ Follicular Hyperkeratosis
- ☐ Oral Lichen Planus

Neurological Symptoms

- ☐ Neuropathy symptoms can include burning, tingling, numbness, vibrations, pinching, stabbing (electric shock type feeling), buzzing, pressure, muscle twitches, a loss of feeling or increased sensitivity to touch.

  Neuropathy symptoms can also include:

  Vestibular dysfunction (dizziness, lack of balance)

  Myelitis (inflammation of the spinal cord)

  Reduced reflexes

  Carpel tunnel syndrome

  Deep sensory loss

  Proprioceptive loss (loss of sense of position in space)

  Dysesthesias (abnormal sensations)

  Feeling like you are wearing gloves or stockings

  Difficulty moving limbs

Frequently dropping items

Walking with a wide stance

Change in bowel habits

Sexual dysfunction

Organ dysfunction

Internuclear ophthalmoplegia

Myelopathies

Paralysis

Acute Paraplegia

Low blood pressure

Dizziness, weakness, fainting

Increased falls

- ☐ Epilepsy
- ☐ Migraines (headaches)
- ☐ Cerebral infarctions (strokes). See stroke symptoms in Chapter 11.
- ☐ Thrombosis (clots)
- ☐ Dementia (see dementia symptoms in Chapter 11)
- ☐ Gluten ataxia has been linked to gluten sensitivity (through Dr. Hadjivassilou's research). Gluten ataxia symptoms can include staggering gait, lack of balance, poor coordination, unsteadiness with standing or walking, increased falls, and dysarthric speech (may be slurred, slow, and difficult to produce and also the pitch, rhythm, loudness, and other voice qualities may change).

  Other symptoms include dysphagia (difficulty swallowing), clumsy exaggerated imprecise limb (arms and legs) movements, difficulty with fine-motor skills (ex. writing, buttoning a shirt, or eating), oculomotor (abnormal eye movements) problems, sensorimotor axonal neuropathy and other peripheral neuropathies.

  As well, dysmetria (inability to judge distance or scale), decreased processing of sensory information, sometimes declining cognitive function, and decreased cerebellar processing of afferent information (information from muscles, joints, movement, visual, auditory, somatosensory, cerebral cortex and midbrain) can occur

- ☐ Some abnormal findings can include abnormal brain waves on electroencephalography (EEG), unusual cerebellar physiology, hypoperfused brain regions, brain atrophy, inflammation, patchy Purkinje cell (out-put neurons) loss in the cerebellum, and progressive multifocal leukoencephalopathy leading to destruction of myelin sheaths that support neuronal impulses. Other findings include lymphocytic infiltration of the cerebellum and peripheral nerves, damage

to the posterior columns of the spinal cord, and widespread IgA deposition around vessels in the brain. As well, brain white-matter lesions or calcifications, likely resulting from autoimmune reactions, calcium deposits, ischemia, vasculitis, or inflammatory demyelination, can occur
- ☐ Myopathies (see symptoms under Musculoskeletal symptoms)

Other Associated Conditions
- ☐ Huntington's Disease/Chorea
- ☐ Ramsay Hunt Syndrome
- ☐ Plummer Vinson Syndrome/Patterson Brown Kelly
- ☐ Stiff Person Syndrome
- ☐ Multiple Sclerosis
- ☐ Amyotrophic Lateral Sclerosis (see 2 studies in neurology chapter)

Psychological And Cognitive Symptoms

- ☐ Learning disabilities
- ☐ Dementia
- ☐ Schizophrenia spectrum disorders
- ☐ Depression
- ☐ Anxiety
- ☐ Mood disorders
- ☐ Personality changes
- ☐ Irritability
- ☐ Apathy
- ☐ Sitophobia (abnormal aversion to food)
- ☐ Obsessional neurosis
- ☐ Anorexia/bulimia
- ☐ Fatigue or hyperactivity
- ☐ Delinquent behavior
- ☐ ADD
- ☐ ADHD
- ☐ Cognitive decline
- ☐ Dementia
- ☐ Autism/Asperger's syndrome (see discussion in psychological chapter)

Musculoskeletal Symptoms

- ☐ Rickets and osteomalacia
- ☐ Soft weak bendable bones could lead to bow legs, pigeon chest, pelvic deformities, deformed skull, and spine deformities (lordosis, scoliosis, and kyphosis).
- ☐ Dental deformities
- ☐ Stunted growth, short stature
- ☐ Dental deformities and cavities
- ☐ Delayed or impaired growth
- ☐ Failure to thrive
- ☐ Bone pain, tenderness
- ☐ Bone fractures, collapsed vertebrae
- ☐ Bone deformities
- ☐ Delayed crawling, sitting, or walking (in infants and toddlers)
- ☐ Osteopenia, osteoporosis
- ☐ Loss of height, low back and neck pain
- ☐ Stooped posture
- ☐ Arthritis, joint pain
- ☐ Muscle cramps, tetany, numbness, tingling, weakness, stiffness, aching, pain, and spasms. Limb weakness.
- ☐ Decreased muscle mass
- ☐ Difficulty lifting objects or doing activities of daily living
- ☐ Change in gait, waddling gait
- ☐ Rachitic rosary (beading of the ribs often seen in rickets)
- ☐ Difficulty moving eyes
- ☐ Decreased mobility
- ☐ Dysphagia (difficulty swallowing)
- ☐ Myopathies
- ☐ Intramuscular hemorrhage
- ☐ Swallowing difficulties (dysphagia)
- ☐ Droopy eyelids
- ☐ Difficulty moving eyes, eye paralysis

Other Associated Conditions
- ☐ Dermatomyositis
- ☐ Polymyositis
- ☐ Inclusion body myositis
- ☐ Rhabdomyolysis

- ☐ Ocular myopathy
- ☐ Muscular dystrophy
- ☐ Neutrophilic myositis
- ☐ Muscular hypotonia of the infant or child
- ☐ Proximal myopathy
- ☐ Generalized myopathy

Reproductive Symptoms

- ☐ Hypogonadism
- ☐ Pubertal delay (failure to develop secondary sex characteristics)
- ☐ Delayed or retarded menarche, (menses, period)
- ☐ Amenorrhea (no menses)
- ☐ Secondary amenorrhea (no period for 6 or more months)
- ☐ Chronic pelvic pain
- ☐ Dysmenorrhea (severe uterine menstrual pain)
- ☐ Heavy menstrual periods (due to low vitamin K)
- ☐ Dyspareunia (intercourse is painful)
- ☐ Vaginal infections
- ☐ Vaginitis (inflamed vagina)
- ☐ Decreased sex drive (decreased libido)
- ☐ Impotence (inability to sustain an erection)
- ☐ Sperm abnormalities
- ☐ Infertility (in men or women)
- ☐ Preeclampsia (high blood pressure in pregnancy)
- ☐ Miscarriages (loss of embryo or fetus)
- ☐ Zygote abnormalities (happens in first stage of development, before new life becomes an embryo, then a fetus)
- ☐ Fetal complications (birth defects, intra-uterine fetal growth restriction, lower birth weight, premature birth)
- ☐ Abnormal bleeding or infections post birth in mother
- ☐ Poor breast milk quality and production
- ☐ Early menopause

Cardiopulmonary Symptoms

- ☐ Cardiomyopathies
- ☐ Idiopathic dilated cardiomyopathy
- ☐ Heart failure
- ☐ Edema (swelling in the tissues can cause weight gain)
- ☐ Angina
- ☐ Abnormal heart rhythms (due to deficiencies)
- ☐ Myocardial infarction (heart attack),
- ☐ Cardiomegally
- ☐ Pericarditis
- ☐ Myocarditis
- ☐ Tachycardia (fast heart rate from anemia, deficiencies, low electrolytes, or low blood pressure)
- ☐ Arrhythmias (from deficiencies or neurological damage)
- ☐ Atrioventricular heart block.
- ☐ ECG and tissue Doppler imaging results were mentioned in 2 studies. ECG changes showed prolonged QT-period with ventricular bigeminus in an adult. Doppler imaging of the heart revealed myocardial systolic wave velocity (of the mitral annulus) was low and the left ventricle had subclinical systolic dysfunction (in children)
- ☐ Hypotension (low blood pressure)
- ☐ Stenosis, occlusions, and aneurysm of the blood vessels could occur due to vasculitis
- ☐ Wet beriberi, acute pernicious beriberi (with a thiamine deficiency)
- ☐ Lung infections
- ☐ Lymphocytic interstitial pneumonia
- ☐ Desquamative interstitial pneumonia
- ☐ Hamman-Rich syndrome
- ☐ Lung abscesses
- ☐ Increased susceptibility to tuberculosis
- ☐ Bronchiectasis
- ☐ Pneumonia
- ☐ Pulmonary hemosiderosis
- ☐ Fibrosing alveolitis of the lung,
- ☐ Pneumococcal septicemia
- ☐ Diffuse pulmonary bleeding
- ☐ Possibly increased risk of lung cancer

- ☐ Asthma symptoms (can be from gluten, or other food allergies)
- ☐ Cystic fibrosis (see discussion in cardiopulmonary chapter)

Vision, Auditory (Hearing), Olfactory (Smell) And Gustatory (Taste) Symptoms

- ☐ Difficulty seeing in a dimly lit room, night blindness
- ☐ Conjunctival xerosis (dryness of the eye)
- ☐ Corneal xerosis (cornea rough, dry, and hazy)
- ☐ Keratoconjunctivitis sicca (dry cornea and conjunctiva)
- ☐ Bitot's spots (pearly foamy patch on conjunctiva and cornea)
- ☐ Keratomalacia (corneal necrosis, corneal ulceration)
- ☐ Corneal scar, formation of corneal opacity (cornea white or clouded over)
- ☐ Xerophthalmia (dry and inflamed eye)
- ☐ Xerophthalmic fundus (white or gray linear or oval opacities in the retina)
- ☐ Blindness
- ☐ Conjunctivitis with corneal vascularization and lens opacity
- ☐ Blepharitis (inflammation of the eyelids)
- ☐ Styes, and eye infections
- ☐ Red (bloodshot) eyes
- ☐ Central retinal vein occlusion may occur if coagulation problems exist
- ☐ Optic neuropathy
- ☐ Optic Neuritis
- ☐ Trigeminal Neuritis
- ☐ Dyschromatopsia (defect in color vision)
- ☐ Foggy, cloudy, or blurred vision
- ☐ Centrocecal or central scrotomas (blind spots)
- ☐ Ocular myopathy
- ☐ Extraocular palsy and nystagmus
- ☐ Tinnitus or ringing in the ears
- ☐ Auditory hallucinations
- ☐ Middle ear infections
- ☐ Loss of hearing
- ☐ Dizziness
- ☐ Anosmia (unable to smell)
- ☐ Hyposmia (decreased detection of odors)
- ☐ Dysosmia (incorrect identification of odors),

- ☐ Parosmia (perception of smell is altered)
- ☐ Phantosmia (false odor detected)
- ☐ Agnosia (can smell, but difficulty in identifying odor)
- ☐ Ageusia (unable to taste)
- ☐ Hypogeusia (decreased taste function)
- ☐ Dysgeusia (taste function is distorted/altered)
- ☐ Decreased appetite (with nausea, vomiting, or decreased ability to taste or smell) or increased appetite (due to malabsorption)
- ☐ Pica cravings (cravings for non-food substances)

Urological Symptoms

- ☐ Chronic prostatitis
- ☐ Interstitial cystitis (bladder pain and altered urination)
- ☐ Bed-wetting in children
- ☐ Stress incontinence
- ☐ Frequency and urgency to urinate, bladder spasms
- ☐ Chronic or recurrent bladder infections
- ☐ Urethritis (inflamed urethra)
- ☐ IgA nephropathy (kidney condition)
- ☐ Nephrotic syndrome (kidney condition)
- ☐ Kidney stones (renal calculus)
- ☐ Active albuminuria (albumin in urine)
- ☐ Proteinuria (protein in urine)
- ☐ Haematuria (blood in urine)

Other Associated Conditions
- ☐ Glomerulonephritis (kidney condition)
- ☐ Mesangial nephritis (kidney condition)
- ☐ Glomerulitis (kidney condition)
- ☐ Membranoproliferative glomerulonephritis (kidney condition)
- ☐ IgA mesangial glomerulonephritis (kidney condition)
- ☐ Immunoglobulin A mesangial nephropathy (kidney condition)
- ☐ Midaortic syndrome affecting infrarenal aorta or renal arteries
- ☐ Renal failure

Some Associated Diseases And Conditions

- ☐ Hashimoto's Disease (Hypothyroidism)
- ☐ Grave's Disease (Hyperthyroidism)
- ☐ Diabetes
- ☐ Addison's Disease
- ☐ Primary Biliary Cirrhosis
- ☐ Down's Syndrome
- ☐ Turner Syndrome
- ☐ William's Syndrome
- ☐ Primary Adrenal Insufficiency
- ☐ IgA Nephropathy
- ☐ IgA Deficiency
- ☐ Alopecia Areata
- ☐ Sjögren's Syndrome
- ☐ Cardiomyopathy
- ☐ Hyperparathyroidism
- ☐ Secondary Hyperparathyroidism (from low calcium)
- ☐ Autoimmune Hypoparathyroidism
- ☐ Hypopituitarism
- ☐ Splenic hypofunction (hyposplenism)
- ☐ Malignancy
- ☐ Vasculitis
- ☐ Antiphospholipid Syndrome
- ☐ Thrombocytopenic Purpura (ITP)
- ☐ Macroamylasemia
- ☐ Systemic Sclerosis
- ☐ Sarcoidosis
- ☐ Crohn's Disease
- ☐ Ulcerative Colitis (Diffuse duodenitis associated with ulcerative colitis)
- ☐ Systemic Lupus Erythematosus
- ☐ Multiple Sclerosis
- ☐ Raynaud's Phenomenon
- ☐ Scleroderma
- ☐ Autoimmune adrenal hypofunction
- ☐ Fibrosing alveolitis

There may be more associated diseases in Chapters 4-14. This may not be a complete list as ongoing research may reveal more associated diseases and conditions.

References for this chapter can be found in the references for Chapters 3-15.

CHAPTER 16
Diagnosis

You Can Be Ruled In, But It Is Difficult To Rule You Out

The tests can help rule you in as having celiac disease (CD), dermatitis herpetiformis (DH) or a non-celiac gluten intolerance, but it is very difficult to entirely rule you out as negative. This can be due to human error, limitations of the tests, and the elusive nature of gluten intolerance. Sometimes, repeated testing is necessary to finally pick up the presence of these diseases.

If the tests yield negative results, you could trial a gluten-free diet to see if it helps to resolve your symptoms. With some individuals, they may experience relief within a few days, others may need to remain on a strict gluten-free diet for a year or more to relieve symptoms (i.e. with neurological). Keep your family doctor informed about your dietary changes and it is prudent to get a referral to a registered dietician to learn about the diet and to ensure that you are getting all of the required daily nutrients.

If symptoms continue while trying the gluten-free diet, review the chapter "What If The Gluten-Free Diet Doesn't Work" to ensure other factors, that may contribute to symptoms, are ruled out and see your doctor for an assessment.

Panel Of Gluten Intolerance Tests

A panel of blood tests and other tests are helpful to diagnose CD, DH, and non-celiac gluten intolerance. The accuracy of the following tests is based on research measuring the sensitivity and specificity of each test. In this situation, sensitivity of a test measures how well the test can identify all the sick people who have CD, DH, or a non-celiac gluten intolerance (without false negatives). Specificity of a test measures how well the test can identify the people who do not have CD, DH, or a non-celiac gluten intolerance (without false positives) [24].

Since none of the gluten intolerance tests have 100% sensitivity or specificity, a gluten free trial may be necessary to truly rule out a gluten intolerance. Prior to the existence of diagnostic tests, doctors used to diagnose based on the evaluation of symptoms and the successful absence or decrease of symptoms with treatment. For example, with gluten intolerance, symptoms would disappear with the maintenance of a gluten-free diet and would reappear with the ingestion of gluten. This would confirm a gluten intolerance. It is important to keep in mind that tests are definitely a useful guide, but the patient's clinical picture (symptom evaluation) must be carefully considered for an accurate diagnosis to occur. Otherwise, undiagnosed patients might suffer unnecessarily.

With gluten intolerance, the tests that provide a useful guide include:

1. IgA and IgG anti-tissue transglutaminase antibody tests

2. Endomysial antibody test

3. Total serum IgA test (important to rule out a deficiency which can cause false negative tests)

4. Total serum IgG test (important to rule out a deficiency which can cause false negative tests)

5. IgA and IgG antibodies against deamidated gluten (good for CD and present in some non-celiac cases if tissue transglutaminase is involved, i.e. gluten ataxia)

6. IgA and IgG antigliadin antibodies

7. Skin biopsy for skin rashes to test for dermatitis herpetiformis The unaffected skin beside (within millimeters of) the lesion should be biopsied, not the lesion itself.

8. Small intestinal biopsies (need several because damage is patchy and easy to miss)

9. Test for IgA deposits against transglutaminase (TG2) on the intestinal biopsy (similar to how a dermatologist will biopsy the skin for IgA deposits, but in this case the intestinal biopsy is examined for IgA deposits against TG2).

   Evidence of this immune reaction in the intestinal mucosa may occur before the changes occur to the small intestinal villi and may be present before the antibodies can be found in the bloodstream of patients. Interpretation requires experience [54,59].

10. Stool testing for IgA and IgG antigliadin antibodies. Enterolab [www.enterolab.com] offers this test. See the website for other tests as well (saliva, etc).

11. Genetic testing

12. A trial gluten-free diet can be tried to see if it relieves symptoms (see discussion in the following pages under "A Trial Gluten-Free Diet".

Blood Testing And Endoscope Issues

Blood Testing Issues

Endomysial antibodies (EMA) and anti-tissue transglutaminase antibodies (anti-tTG) tend to correspond with the severity of intestinal damage. Therefore, if the intestinal damage is minimal or the person has a non-celiac gluten intolerance with no bowel damage, these tests may be negative. With EMA, the analysis of results can be subjective so a lab error may produce a false negative result [1,3,7,9,11,60].

With anti-tTG, the type of tissue transglutaminase used in the blood test (to see if our serum antibodies react) is also important. Human tissue transglutaminase is best. Therefore, to help increase the specificity of the anti-transglutaminase antibody test, it is advisable to make sure the tissue transglutaminase (tTG) is human tTG, not guinea pig liver tTG if possible [62].

With the blood tests, false negatives can occur due to immunoglobulin subclass deficiencies, a very young age, hemolysis (breakdown of red blood cells) and/or sensitivity and specificity limitations with the test. The blood tests are not 100% accurate [3,8,20,25,46,57,60]. The sensitivity and specificity of many of the tests can be viewed online at

www.csaceliacs.org/SensitivitySpecificity.php.

Two immunoglobulin subclass deficiencies that can cause false negatives include IgA and IgG antibody deficiencies. IgA deficiency is 10-15 times more common in people with celiac disease than in people without any medical problems. An IgA deficiency may cause a false negative in any of the IgA tests (i.e. IgA anti-tissue transglutaminase, IgA antigliadin antibody tests, etc). If an IgA deficiency is present, then an IgG anti-tissue transglutaminase antibody test (and other IgG tests) with total serum IgG would be helpful. It is important to include a total serum IgG because an IgG deficiency could cause false negatives in any of the IgG tests (i.e. IgG anti-tissue transglutaminase antibody, IgG antigliadin antibody tests, etc) [3,11,20,27,46,47].

Immunosuppressive drugs may also suppress antibody production and affect IgA and IgG levels. This could give false negative results in any of the tests that measures IgA or IgG, including the stool tests mentioned below.

Antibodies against deamidated gluten is another test that should be added to the screening process. This test measures the antibodies that are reacting against the gluten once it has been altered by transglutaminase (deamidated gluten). This is described in more detail in chapter 2. This type of antibody might be positive before measurable tissue damage occurs. It is a very valuable addition to the panel of gluten intolerance blood tests. [10,22,23].

See discussion about antigliadin antibodies in the following pages. It is discussed separately due to the variety of opinions around its use.

Endoscope Issues

To help rule out celiac disease in an adult, generally an upper endoscopy with multiple biopsies (4-6 or more from the distal duodenum) to investigate small intestinal involvement is completed. I worry that positive biopsies could be missed with this approach. In some patients, it may be necessary to get a duodenal bulb biopsy as well to help rule out CD. One study found a positive biopsy result for CD in the duodenal bulb (just under the stomach) of an adult [55]. Another study suggested that sometimes celiac disease can only be diagnosed with biopsies from the duodenal bulb in adults when there isn't any damage in the duodenum [56].

This makes sense. If the intestinal damage is just beginning, then it may not have extended into the duodenum (area distal to duodenal bulb) to the area where biopsies are generally taken. Unfortunately, the duodenal bulb area is often avoided because Brunner's glands or peptic changes may make it difficult to see the damage when the biopsy is being analyzed. Another consideration: It may be necessary to also biopsy the jejunum (area below duodenum) since there have been reports of patients who have positive jejunal biopsies with negative duodenal biopsies [58,71]. Overall, for adults, it is reasonable to suspect that biopsies from the duodenal bulb, duodenum, and the jejunum may be needed to help rule out CD.

For children, a recent study (2010), found that 4 biopsy samples obtained from the duodenal bulb (near stomach) and 4 from the descending duodenum offered a better chance of diagnosing CD. In their conclusions, they suggested that these 8 biopsy specimens may help to improve the chances of locating the patchy intestinal damage and may improve diagnosis. Sometimes, the bulb damage may be present with no duodenal damage [53]. Two other studies highlighted the importance of doing duodenal bulb biopsies in the pediatric population as well [12,57]. Like adults, it may be necessary to obtain biopsy specimens from the duodenal bulb, duodenum, and perhaps even the jejunum to catch all cases of CD.

During the biopsy procedure, the patient is generally sedated, then a scope is passed in through the mouth, down the esophagus, through the stomach and into the upper intestine where the biopsies are taken. Although this procedure may sound unpleasant, I was sedated and didn't experience any discomfort.

With an upper endoscope, false negatives can occur due to the patchy nature of the intestinal damage, incorrect slide preparation, or an inexperienced interpretation of the biopsies. A lab and pathologist who is experienced with slide preparation and interpretation for CD will help to decrease the risk of false negative results [1,3,7,9,11,46,47,60].

A new type of scope called endomicroscopy can help decrease the risk of missing the patchy damage. This scope has a built in microscope that can examine the small intestinal villi and possibly diagnose celiac disease during the endoscopy procedure. The microscope also allows the gastroenterologist to take targeted biopsies of the affected areas which helps to ensure the damage will be detected [13].

If the scope and biopsies yield negative results, the doctor may also order a capsule endoscopy. With this test, the patient swallows a small capsule that contains a tiny camera. As this camera moves through the gastrointestinal tract, it takes pictures which might unveil an abnormality. This can allow the gastroenterologist to see parts of the bowel that are difficult to access with scopes. As well, a colonoscopy may also be ordered to investigate the ileum and colon for other diseases [52].

The Value Of Antigliadin Antibodies: A Difference Of Opinion Prevails

IgA and IgG antigliadin antibodies may be helpful (in adults, children, and babies) to identify if increased intestinal permeability has allowed gluten to leak in through the tight junctions between the intestinal epithelial cells. Presence of these antibodies demonstrate that an immune reaction has occurred. This interaction with the immune system could lead to tissue damage and many symptoms [2,4,5,8,16-19,26,36,72].

According to some doctors, an elevated IgA and/or IgG antigliadin antibody level definitely indicates that a gluten intolerance does exist and that the patient will benefit from a strict gluten-free diet. Other doctors feel that antigliadin antibodies are not accurate for diagnostic testing and shouldn't be relied upon. This difference of opinion has led to a distinct difference in diagnostic practices. The reason for this variation in opinion will be outlined in the following pages.

Why Do Approximately 10-20% Of The Healthy Population Have Antigliadin Antibodies?

Many doctors feel that the IgA and IgG antigliadin tests are not that accurate since 10-20% of the apparently healthy public have these antibodies. Doctors who favor antigliadin testing feel that this 10-20%, of apparently healthy individuals may have an early stage, latent or silent gluten intolerance with little or no symptoms [4,5]. This makes sense, many people with latent or silent celiac disease are asymptomatic or have vague symptoms. For years, my mother and I had very vague symptoms. Our doctors, mistakenly, thought we were healthy.

Has The Antigliadin Antibody Test Been Judged Unfairly?

A second issue, some doctors feel the antigliadin test has been judged unfairly because it has been compared to the endomysial antibody (EMA) test and the IgA anti-tissue trans-glutaminase antibody (anti-tTG or ATA) test for accuracy. The anti-tTG and EMA results generally parallel the amount of small intestinal damage present (evident in the biopsy). Whereas, the IgA and IgG antigliadin antibody test measures whether the immune system is reacting to ingested gluten. Therefore, the antigliadin antibodies would be positive as soon as the gluten enters the body and the immune system reacts. The anti-tTG and EMA may not be positive until damage has occurred to the small intestine [4,5].

When you look at how the accuracy of antigliadin antibodies has been judged, it doesn't really make sense, since antigliadin antibodies are measuring the initial immune reaction, not the end stage damage. Comparing the accuracy of these tests to the gold standard (a positive intestinal biopsy result), which measures the end stage damage, isn't really fair. It is ideal to diagnose a condition before any damage occurs.

Are Antigliadin Antibodies Found In Other Autoimmune Diseases?

A third issue, IgA and IgG antigliadin antibodies have been found in some other autoimmune diseases and other conditions [28-39], so some doctors feel it is not that accurate or specific for celiac disease or gluten intolerance. Other doctors and health professionals feel that these other autoimmune diseases may be caused by a gluten intol-erance so the presence of antigliadin antibodies in these patients should not rule out the accuracy of this test. For me, this makes sense since all the systems of the body can be affected with gluten intolerance. Therefore, other autoimmune diseases, with their multisystem symptoms may have a connection to gluten.

My Thoughts

After reviewing the reasons behind this difference of opinion, I am suspecting that the IgA and IgG antigliadin tests may be quite useful. I think it is important to do all of the tests for celiac disease (along with other gluten intolerance tests) and equally as important to include IgA and IgG antigliadin antibodies. Not including these antibodies could potentially place a patient at risk for many complications.

Some doctors may be reluctant to order antigliadin antibodies because they feel there are better tests to diagnose celiac disease and dermatitis herpetiformis. Unfortunately, they often don't acknowledge that this test could be valuable to test for a non-celiac gluten intolerance. Some other doctors do include the test in the celiac screening, but don't take a positive result seriously unless the intestinal biopsy or skin biopsy is positive (the gold standard approach). This is disheartening because gluten intolerance can lead to damage in many areas of the body, without any bowel damage, so with the gold standard approach, many patients could be left undiagnosed. Only, the patients with obvious celiac disease or dermatitis herpetiformis diagnostic findings would get a diagnosis. Individuals with a non-celiac gluten intolerance or latent celiac disease would be left to suffer.

Many doctors still do not recognize non-celiac gluten intolerance and the importance of having tests designated for its diagnosis. This is unfortunate because many patients are suffering from non-celiac gluten intolerance. Acknowledging and testing for this condition could significantly decrease the suffering and save health care dollars.

As a primary prevention technique, antigliadin antibodies may also be beneficial to help diagnose celiac disease or DH before the damage occurs. Antigliadin antibodies may be positive before damage is evident in the intestine or elsewhere [4,5]. Too often, the focus is only on diagnosing CD and DH once the damage occurs, not before.

Doctors who inform their patients that a positive antigliadin test isn't conclusive and that she/he should continue eating gluten may be taking a big risk. Diagnosis could be delayed by disregarding the results and this could put these people at risk for villi damage, skin damage, nerve damage (i.e. gluten ataxia and other nerve problems), organ damage, more autoimmune diseases, food allergies, cancer, death, and many other complications that were discussed in the previous chapters.

I believe the IgA and IgG antigliadin antibody test could be of great value and that many doctors should re-examine its use for early diagnosis. Antigliadin antibodies may be the best EARLY test available for measuring all forms of gluten intolerance. The other tests just help to define what area of the body is being damaged, once the damage occurs. Ideally, this test along with testing for celiac disease and other tests (to investigate other damage) can help to identify a gluten intolerance and the type of damage that has occurred.

Checking intestinal biopsies for IgA deposits against transglutaminase 2 can be a useful early test as well since this reaction might occur before antibodies are in the blood stream.

According to Enterolab (www.enterolab.com), stool tests for antibodies may be positive before blood tests are positive. There are blood tests, saliva tests and stool tests that test for the presence of IgA and IgG antigliadin antibodies. An IgA and/or IgG deficiency or immunosuppressive drugs could cause a false negative result.

During my undiagnosed years, I likely would have tested positive for antigliadin antibodies, however, I may have tested negative for anti-tissue transglutaminase or endomysial antibodies if my bowel wasn't damaged enough to have a positive result.

Tests To Consider For Gluten Ataxia And Neurological Issues

Anti-tissue transglutaminase 2 antibodies (anti-TG2) are involved in CD, anti-tissue transglutaminase 3 antibodies (anti-TG3) are involved in DH and anti-tissue transglutaminase 6 (anti-TG6) antibodies are involved with gluten induced neurological issues. Therefore, it is valuable to add IgA and IgG anti-tissue transglutaminase 6 to the panel of blood tests when neurological issues are involved [1,3,4,54].

Dr. Hadjivassiliou's Recommendations

A 2010 article by Dr. Hadjivassiliou (neurologist) and his colleagues recommended testing for IgA and IgG antibodies against deamidated gluten, IgA and IgG antigliadin antibodies, IgA and IgG anti-tissue transglutaminase 2 antibodies plus it suggested doing a small intestinal biopsy if one of the blood tests are positive. Positive blood test results can indicate that the patient has a gluten sensitivity, even if the scope doesn't yield positive biopsy results (The scope just clarifies whether intestinal villi damage is present). The article mentioned that this provides a good start to investigate a gluten sensitivity [54].

If these results are negative, then the article suggested testing for anti-TG6 along with genetic testing. The anti-TG6 test may be difficult to find. I noticed online that Elisa-kits are available from www.zedira.com (in Germany) for anti-transglutaminase 6 IgA and IgG antibodies. If the anti-TG6 is negative, then the article recommended a test for IgA deposits against transglutaminase 2 on an intestinal biopsy (explained more under the list of tests in the panel). Anti-TG3 might be useful as well (to check for skin involvement). The article mentioned that IgG types of blood tests would be helpful if an IgA deficiency exists [54].

Due to the possibility of false negatives with blood tests, I think a small intestinal biopsy may still be valuable if the blood tests are negative. The addition of the EMA and other blood tests to check for IgA and IgG antibody deficiencies would be useful as well since this could affect the validity of the suggested blood tests.

Dr. Marios Hadjivassiliou (Neurologist), Department of Neurology, Royal Hallam-shire Hospital, Glossop Road, Sheffield S10 2JF, UK. Phone: 0114-271-2502.

Discuss www.zedira.com with your doctor before ordering as the test might be available at your lab, and do investigate, because I haven't used this service or company before

Do I Need To Be Eating Gluten For The Tests To Be Accurate?

Initiating a gluten-free diet prior to testing can cause false negative test results (except for genetic tests) so it is important to keep eating gluten until the testing is complete. The antibody levels generally go down with a gluten-free diet (unless you are accidentally eating gluten) so this can cause false negative tests. Consult your doctor about this.

What If I Am Already Consuming A Gluten-free Diet? Would Genetic Tests Or A Gluten Challenge Help With Diagnosis?

Genetic Tests

If you have been consuming a gluten-free diet for awhile and the blood tests are negative, genetic testing may be helpful to investigate whether you carry the genes for celiac disease. This can be done through a mouth swab or a blood test.

95% of people with celiac disease carry class II molecules HLA DQ2 and HLA DQ8. The problem is that 30-40% of the general population have these genes and only 1% get celiac disease. In other words, the presence of these genes means that you have a higher risk of developing celiac disease, but it doesn't mean that you will get it for sure [43-45].

There are other genes that may be involved as well (that other 5%) so a negative result doesn't conclusively rule you out. There have been cases of people with biopsy proven CD who lack the DQ2 or DQ8 genetic predisposition for CD [43-45].

As well, some labs may not test for both alpha and beta subunits of the DQ molecule in their genetic testing. A lab might only test for one subunit which might miss the presence of a DQ2 or DQ8 predisposition to CD. Ask your lab if it does the full test [44,45].

Another issue, you may have a non-celiac gluten intolerance, the genes associated with this are not well known. Dr. Marios Hadjivassiliou (Neurologist) in the UK identified that DQ1 seems to be involved, further research may unveil many other genes [4,5]. In an article by Dr. Scot Lewey, he mentioned that Dr. Kenneth Fine at Enterolab is finding many patients with positive fecal gliadin have a variety of genes [45].

It may be difficult to rule out a gluten intolerance with a genetic test since there are continuously new genes being associated with gluten intolerance. Further research will help to confirm all of the genes that are involved and may help to clarify how accurate genetic testing is for identifying or ruling out a gluten intolerance. Currently, I believe genetic tests are helpful, but cannot conclusively rule out a gluten intolerance.

Gluten Challenge

Your doctor may want you to do a gluten challenge to see if it will induce symptoms and help with diagnosis. This challenge includes eating a specific amount of gluten daily for a certain period of time with the hope that antibodies will elevate and the resulting damage may be sufficient enough for diagnosis to occur.

The gluten challenge is not 100% effective. Remember that false negatives can occur with the tests and, in some people with a gluten intolerance, the damage may take years to develop. Continuing a gluten challenge for this length of time could place a patient at risk for permanent immune related damage and other complications.

With a gluten challenge, IgA and IgG antigliadin antibody testing along with testing for IgA deposits against transglutaminase (TG2) on the intestinal biopsy are helpful and should be added (along with the other tests) at the end of the challenge to help rule out a gluten intolerance. As discussed, the results in these two tests may be positive before the other tests show a positive result.

The need for a gluten challenge is something to discuss with your doctor. For some, this could make them very ill to the point of being hospitalized. The risk may outweigh the benefits so discuss this option carefully with your doctor. If a gluten challenge makes you quite ill, your doctor may choose to encourage a gluten-free diet without the testing, especially if the symptoms returned with the ingestion of gluten and a gluten-free diet relieves your symptoms. Overall, I suspect that the clinical picture is worth more than a positive test. No gluten equaling no symptoms is pretty good evidence.

How Does The Doctor Or Dermatologist Test For Dermatitis Herpetiformis (DH)?

Endomysial antibodies and anti-tissue transglutaminase antibodies might be negative in DH since they tend to correspond with the severity of intestinal damage in CD, not the severity of skin damage. Antigliadin antibodies would likely be positive since this test corresponds with the initial immune reaction to gluten and can be present prior to intestinal or skin damage. However, even this test can have false negatives [1,7,11,16,60].

The unaffected skin beside (within millimeters) the lesion should be biopsied, not the lesion itself. The inflammation in the lesion may make it difficult to see the initial immune factors responsible for DH. A skin biopsy that is positive for DH indicates that a strict gluten-free diet should be started, even with a negative intestinal biopsy [40].

If the skin biopsy and intestinal biopsy are negative, but the rash appears to occur after gluten consumption (can be up to many days), then talk to your doctor about repeating the biopsies (could have missed the intestinal damage or IgA deposits in the upper papillary dermis of the skin). A non-celiac gluten intolerance and/or food allergies may also be responsible for skin symptoms [15,40,42,69].

What If The Blood Tests Are Positive, But The Intestinal Biopsy Is Negative?

An upper endoscopy will help your gastroenterologist to see if villus flattening has occurred. Currently, the endoscope with biopsies is only good for diagnosing celiac disease, a negative result does not rule out DH or a non-celiac gluten intolerance.

If one or all the blood tests are positive, but the intestinal biopsy is negative, then it is possible that the biopsies missed the patchy intestinal damage or the villi haven't flattened yet. With latent CD, villus atrophy may not present for years (only the blood tests may be positive). As well, the interpretation of the biopsies is very subjective so an inexperienced pathologist who isn't knowledgeable about celiac disease may misinterpret the results. An additional concern, the biopsied tissue has to be orientated right on the slide for accurate interpretation to occur [1,3,7,9,11,46,47,60].

If the intestinal biopsy is negative, consider asking your doctor to recheck the biopsy specimens that were taken in the endoscopy to see if any errors in the interpretation have been made. You could also discuss further testing (more biopsies) with your doctor.

Another consideration: You can ask your doctor to look into testing for IgA deposits against transglutaminase (TG2) on the intestinal biopsies that have been taken (similar to how a dermatologist biopsies the skin for IgA deposits, but in this case the biopsied mucosa is examined for IgA deposits against TG2). This immune reaction in the intestinal mucosa may occur before the changes occur to the small intestinal villi. Therefore, this test may help to provide some confirmation. An experienced lab is recommended for an accurate result.

What if the intestinal biopsy is negative, but the antigliadin antibodies are positive? As discussed previously, the presence of antigliadin antibodies in the blood or stool helps to confirm that a gluten intolerance exists even in the absence of small intestinal damage. This test tends to be positive before the intestinal villi damage occurs.

A final consideration: A trial gluten-free diet can be tried to see if it relieves your symptoms. If the gluten-free diet doesn't work then see Chapter 20, "What If The Gluten-Free Diet Doesn't Work" and Chapter 21, "Could A Grain-Free, Specific Carbohydrate, Paleolithic, Or Elimination Diet Be Helpful". In this situation, consult your doctor and a registered dietitian (who are preferably knowledgeable about gluten intolerance) for advice.

Should I Get My Relatives Screened?

Once you are diagnosed, screening relatives for celiac disease and dermatitis herpetiformis is recommended since these diseases can run in families. For example, in my family, my mother, my daughter, and I have celiac disease.

With non-celiac gluten intolerance, the genetic link is less clear. It is reasonable to suspect that it could run in families, similar to celiac disease so testing relatives is likely beneficial.

Would A Celiac Home Test Be Helpful?

In British Columbia, Canada (where I live), the IgA anti-tissue transglutaminase test is currently covered by our government's medical plan, but in other provinces or countries, it may not be covered. If you live in an area where your medical plan doesn't cover this test, the tests are not readily available to you by the doctor or the cost is too expensive for you to afford, then consider the celiac home test from 2 G Pharma [www.2gpharma.com].

This test measures the presence of IgA anti-tissue transglutaminase antibodies in your blood. Transglutaminase is an enzyme that has an affinity for undigested gluten and deamidates (alters) it into a form that is toxic for those with the genetic predisposition for celiac disease. The immune system reacts, antibodies are created, and these antibodies tag transglutaminase for destruction (see under pathophysiology).

Procedure For Testing

For this test, you will need to obtain a fingertip blood sample with the small sterile lancet that is supplied in the package. According to their website, the results are apparent within 10 minutes with a yes or no. There is a video with instructions available at the 2G Pharma website.

If your result is positive, continue eating your regular gluten containing diet, print out the 2G Pharma's "Dear Doctor Letter" for your doctor to help explain the test results, and see your doctor (I suggest taking the test with you as well) as soon as possible. Maintaining a gluten containing diet until all tests are complete can help prevent false negatives.

The doctor can do further testing and make appropriate referrals for blood testing, other diagnostic tests, and to other professionals. As well, talk to your relatives about screening (since their risk has increased with your diagnosis) and request that your physician take steps to screen your children.

False Negative Result Is Possible

There are a number of reasons why this test may give a false negative result. If an individual has an IgA deficiency, then a false negative test result could occur. In this situation, an IgG anti-tissue transglutaminase antibody test could be used (as long as you don't have an IgG deficiency).

Secondly, this home test (IgA anti-tissue transglutaminase) result tends to parallel the amount of intestinal damage present. If you have a gluten intolerance with very little or no bowel involvement, then the result could be negative.

Thirdly, some individuals have latent celiac disease and the test may show a negative result a few times before there is enough bowel damage (and antibodies) to show a positive result.

Fourthly, with very young children, this test might be negative since they may not have high enough antibody levels to show up on the test yet.

Fifthly, for an accurate result, the person using the home test should be eating gluten regularly. The antibodies necessary for testing may not be present if gluten is not being consumed.

Overall, I believe this home test can help rule you in (as having celiac disease), but it can't entirely rule you out. A complete panel of blood tests (see previously) along with an endoscopy is helpful to test for celiac disease.

Could Stool, Saliva, Or Urinary Peptide Testing Be Helpful?

As with the other previously mentioned tests, you can be ruled in as having a gluten intolerance with the following tests, but it is difficult to rule you out. There are a variety of factors that can cause false negative test results. Diagnosing gluten intolerance is not an easy task.

Stool And Saliva Tests

Some doctors feel that more research needs to be done into the accuracy of stool and saliva testing for antibodies. Other doctors use it regularly and feel that their patient's have benefited from its use. As with the other tests, my concern is that false negatives could occur and this could lead someone to mistakenly believe that they don't have a gluten intolerance.

Ideally, along with the stool and saliva tests, I feel that the full panel of tests is helpful to assess for a gluten intolerance and to assess the type of damage that has occurred. A trial gluten-free diet is helpful as well. No gluten equaling no symptoms is quite convincing proof.

There is a local naturopathic doctor here in Vancouver who uses the stool tests for his patients. He has had good results with the implementation of the gluten free diet following positive test results. His clinical findings with patients are very interesting and help to provide confirmation that the use of the stool and saliva tests can be quite beneficial. I guess in the end, the real proof is the resolution or relief of symptoms.

Vancouver ND: Dr. Arjuna Veeravagu, ND, located at 487 Davie Street, Vancouver, BC, Canada. I have had the pleasure of meeting Dr. Veeravagu. He is very approachable, professional and knowledgeable about gluten intolerance. He offers blood tests, saliva, and stool tests.

Phone: 1-604-697-0397

Website: www.sageclinic.com

About Dr. Veeravagu: www.sageclinic.com/drveeravagu.html

A company owned by Dr. Kenneth Fine, Enterolab, will test your stool or saliva for antibodies. Dr. Fine's website can be found at www.enterolab.com.

FAQ page: www.enterolab.com/StaticPages/Faq.aspx

Urinary Peptide Tests

This urine test checks for the presence of gliadorphin (gluteomorphin), and casomorphin in the urine. These are opiate peptides found in gluten (protein in wheat, rye, barley and oats) and casein (protein from dairy). Studies have found that some people can have neurological and psychological symptoms from these two peptides since they appear to have addicting morphine like effects in some individuals. This may be due to a decreased ability to break down opiate peptides during digestion. Interestingly, some people can actually experience withdrawal symptoms when they stop eating these foods [48-50].

I have met a few people who have benefited from this test. For example, a mother did this test for her daughter and it came back positive (other tests were negative). Eliminating gluten and dairy from her daughter's diet improved her child's mood, academic abilities, and relieved her gastrointestinal and eczema symptoms. Her daughter was previously diagnosed with attention deficit attention disorder (ADHD).

Urine peptide testing is available at Great Plains Laboratory

www.greatplainslaboratory.com/home/eng/peptide.asp.

The test can be ordered from there or a naturopathic doctor can generally arrange for this test to be done. This site has a printable brochure with information about peptides.

A Trial Gluten-Free Diet

There can be many reasons for implementing a trial gluten-free (GF) diet. Some or all of the tests may not be available in your country, you may not be able to afford the tests (may not have insurance or medical coverage in certain countries) or you may have had the tests with inconclusive results. As well, there may be many underlying reasons for false negative test results so negative results may not be valid, strengthening the need for a trial GF diet. As mentioned earlier, you can be ruled in, but it is difficult to rule you out.

If symptoms are relieved with a GF trial, then that provides fairly concrete proof that the symptoms are likely related to diet. With this approach, consider trying a gluten–free diet for 6 months to a year (or more) to see if it provides relief before giving up the trial. With some people, their neurological symptoms or cystitis can take months or up to a year or more to completely resolve. Sometimes, the damage is permanent and doesn't resolve, but doesn't progress either.

If the gluten-free diet doesn't work then see Chapter 20, "What If The Gluten-Free Diet Doesn't Work" and Chapter 21, "Could A Grain-Free, Specific Carbohydrate, Paleolithic, Or Elimination Diet Be Helpful".

With a trial gluten free diet, consult your doctor and a registered dietitian (who are preferably knowledgeable about gluten intolerance) for advice. The dietitian's advice can help to prevent complications resulting from accidental gluten exposure and lesson the risk of experiencing nutrient deficiencies. An overall assessment by a physician is important to rule out other causes of your symptoms.

A social worker may be able to help you find some financial help if you can't afford the tests.

Concerns With Starting A GF Diet Without The Testing

It is advisable to be screened for a gluten intolerance for a variety of reasons. It is important to have an overall assessment by a physician when you have medical symptoms. It allows a doctor to not only test for a gluten intolerance, but to test for other diseases or medical conditions as well.

Once diagnosed, your doctor will likely refer you for other testing (i.e. bone density test and tests for nutrient deficiencies, etc), follow-up tests, and give referrals to other specialists. Life threatening nutrient deficiencies can be treated promptly and tests can be done to rule out cancer. With CD or DH (and sometimes with non-celiac gluten intolerance), multiple nutrient deficiencies may be present and this could be life threatening if not treated promptly. I do worry that people who refuse the testing (or can't afford the tests) might be at risk for many complications and may not get the follow-up support from their physicians without a diagnosis.

A doctor's diagnosis will also help eliminate self doubt that may occur later in life (with a self diagnosis) and may be necessary to claim some of your gluten-free products, if your government offers that type of program.

An additional concern, once you are gluten-free, it makes it more difficult to test you for a gluten intolerance in the future. The antibody levels generally go down with a gluten-free diet so this can cause false negative tests in the future. For testing, you would have to do a gluten challenge (eat gluten) for an extended period of time to induce symptoms and detectable damage. No one is ever excited about doing this because it may trigger the onset of unpleasant symptoms again. For all the reasons above (and more), I believe it is ideal to get all of the testing and an overall assessment by your physician before starting the gluten-free diet.

Could Other Allergies Or A Food Intolerance Be Causing My Symptoms?

Like gluten intolerance, other food allergies and or a food intolerance can contribute to a wide variety of symptoms that can be vague or obvious. Unfortunately, there are doctors that are not aware that reactions to food may be connected to their patient's symptoms. Too often, the presence of food allergies and food intolerance is not investigated or acknowledged.

There are five classes of antibodies that are present in our bodies, IgA, IgD, IgE, IgG and IgM. Unfortunately, for many patients, only the IgE mediated food reactions are investigated since this type of allergy is well researched and acknowledged amongst allergists.

Some other people are lucky to have the IgG mediated food reactions investigated as well. This may have been offered during a naturopathic or chiropractic consultation. IgG is often chosen because IgG (as subtypes IgG1, IgG2, IgG3, and IgG4) is the most abundant antibody class in the blood and it has high specificity toward antigens (i.e. allergenic foods).

Testing for IgA antibodies against foods is valuable as well. IgA antibodies protect the mucosal membranes in the respiratory tract, the gastrointestinal tract, the reproductive tract, the urological tract and can be found in the blood. IgA antibodies are the most abundant antibody class in the body and are quite efficient at binding antigens with up to four antigen binding sites (IgG only has two). With this in mind, it is reasonable to suspect that these antibodies can react to various foods, just like IgA antibodies react to gluten. There are blood tests available that can check for this type of reaction [42,69].

It is important to recognize that false negatives can occur with these blood tests, just like the gluten intolerance tests. An elimination diet is sometimes used to help identify foods that are causing a reaction or to confirm the results of the blood tests. Discuss this further with your doctor [42,69].

More research will help to reveal how IgD and IgM may be involved with food reactions. Immature B cells have IgM antibodies on their surface and once mature, these cells also carry IgD antibodies on their surface. IgM antibodies are very involved in the early stages of a reaction. In fact, IgM predominates in early reactions to perceived invaders before IgG (or other antibodies) are involved and is very efficient at activating the complement cascade (other chemicals) to help with attacking an invader. Unfortunately, with IgD, the function is less clear. IgD can activate basophils and mast cells to produce antimicrobial factors so it appears to be involved in the early stage of a reaction. Overall, more research into the function of IgM and IgD antibodies may lead to other tests that can identify early reactions to food molecules. These two antibodies may contribute more than we realize.

Extra Information: When the mature B cells (with IgD and IgM on their surface) encounter an invader, they become activated. Then daughter cells (of the B cells) can class switch from IgM to IgA, IgG, or IgE antibody classes as needed by the immune system.

In my experience, the allergist often only tests for IgE mediated reactions during a consultation and offers the elimination diet to help identify other allergies. Whereas, a naturopathic doctor usually investigates the other forms of food reactions through the use of blood tests (might use an elimination diet as well). This may vary from country to country, so clarify what tests your allergist and naturopathic doctors can do for you.

With blood tests, keep in mind that you may be reacting to something not included in the tests. This could be a food dye, an additive, or an allergy to something else in the foods. It may be helpful to have the allergy testing done first, then try an elimination diet to confirm the blood test results and to further clarify other offending foods or additives [42,69]. You can discuss this with your naturopathic doctor or allergist, they should be able to provide resources and guidance for you.

It is also possible to have an intolerance to a food due to a lack of enzymes. If a digestive enzyme is diminished or absent, then the food (or part of the food) may sit undigested in the bowel. As the food ferments, it can cause a variety of symptoms. For example, lactose intolerance can lead to a variety of gastrointestinal symptoms. Ask your doctor for testing to investigate this possibility. Enzyme supplementation may be necessary.

I happen to have both an intolerance to gluten and an IgE mediated allergic reaction to wheat (one of the grains with gluten). As well, I have other food allergies and I seem to react to the foods that contain lectins.(see Chapter 21 for more).

A Concern: I have met patients who, previous to their gluten intolerance diagnosis, have had allergy testing through an allergist (IgE mediated) that was negative so they believed their symptoms were unrelated to diet. Later, they discovered that they had celiac disease, DH, or a non-celiac gluten intolerance. Since the reaction in these diseases wasn't IgE mediated, it was missed with the skin prick tests the allergist used. Gluten intolerance is IgA and IgG mediated. Unfortunately, they all suffered for awhile before this connection was made and a diagnosis occurred.

Doctors May Have Different Approaches With Diagnosis

I have noticed that there is a difference in diagnostic practices with different medical doctors, naturopathic doctors, and chiropractors. As a result, some of the tests, mentioned in this chapter, may not be ordered due to the doctor's preference.

Some doctors may only test for celiac disease (CD) or dermatitis herpetiformis (CD) with the belief that non-celiac gluten intolerance is an invalid diagnosis or unreal possibility. For the patients who have a non-celiac gluten intolerance, this approach can leave them feeling confused, frustrated and still suffering unnecessarily. These doctors can be useful to help rule out CD or DH, but the use of other doctors to test for a non-celiac gluten intolerance along with a trial gluten-free diet should be considered as well.

Keep in mind that some of the tests mentioned previously can be ordered by the patient.

Other doctors may prefer to test for a gluten intolerance without clarifying whether intestinal damage has occurred (i.e. celiac tests and a scope). The thought behind this approach is that the gluten-free diet will heal all the damage (caused by gluten) in the body so further clarification is not needed. Generally, vitamins are recommended to compensate for any deficiencies and the gluten-free diet is taught to the patient. Follow-up care is provided by the doctor who diagnosed the gluten intolerance. For many, this approach can send them on a path of recovery.

Having said this, I would like to point out that the celiac tests may still be beneficial even though a gluten intolerance has already been identified. Follow-up scopes, blood tests, and other referrals are generally done on a patient with a celiac diagnosis to ensure the healing is progressing, and that life threatening nutrient deficiencies are identified and treated promptly. An endoscopy and other tests can also help to identify any other complications early (i.e. cancer, etc). If abnormalities are found, treatments can be started right away and not be delayed.

Another concern, many people with celiac disease can still have small intestinal damage years after starting a gluten-free diet. This may be due to accidental ingestion of gluten, the presence of other food allergies (to the gluten-free grains or other foods), or exposure to other agents that may negatively affect the intestinal villi (see more in Chapter 19, "Celiac Disease, Helping The Villi Heal" and Chapter 20, "What If The Gluten-Free Diet Doesn't Work"). Additional follow-up and tests afforded with a celiac diagnosis may help to monitor for this potential complication. Steps can be taken to identify the cause and treatment can be started.

Keep in mind that it is better to do celiac blood tests and an endoscope while you are ill (and still eating gluten) because this will provide a higher likelihood of detecting intestinal damage. Once you are gluten-free, the antibodies (that are measured in the testing) begin to decrease and the bowel begins to heal. Therefore, testing after the initiation of a GF diet significantly increases the chance of a false negative result.

It is prudent to be aware of all your options so that you can make informed choices. The information in this book can provide you with the basic knowledge required to create a co-active plan (with your doctor) for diagnostic testing and to create a plan of care for healing that is unique to your needs. In the end, it is your choice to make.

Caution: I am not a physician, I am a registered nurse. The previous discussion about tests is a guide to be reviewed with your family doctor and your specialists.

CHAPTER 17
My Gluten-Free Diet

A gluten-free (GF) diet is the treatment for celiac disease (CD), dermatitis herpetiformis (DH) and a non-celiac gluten-intolerance. A GF diet consists of foods that are free of the grains wheat, rye, barley, and some types of oats (see discussion about oats). When I first realized that I needed to eat gluten-free, I thought, "that doesn't sound too difficult, I don't really like bread and pasta anyway". I didn't realize how traces of gluten are in many packaged foods disguised as other names, such as spelt, triticale, malt flavoring, farro, or kamut (see other keywords). Once I did some research and saw a registered dietitian, my GF reality settled in. Even though it initially seemed overwhelming, I embraced the diet knowing it was my only chance to finally feel healthy and I felt lucky to know what was causing all of my symptoms.

The first question most people with a gluten intolerance ask is "What can I eat?". For me, it makes sense to start with all the foods that are naturally GF such as fruits, vegetables, nuts, seeds (GF seeds), unprocessed natural meats and fish, eggs, natural seafood, sea vegetables, beans, and lentils. These foods are full of nutrients which your body requires to help heal yourself. For years, doctors have been telling us to eat more of these foods, so now is your chance to make a healthy transition to a GF diet. Then, branch out to other GF products such as GF pasta, GF multigrain bread, GF waffles, and all of the other products available out there. I was diagnosed 6 years ago and not much was available in our local grocery stores. Now that has changed, I am continually finding new products for my family.

Overall, I tend to discourage the use of unhealthy processed foods. I feel that if my family consumes these foods in great quantities, we may risk having nutrient deficiencies, since many GF processed products are not very nutritious and many are not fortified with nutrients. Generally, processed foods contain a lot more chemicals, preservatives, and flours that are low in nutrients.

When I require a processed GF product for my family, I always check for the presence of nutritious GF grains such as amaranth, quinoa, chickpea, teff (see list for other healthy flours) or other healthy ingredients on the label [30]. There are some healthy GF processed products that contain these ingredients.

I eat a wide variety of healthy, unprocessed, natural foods to help my body get a wide variety of nutrients. My body needs all the help I can offer to it by eating wholesome nutritious foods. As well as being nutritious, eating natural foods saves money since processed GF foods are usually expensive. Although, I appreciate the availability of these foods, I only buy processed food as a treat, when I am traveling, or to stock my earthquake kits.

Extra Note About Fortified Foods

Processed foods get fortified with nutrients for a reason, they don't naturally have a healthy level of vitamins and minerals so the products need to be fortified. For me, it make sense to eat foods that naturally have these vitamins and minerals.

Healthy foods such as fruits, vegetables, nuts, seeds, unprocessed natural meats and fish, eggs, natural seafood, sea vegetables, beans, lentils, and healthy nutrient dense flours do not need to be fortified with vitamins and minerals like processed foods. That is because these foods are naturally nutritious and provide the best sources of food for healing and for the GF diet.

My Safe Foods

My family consumes the foods, in the safe categories below, as long as they haven't been cross contaminated while growing, processing, transporting, or packaging the food. Sometimes the product will have a gluten-free label, other times I have to check with the manufacturer.

My current diet is more restricted than the gluten-free diet. I eat a paleolithic diet due to my other food sensitivities. This is discussed more in Chapter 21 under "A Paleolithic Diet". My three children consume a gluten-free diet.

Natural Foods I Consume In Large Quantities

The more natural foods I eat from this category, the better I feel. These fresh natural foods are nutrient dense, many are high in fiber, and have a low risk of any cross contamination unless seasoning has been added, the food was contaminated with gluten containing foods that are close by, or the food has been processed in some way [30].

- Fruits and vegetables
- Nuts (nut flour is very nutritious), seeds (as long as it isn't wheat, rye, or barley)
- Unprocessed natural meat and fish
- Natural seafood, sea vegetables

- Beans (bean flours are very nutritious), lentils
- Peas (pea flours are nutritious)
- Plain coconut
- Eggs
- Fresh herbs
- Seaweed (I eat kelp and dulse)

Currently, I don't eat beans and peas since I seem to react to these foods

Nutritious Grains And Flours That I Use Regularly For My Family

I look for these flours on the labels of processed foods and cook or bake with them to increase nutrition and fiber [5,30].

- Quinoa
- Teff
- Millet
- Brown rice
- Buckwheat
- Chickpea flour, garbanzo bean flour
- Fava bean flours
- Flaxseed flour
- Other pea and bean flours
- Nut flours
- Sorghum
- Rice bran
- Amaranth
- Manioc flour (Cassava)
- Coconut flour (high in fiber)
- Please see the following information about pure uncontaminated oats under "My Thoughts About Pure Uncontaminated Oats".

Less Nutritious Grains And Flours That I Use As A Treat For My Family

My family consumes processed foods with these flours (without nutritious grains added) just as a special treat due to their low nutrient value [30].

- Tapioca flour and starch
- Potato starch
- White rice

- Arrowroot flour
- Corn flour, cornstarch, and cornmeal can be used, but we don't use it due to a corn allergy
- Potato flour
- Rice polishings
- Rice starch

Gums I Utilize For Baking

I use two different types of gums to help my baked products trap air when they are rising and it helps to bind the baked product together. I ensure my gums are free from gluten contamination before purchasing.

There are other usable gums that are not included in this list. At the end of this chapter, there is a list of websites that discuss the GF diet and a list of gums can be found at some of these websites such as www.celiac.ca.

- Guar gum
- Xanthan gum

Essentials I Use For Baking Or Cooking

With these ingredients, always check to ensure there are no additives that may be derived from gluten.

- Baking soda
- Baking powder
- Gluten-free yeast (not brewer's yeast)
- Cream of tartar
- Brown (I use Demerara) and white sugar
- Gelatin
- Salt and pepper
- Yeast
- Olive oil, safflower oil, coconut oil, nut oils
- Milk, cheese, butter, and other dairy (Always check to make sure it is gluten-free. It may have had some gluten added.)
- Psyllium
- Distilled vinegar (not malt vinegar)
- Molasses
- Fresh spices and herbs (ensure dried or processed are gluten-free)
- Ground mustard

Unsafe Foods (Containing Gluten)

Key Ingredients I Avoid

There are many ingredients that are derived from grains containing gluten. Be careful to check every ingredient on the label each time you purchase a product and contact the manufacturer to ensure it is gluten-free.

There may be additional ingredients (not listed here) that contain gluten. Research is continuously revealing more information. The list below includes the foods and ingredients I avoid in my gluten-free diet. A consultation with a registered dietitian who is knowledgeable about the gluten-free diet can provide a comprehensive review of the diet and can provide you with updated information [6-15].

Ingredients That Contain Gluten (NOT Gluten-free)

- Wheat (all forms)
- Rye (all forms)
- Barley (all forms)
- Contaminated oats (all forms). See the following information about oats under "My Thoughts About Oats"
- Kamut
- Emmer
- Chapatti flour (Atta)
- Brewer's yeast
- Farina
- Semolina
- Spelt (other names Farro, Faro, Dinkel, or Dinkle)
- Fu
- Bulgur
- Couscous
- Durum
- Einkorn
- Malt (all forms from gluten containing grains)
- Seitan
- Triticale
- Graham flour

Caution: The gluten-free information above discusses the gluten-free diet I use for my children (I follow a paleolithic diet). Please clarify and confirm all content with a registered dietician who is knowledgeable about the gluten-free diet. I am not a registered dietitian (RD), I am a registered nurse (RN).

My Thoughts About Oats

The Canadian Celiac Society stated (Aug. 20th 2007) that studies show that pure uncontaminated oats are safe in the amounts of 50-70 grams per day for adults and 20-25 grams per day for children [2]. However, in the studies, the oats were pure and uncontaminated, each study size was small, and the amount consumed was limited. As well, some patients reacted to the ingested oats. For these reasons, I personally feel I would like more research just to be sure [1-3,23-25,28,29,33,36].

Some individuals may be react to oats because of cross contamination issues (while growing, processing transporting, or packaging), although, the individuals in the studies appeared to be eating pure uncontaminated oats. The type of tests used to detect gluten in oats, and the accuracy of the tests could influence how pure the oats really were in the studies. Inaccurate testing could lead to immune reactions due to gluten contamination. Further studies will help to clarify this possibility.

In the studies, the presence of an oat allergy may be the underlying reason for a reaction. This could be the reason why some people with celiac disease do not tolerate even a small amount of oats [34,35]. As well, perhaps there is something else within the oat grain that these individuals are reacting to (i.e. lectins or another protein). Future research will help to reveal the exact cause and this may help to alleviate my concerns.

My daughter (with CD) and I don't eat oats. I would like to see larger studies before I take that step. Until I have more information, I feel healthier without this grain in our diet. In the future, larger studies with larger doses of pure uncontaminated oats will help to clarify whether my worries are valid. For now, there is still much debate around this issue. Different countries have different statements and recommendations.

If you choose to eat pure uncontaminated oats, it is prudent to let your doctor (and specialists) know, get regular blood tests (antigliadin antibodies, anti-tissue transglutaminase antibodies and IgA levels) done (and perhaps a scope) to check for a reaction. As well, if you are newly diagnosed, it makes sense to wait until your bowel has healed, your symptoms are gone, your antibodies have returned to normal and you are well established on the gluten-free diet before adding oats (at least past 1 year). It will be easier to catch a reaction if you wait to reach these milestones first [1-3,23,25,28,29,36].

An extra consideration: The risk of oat sensitive enteropathy (damage in the bowel) can be increased with the presence of elevated antigliadin antibodies since it may promote anti-avenin (in oats) antibodies. As discussed, elevated antigliadin antibodies can be found in people with a gluten intolerance. Therefore, the risk of a reaction to oats might be a significant problem in this population, especially while the antigliadin antibodies are elevated [36]. Waiting until antigliadin levels return to normal and testing for an oat allergy before introducing oats seems like reasonable measures to lesson the risk of a reaction.

Keep in mind that the methods of checking for a reaction are not fool proof since false negatives can occur with all the tests. Undetected damage could put you at a higher risk for complications such as cancer, nutrient deficiencies, or other autoimmune damage. I personally have to be absolutely sure before I introduce oats and feel that introducing oats to my daughter at this point might be risky. For others, it is an individual choice and it may add extra nutrients to the gluten-free diet if no reaction occurs.

If you choose to consume oats, then buy your oats from a reputable company that will guarantee that there is no cross contamination with wheat, rye or barley. In Canada, pure uncontaminated oats (according to their website) are available at www.creamhillestates.com and www.onlyoats.com. If you choose to purchase pure uncontaminated oats, ask the companies if they use the R5 ELISA test (with a hordein standard for barley) since it tests for the presence of wheat, rye, and barley. Some tests do not test for all three of these grains.

There are guidelines available for the introduction of pure uncontaminated oats at the Canadian Celiac Association website:

www.celiac.ca/Articles/PABoatsguidelines2007June.html.

Thirty Gluten-Free Diet And Health Tips

Below, I have included 30 tips to help ease the transition to a gluten-free diet. At the beginning, it can seem overwhelming, but with time you will learn the diet, will find some wonderful recipes, and will find the gluten-free products and restaurants that will help normalize your daily routines. For now, take a deep breath, use your resources (i.e. support group, dietitian, etc), read my suggestions below and take one day at a time. You are not alone, there are many others currently out there making this same dietary adjustment and there are many others yet to be diagnosed.

Once everyone is diagnosed, life will be much easier for all of us who are affected by gluten. The increased demand for products will encourage restaurants, companies, and grocery stores to sell more GF products and meals. Even now, I have noticed that there are many more products and GF restaurants/bakeries available than there were six years ago, when I initially started the GF diet. Try to think positive and look forward to a healthy future.

Top Tip: See a registered dietitian (who is knowledgeable about gluten intolerance and the diet) to review the GF diet. This should save you a fair amount of time because she/he can tell you where GF products are available locally and can provide accurate knowledge about the GF diet. This can help decrease the risk of exposure to gluten.

You may have additional issues (high blood pressure, diabetes, etc) that may require dietary changes so inform your dietitian about any additional medical conditions. As well, take your blood test results with you so the dietitian can see your deficiencies and recommend foods high in those deficiencies.

1. Unfortunately, beverages and foods may be thickened, stabilized, or seasoned with wheat, rye, barley, oats or derivatives of these grains. Gluten containing grains may also be used as fillers. I check all labels and call companies to ensure everything is gluten-free.

   Deli meats, some bacon, and processed sea food can often contain various forms of added gluten which is a problem. Check labels very carefully and check with the manufacturer if it doesn't say gluten-free.

2. I ensure all of my flour is really gluten free and that it hasn't been blended in with another flour. Check to make sure it hasn't been contaminated while growing, packaging, transporting, or processing.

   Be aware that flour (or other foods) from a bulk bin could be contaminated.

3. I check to make sure all of my spices, salt, and pepper is really gluten free with no cross contamination.

4. I watch out for malt which is used in cereals and other products as a flavoring. Malt can be made from barley.

5. Also be careful, because soy sauce and bouillon cubes generally have wheat in them. I have found gluten-free bouillon cubes and soy sauce in various markets and health food stores in Canada and the USA.

6. I'm careful with dried fruits, there may be added gluten sprayed or dusted onto it. Check with the manufacturer.

7. Food that is hydrolyzed or modified may contain gluten. I always check with the manufacturer.

    For example, sometimes, frozen turkeys or frozen chicken can be injected with hydrolyzed vegetable protein (HVP) to make the meat look more plump. Unfortunately, HVP can have gluten in it. Check with your local manufacturer to ensure that HVP hasn't been added. The local manufacturer I called said that fresh chicken and turkey that hasn't been previously frozen is okay. Check with your local manufacturer, it may vary in different areas.

8. When I am eating out, I call the restaurant ahead of time and I talk to the chef when I arrive to make sure there is no chance of cross contamination. My food should be prepared by staff with clean freshly washed hands, fresh gloves, and a fresh apron.

    As well, food should be made in a separate GF area with designated bowls, pots, pans and mixers, strainers, and spoons, etc, to lesson the risk. I also ask whether they use the same oil to fry my foods as they do for other gluten containing foods. Clean oil is required.

    I avoid any seasoning or additives, and I generally ask the chef to use olive oil to cook. Natural foods with no additives are fairly safe. Be aware that cross contamination can also occur if there is any air born gluten from flour that is being used in the restaurant.

    Some websites that can be resources while traveling or eating out include:

    www.bobandruths.com,

    www.glutenfreerestaurants.org,

    www.glutenfreeonthego.com,

    www.glutenfreetravelsite.com, and

    www.theceliacscene.com.

    Other websites are listed in Chapter 30, "Support For A New Lifestyle" and there are guidelines for restaurants at

    www.gluten.net/downloads/print/GFKitchen.pdf

    that you can take with you to show the restaurant staff.

9. Beer has gluten in it (made from barley). There are companies that make gluten-free beer, such as

www.bardsbeer.com,

www.rvbrewery.com,

www.gfbeer.com.au, or

www.lesbieresnouvellefrance.com/home.

There are likely others as well. Search each site for the section that talks about their GF beer to ensure that you are purchasing a designated GF product. Also check with each company to ensure their beer is truly gluten-free with no cross contamination.

10. I have run into sales people (and others) who have told me false information. Knowing my list of safe foods has saved me from being misled.

I have also had sales people tell me that something is gluten-free and upon investigation, I find that it isn't. I always check to make sure it is gluten-free by checking with the manufacturer.

11. I have encountered sales people (and others) that say "a little gluten likely wouldn't hurt me". This is, of course, false, a little gluten can hurt me. I maintain a strict gluten-free diet to decrease the risk of cross contamination and to maintain my health. This does take some work, but is well worth the effort.

12. Sometimes, according to the ingredient list, a product may appear gluten-free. To verify, I call the company and ask to speak to the area of the company that manufacturers the food or the manager. I ask the company if there is any chance of cross contamination on any of their machines while processing or packaging. I also ask whether there is any chance of cross contamination while growing or transporting the GF ingredients they use.

I always investigate every ingredient on the label (and what it is made from) with the company to make sure there are no traces of gluten. While learning the GF diet, I kept my list of safe GF ingredients and list of unsafe foods handy as a checklist.

I always inform the company that I have celiac disease and that I will get very ill from even a trace of gluten (wheat, rye, barley, and contaminated oats) to ensure that they understand the importance of accuracy.

I ask for a written copy of their answer (e-mail) to keep on file. I feel it is likely checked out more thoroughly if they put it into writing, although this isn't guaranteed. Therefore, I will question them if I have a reaction. An at home test kit can be used to test for the presence of gluten in foods.

13. I have been in vitamin stores a few times recently and noticed there is a product that claims you can tolerate small amounts of gluten if you take the pills with meals. I am not aware of any product that can currently do this without eliciting an immune response in individuals with a gluten intolerance. With this type of medication, the ongoing risk for complications would be high if ingested gluten caused an immune reaction. I would bring this type of product to the attention of your local celiac association so that they can look into it and show anything like this to your doctor and specialists for approval before using it. I personally wouldn't take the risk.

    In the future, even if a medication or herb is approved for this type of use, I don't feel I need any medications or herbal supplements since a strict gluten-free diet is working well for me. I don't feel that I need a treatment since I view my immune system as healthy. Chapter 29, "Is Our Immune System Really Abnormal" discusses my thoughts more.

14. A product that the manufacturer said is gluten-free last month may not be this month if they changed their ingredients or way of processing. I always recheck the ingredients on the label each time I buy it and I periodically recheck with the manufacturer.

15. A gluten-free label on something doesn't always mean it is gluten-free. There have been cases of manufacturers contaminating their products. If you have symptoms after eating a product (some people don't have symptoms so please don't depend on this) or if you just want to verify it is gluten-free then talk to the company. I call the company and ask what it does to guarantee its products are GF. Does it have an outside source test their products. You can also use home test kits to check the product for the presence of gluten.

    The Gluten-Free Certification Organization (GFCO) at www.gfco.org provides a program that will certify companies. It is run by The Gluten Intolerance Group (GIG). You can do searches for GF companies that have been certified on this site.

16. My kitchen at home is 100% gluten-free since my husband, my children and I all consume a GF diet. I have a new fridge, stove, counter top, etc so it really doesn't have a trace. We just happened to be replacing these item when I was diagnosed.

For others, a thorough cleaning is necessary to lesson the risk of trace amounts of gluten remaining there. This may be difficult if others in the home are eating gluten. Following the guidelines for restaurants at

www.gluten.net/downloads/print/GF Kitchen.pdf

may be helpful to set up a designated area in your kitchen for GF cooking. Having your own jars of jam, peanut butter, and your own toaster, pots, pans, etc, can also help to lesson cross contamination.

A registered dietician who is knowledgeable about the gluten-free diet can give you comprehensive advice about avoiding cross contamination in this situation.

17. When my children were young, I was surprised to learn that their play-doh had gluten in it. This was a problem because they would get play-doh under their nails and on table surfaces so this caused cross contamination. I went to an art store and purchased gluten-free clay for them to mold instead.

    There are companies that advertise gluten-free play-doh:

    - Aroma Dough [www.aroma-dough.com/kids-products.htm] and
    - Mama K's Aromatic Play Clay [www.etsy.com/shop/MamaKs]

18. I check all of my vitamins and supplements to make sure that they are gluten free. I don't take any regular medication, but I checked the medications in our first aide cupboard. A resource is www.glutenfreedrugs.com.

19. I check my cosmetics to make sure they are gluten-free.

20. I buy my food from our local grocery stores (they all have a GF section), local farmers, health food stores, fresh fruit and vegetable markets, and I grow some food in my organic garden.

21. I am extremely careful at bakeries that claim to have GF products. I meet with the manager and ask how food is prepared. I listed some of the questions I ask.

    - Is food with gluten prepared in same facility? If the answer is yes, this increases the risk of cross contamination
    - Is the gluten-free food made in a room designated for gluten-free cooking only? Does the room have a stove, pans, cookware, and spoons that are only used for cooking gluten-free? Can I see the room?

- Do they ensure that all ingredients are free from gluten contamination during growing, processing, transporting, and packaging and baking?

- Is the GF baked product displayed in the same display cabinet as other gluten foods? If the answer is yes, then I won't buy the product because the risk of cross contamination is too high.

- Is there any chance for cross contamination? Do they wash their hands, change their gloves, and apron before handling my GF product?

- I personally want to see the set-up. Do they test the final product for gluten?

I do ask lots of questions. With a reaction, I can loose time with my family, time at work, etc. Any bakeries/companies offering GF products need to take it very seriously.

22. I use olive oil to cook most of my food (there are many different types with various natural olive flavors). I enjoy the flavor, it is very healthy, and it is a natural anti-inflammatory [32]. As discussed previously, there many other oils you can use, this one is my favorite.

23. I try to eat many foods with omega 3 fatty acids, such as walnuts, salmon, pumpkin seeds, and I use cod liver oil. I also avoid anything with trans-fats. All of my herbs are fresh (better flavor and likely healthier) when possible.

    If you use cod liver oil, ensure that you are not consuming too much vitamin A and D. This may happen if you are consuming other vitamins as well. Check with your dietitian, doctor and pharmacist.

24. Since I had anemia when I was diagnosed, I took iron pills (as recommended by my doctor). To enhance absorption I took my iron with a vitamin C tablet or with a food high in vitamin C such as an orange.

    I also avoided taking my iron at the same time as my calcium supplements or dairy since calcium can decrease the absorption of iron. I would space calcium and iron at least 2 hours apart.

25. With my fat soluble vitamins (A, D, E, K), I added a fat such as fish oil or cod liver oil to enhance absorption. If you choose cod liver oil, be careful, this along with a multivitamin may provide too much vitamin A and D which could be toxic. Discuss this with your pharmacist, doctor, and registered dietitian.

26. Upon diagnosis, I took GF liquid vitamins since this type of vitamin is easier to digest and poses less risk of passing by the area of prime absorption in the intestine. Be careful with supplements, toxicities can occur with over supplementation and this can lead to permanent damage. Check with your doctor and your registered dietitian for appropriate dosages.

27. To support my immune system, I take vitamin D (immune modulator), vitamin A (i.e. vitamin A and D are in cod liver oil), a multivitamin, probiotics, omega 3 foods and ensure that I eat healthy proteins throughout the day as well as a wide variety of other healthy foods.

    Please see the discussion under Chapter 20, "What If the GF Diet Doesn't Work", 3rd recommendation for more information and concerns about probiotics.

28. Initially, I avoided lactose or took lactase supplements with dairy until my intestinal villi healed since I was lactose intolerant. Once my villi healed (and could produce enzymes), I didn't appear to have a lactose intolerance any longer.

29. There are many gluten-free cookbooks available online, at bookstores and sometimes at used bookstores. There are also many blogs and websites with recipes, such as

    www.glutenfreegoddess.blogspot.com,

    www.glutenfreegirl.blogspot.com,

    www.glutenfreehomemaker.com,

    and I have shared some of my family's favorite recipes at

    www.celiacnurse.com/category/recipes.

    In Chapter 28, "Support For A New Lifestyle", I included many other resources (books, blogs, etc) that may be helpful.

30. Various registered dietitians have written books about the GF diet. For example, Shelley Case's book "Gluten-Free Diet" is very comprehensive, a great guide and can be found at www.glutenfreediet.ca. Tricia Thompson also has four books, "Celiac Disease Nutrition Guide", "The Gluten-Free Nutrition Guide", "Easy Gluten-Free" and "The Complete Idiot's Guide To Eating Gluten-Free" at www.glutenfreedietitian.com. I have found other books online and at local book stores.

The gluten-free information above discusses the gluten-free diet I use for my family. Please clarify and confirm all content with a registered dietitian who is knowledgeable about the gluten-free diet. I am a registered nurse, not a registered dietitian.

I recommend waiting until the testing is complete before initiating a gluten-free diet because it may create a false negative. Discuss this with your MD or specialist.

Consult your MD, Registered Dietitian, or other medical specialists involved in your care to determine which nutrients should be supplemented and to identify appropriate dosages for you. Review your symptoms and everything in this book with a medical doctor and your specialists before you make any changes.

Some Websites That Discuss The GF Diet

1. Registered Dietitian, Shelley Case's Book and Blog.

   Book: Gluten-Free Diet, A Comprehensive Research Guide. Case Nutrition Consulting, Inc, 2008.

   Blog: www.glutenfreediet.ca

2. Gluten Free Dietitian, Tricia Thompson has a website and four books.

   Books: "Celiac Disease Nutrition Guide", "The Gluten-Free Nutrition Guide", "Easy Gluten-Free" and "The Complete Idiot's Guide To Eating Gluten-Free".

   Blog: www.glutenfreedietitian.com

3. Registered Dietitian, Betty Kovaks, MS RD.

   MedicineNet.com:
   www.medicinenet.com/celiac_disease_gluten_free_diet/article.htm

4. The Gluten-free diet. Gluten Intolerance Group of North America (GIG)

   Site: www.gluten.net/diet.php#allowed

5. Canadian Celiac Association www.celiac.ca

   Also has a pocket dictionary for the GF diet available for purchase.

6. www.americanceliac.org [USA]

7. www.csaceliacs.org [USA]

8. www.celiaccentral.org [USA]

9. www.coeliacsociety.com.au [Australia]

10. www.coeliac.ie [Ireland]

11. www.coeliac.co.uk [UK]

12. www.celiac.com - Click on "Safe Gluten-Free Food List/Unsafe Foods And Ingredients" in left hand column.

13. www.americanceliacsociety.org [USA]

14. www.celiac.org

15. Children's Hospital Boston

    Celiac Patient Education Information: Safe And Unsafe List Of Grains And Flours. www.childrenshospital.org/clinicalservices/Site2166/mainpageS2166P12sublevel5 0Flevel39.html

16. Gluten-Free Diet Guide for Families. Children's Digestive Health And Nutrition Foundation www.cdhnf.org/wmspage.cfm?parm1=40

17. Celiac Center at Beth Israel Deaconess Medical Center, Harvard Medical School.

    PDF: Following a Gluten-Free Diet.

    www.bidmc.org/CentersandDepartments/Departments/DigestiveDiseaseCenter/C eliacCenter.aspx

My Weight Gain And Other People's Weight Loss

Initially, when I started consuming a gluten-free diet, I looked for breads, pastas, muffins, and cakes that I could eat. I was really enjoying eating these foods and I didn't realize how fast I was gaining weight.

Within 1 and ½ months I gained 22 pounds which was remarkable for me. For likely the first time in my life, I was absorbing most of my food. Some of the weight gain was needed, but not quite this much. I was surprised and had nothing to wear but big loose dresses.

This presented another issue, in addition to learning the GF diet, I had to learn how to eat all over again. I realized that I was not hungry all the time and I didn't need to eat constantly any longer. As well, I focused less on GF processed foods and more on eating foods that are naturally healthy. These healthy foods included fruits, vegetables, nuts, seeds (GF seeds), unprocessed natural meats and fish, eggs, natural seafood, sea vegetables, beans, and lentils, and the use of nutritious GF flours. This dietary change and exercise helped me to decrease my weight.

As time passed, I discovered that I had other food allergies. This limited my diet to the point where it became paleolithic, I discuss this further in Chapter 21 under "A Paleolithic Diet". A paleolithic diet helped me to remove other symptoms that were affecting my health. I also found that this diet makes it very easy for me to control my weight since it is fairly low in carbohydrates.

There are other people that are overweight when they are diagnosed. I have talked to a number of people that seem to loose weight once gluten-free. Perhaps, this is due to an increased focus on the foods they eat, a shift to more natural foods, the effect of decreasing the inflammation in their body, or the positive effect of eating gluten-free on their thyroid and metabolism. Additional heart, kidney, or liver issues may also add to weight gain while undiagnosed. A GF diet may not correct this if permanent damage is present.

Claiming Your GF Foods

Check to see if your government has a service to reimburse the additional cost of buying GF foods. In Canada, see the Canadian revenue agency website:

www.cra-arc.gc.ca/tx/ndvdls/tpcs/clc-eng.html

Your local support group can provide guidance with this.

Test Kits To Check Food (Optional)

Test kits can be used to check questionable food for the presence of gluten. These kits can be quite helpful if you travel, eat out frequently, or would like to check your baking supplies (i.e. flours) for cross contamination.

There are a variety of test kits that can be found online. For example, EZ Gluten test strips are available from 2G Pharma Inc. According to their website at www.celiachometest.com, this test is 99% accurate in detecting the presence of gluten in foods to levels as low as 10 parts per million (ppm). Individual ingredients or finished and cooked products can be tested for the presence of gluten.

In the EZ Gluten® Test, a food sample is added to the gluten extraction solution, and then mixed. A few drops of the sample extract are placed into a test tube. The EZ Gluten® test strip is placed into the test tube and allowed to absorb the sample extract. After 10 minutes, the test strip can be read visually for the presence of gluten in the sample.

Please follow the instructions provided with your test kit.

It can be difficult to ensure your food is GF while traveling, unless you bring your own food or just eat basic paleolithic styled foods. It is nice to broaden one's GF choices. I can see how the use of test kits can help to decrease the risks associated with eating out.

CHAPTER 18
Thirty Lifestyle Tips To Help Ease The Transition

Finally, you have a diagnosis that makes sense and the treatment, a healthy gluten-free diet, actually relieves your symptoms with out side effects. Fantastic! It feels great to make progress, but are there other steps you can take to speed up your healing and help decrease any potential complications? I believe there are and have listed 30 additional tips below to help ease your transition to a gluten-free lifestyle.

Once diagnosed, I learned several tips from other fellow gluten intolerant people who shared their stories, from my doctors, my own trial and error, and through literature reviews and research. It can seem a bit overwhelming at the beginning, but with time, living gluten-free will just become a natural part of your life. For me, a gluten-free diet (now paleolithic) along with other interventions equaled a new increased quality of life, a life worth celebrating!

30 Tips

1. Blood tests helped my doctor and I to clarify my anemic status, potential nutrient deficiencies, and screen for some co-existing autoimmune diseases. This helped my doctor to identify the type of supplements necessary to correct my deficiencies and to order other follow-up tests.

    Upon diagnosis, my initial screen included a complete blood count, liver enzymes (ALP, AST, ALT, Bilirubin), fasting blood sugar, thyroid tests, phosphorus, calcium, magnesium, vitamin B-12, folic acid (folate), total protein, albumin, calcium, BUN, creatinine (to check kidneys), electrolytes, ferriton (iron) level, erythrocyte sedimentation rate (to assess inflammation), and C-reactive protein (to assess inflammation). This was a great start. Additional blood tests for vitamins A, D, E, K, B Complex (esp. B-1,B-6), copper, and zinc would have been helpful as well [4-10,13].

2. I had a bone density test to check the health of my bones. Malabsorption issues and autoimmune factors can lead lead to weak, fragile, unhealthy bones (i.e. osteoporosis). This was discussed in Chapter 8. Discuss this test with your doctor.

3. Ask your doctor about a referral to a registered dietitian who is knowledgeable about gluten-intolerance and the gluten-free (GF) diet. This is discussed in more detail in Chapter 17, "My Gluten-Free Diet". Also, review my 30 gluten-free diet and health tips located in Chapter 17.

4. Talk to your doctor about screening your children for celiac disease and gluten sensitivity since it can run in families. Tell your first degree and second degree relatives to ask their doctor about screening.

5. Consider asking your doctor for a referral to an allergist or see a naturopathic doctor to check for allergies (read more in the diagnostic chapter). Reactions to foods may be an underlying reason for ongoing symptoms once on a GF diet.

6. A local support group can help emotionally since you will meet others who face the same issues as you. People from your support group can help you to problem solve, find gluten-free products, try new recipes, locate knowledgeable dietitians, and find great local gluten-free restaurants.

7. Start cooking and baking as a new hobby. Creating your own food can be very enjoyable and this will help to provide a wider variety of GF foods to enjoy. Find some new gluten-free cookbooks or go to the blogs mentioned in Chapter 17 for recipes. Chapter 30 has a list of blogs as well.

8. Try to think positive. We are lucky that we have a treatment that doesn't involve drugs and fortunately we have a diagnosis. Many are still undiagnosed and suffering.

For me, it helps to focus on the benefits of my good health and to visualize an encouraging future. In my ideal future, all the undiagnosed people with CD, DH, and non-celiac gluten intolerance will be diagnosed and the medical profession will be very knowledgeable about the full spectrum of gluten intolerance. As well, there will be abundant restaurants with prolific GF choices on their menus, GF products will outnumber gluten containing products in grocery stores, and living gluten-free will be the norm, rather than an unusual way of life.

For me, this positive way of thinking helps me to cope and work towards an easier future for myself and my children.

In Chapter 30, "Support For A New Lifestyle", there many resources that may be helpful for this adjustment in lifestyle.

9. Consider creating a disaster kit full of gluten-free products (and water) for your home and another kit for your vehicle. If you have children, then make up a gluten-free emergency kit for their teachers to have as well. Everyone should have this whether they eat gluten-free or not. However, I believe it is even more important when you live gluten-free since it may be more difficult to find gluten-free food during a crisis.

    I have a container full of non-perishable gluten-free food items, a big bag of brown rice that I buy from a local mill, camping fuel, a Coleman stove, a tent, lots of water, a water purifier, and some first aide supplies for our emergency kit. I replace the supplies before their expiry date so that I can use them up and avoid wasting any food.

10. Keep your favorite gluten-free snacks in your purse, bag, and car (non-perishable) for times when GF food may not be accessible.

11. With children, keep treats in their backpack and in the school freezer. I put ice cream and frozen treats in the freezer in the spring, and I keep cupcakes in there all year round.

    My children and the teachers are aware of this supply and it gives my children a sense of control when they need GF food that will equal what the other kids are receiving. It is good for their self esteem to have control and to have options. I also ask the teacher to notify me if there is going to be any food related activities in the classroom.

    My children participate in mixing and preparing the foods we eat. Occasionally, we take cookies or cupcakes to school to share with others. My kids have enjoyed sharing their food with their classmates and this has boosted their view of the diet since the other kids have given them many complements. I make something that I know the other kids will love to decrease the risk of negative comments. We always check with the teacher first in case there are other food allergies in the classroom.

12. When my children attend a birthday party, I provide all of their food (pizza, cake, etc). I ask if there is going to be any ice cream, pinatas, or gift bags with treats, etc at the party so that I can prepare the same for my children.

13. At the beginning of every school year, I talk to the principle and staff about my children's dietary and health needs. If gastrointestinal symptoms are still present, let the teacher know your child needs bathroom breaks ASAP when requested.

    Also review Chapter 20, "What If The Gluten-Free Diet doesn't Work?" if gastrointestinal symptoms are still present.

14. Read about CD, DH, and non-celiac gluten intolerance. Empower yourself so that you can manage your health well and have meaningful discussions with your doctor.

    I listed some helpful books in Chapter 30, "Support For A New Lifestyle".

15. Consider setting up "Google Reader" on your computer to receive new news about gluten intolerance, gluten-free recipes, etc. This will help you keep up with the latest news.

16. View some helpful videos on You-Tube by Dr. Peter Green from The Celiac Disease Center at Columbia University. There is a video series on there that discusses celiac disease and the gluten-free diet. You can find it by entering his name and celiac disease in the search bar.

17. Exercise helps with keeping a positive outlook and can help to keep you healthy. Always check with an medical doctor before starting an exercise program, just in case there are any concerns. Some people may be too ill or have heart problems such as cardiomyopathy. They may require a specialized rehabilitation program. Everyone has individual needs.

18. Get enough sleep every night and try to include some relaxation activities in your life. I understand this can be very hard to achieve, but try to make some changes to allow for this as it may help decrease the stress associated with adjusting to a new lifestyle.

19. Keep your doctor informed about any new or persistent symptoms. See Chapter 20, "What If the GF Diet Doesn't Work" for recommendations to discuss with your doctor. Chapter 21 may be helpful as well.

20. If you have intestinal villi damage, review Chapter 19, "Celiac Disease: Helping The Villi Heal", for recommendations to discuss with your doctor. The use of probiotics is discussed in Chapter 20.

21. Keep a file for ongoing blood test and other test results. As well, keep a medical diary and write down everything your doctors have said to refer to later. This will be helpful if your doctor goes on vacation and you have to see a different doctor. You will have a personal history to provide to the doctor at a walk in clinic or at the emergency room.

22. If you are ill and in the hospital, then review some tips from the Gluten Intolerance Group Of North America (in the US) at www.gluten.net. Go to their site and type in hospitals in the search bar, then look for "Hospitals Made Safe-Gluten". In this PDF, they have a number of suggestions to help with a safe GF hospital stay and also include sample letters to the hospital staff, the nurses, dietitian (with menu suggestions), and the pharmacist.

23. Have you been vaccinated against Hepatitis B? Studies have found that some people with undiagnosed celiac disease don't produce antibodies and memory cells (immune cells) to the hepatitis B virus after vaccination [1-3].

    Talk to your doctor about having blood tests done to check for the presence of hepatitis B surface antibodies. If you are hepatitis B surface antibody positive, then your immune system has reacted appropriately to the immunization [1-3].

24. Review Chapter 21 about the use of grain-free, paleolithic, specific carbohydrate, and elimination diets. These therapeutic diets may be helpful for persistent symptoms that cannot be resolved by the doctors. Discuss any therapeutic dietary changes with your doctor.

    Naturopathic doctors and dietitians are generally more aware of these therapeutic diets than medical doctors.

25. Ask your doctor about a follow-up endoscopy to check intestinal healing (especially with ongoing symptoms). It is important to know whether the intestine has healed completely.

    For celiac disease, The Celiac Disease Center at Columbia University (USA) website, recommends a follow-up biopsy at 2-3 years after diagnosis to check small intestinal health. It mentioned that some doctors do a second endoscope at 6 months after diagnosis, however, this may not be necessary unless complications are occurring and/or there is difficulty with the gluten-free diet [10]. Discuss this with your doctor. This recommendation can be found at

    www.celiacdiseasecenter.columbia.edu/C_Doctors/C07-Management.htm

According to a couple of studies, many Celiacs still have some intestinal damage and nutrient deficiencies even though they are eating gluten-free. There can be many reasons for this such as poor food choices, the selection of processed foods that are not fortified, or accidental ingestion of gluten. An endoscope will help to clarify if ongoing intestinal damage is occurring [11,12].

It is very important to make healthy food choices and to follow a strict gluten-free diet. Buying healthy foods that are dense in nutrients is helpful as well.

Chapter 20, "What If The Gluten-Free Diet Doesn't Work" reviews many possible causes for persistent bowel damage and symptoms (i.e. could be getting accidental gluten, could have food allergies, nutrient deficiencies, etc).

26. The Celiac Disease Center at Columbia University (USA) website also recommends that antibody levels should be checked every 6-12 months until normal (might take up to 3 years). Then annual checks may be helpful to monitor for any immune reactions [10].

    Sometimes, gluten can be ingested accidentally, elevated antibody levels may help to reveal that this is happening. Although, this isn't 100% effective for monitoring due to the false negatives that can occur. Discuss this with your doctor. This recommendation can be found at

    www.celiacdiseasecenter.columbia.edu/C_Doctors/C07-Management.htm

27. Ask your doctor to monitor your cholesterol levels. Once the bowel heals it can absorb food and cholesterol levels may go up, especially if the foods consumed are heavily processed. Talk to your registered dietitian about implementing a healthy diet [8-10].

28. Monitor for any signs of cancer (especially while the bowel is healing). Discuss symptoms and tests with your doctor. Ask about stool tests to check for the presence of blood [7-10].

29. Make sure all cosmetics are gluten-free. Some can contain gluten.

30. Go through all of your medication with your doctor, pharmacist and the companies to ensure it is gluten-free.

    Extra Tip: *Read the information about probiotics in Chapter 20, What If the Gluten-Free Diet Doesn't Work", recommendation #3. Also read recommendation #5 about pancreatic insufficiency.*

As always, I recommend that you review all of these tips with your medical doctor and specialists before you make any changes.

CHAPTER 19
Celiac Disease: Helping The Villi Heal

In many individuals with Celiac Disease (CD), the small intestinal villi, responsible for absorbing nutrients, becomes damaged, creating a flattened mucosal surface (villous flattening). Autoimmune reactions to ingested gluten cross-react with intestinal villi and create this damage. The resulting malabsorption, possible development of allergies, and opportunistic intestinal infections may further complicate villi health [5,16]. In this Chapter, 10 facts about intestinal villi and 10 steps you may take to improve villi health will be discussed.

What Are Intestinal Villi?: Ten Facts

1. Small intestinal villi are finger-like projections that are each approximately 1mm in length. Millions of villi cover the circular folds of the small intestine. These small intestinal folds are valuable because the folds increase the intestinal surface area that is available to interact with and absorb nutrients. As well, smooth muscle within each villus help it to lengthen and shorten which allows the villi to inter mix with the nutrients in the intestinal lumen for optimum absorption. Enzymes on the villi's surface assist with digestion [1,2,5,16-18].

2. The outer layer of each villus consist of columnar shaped epithelial cells that have absorptive abilities. Nutrients are absorbed through these epithelial cells into the core of each villi and enter into the bloodstream through the blood capillaries within each villus. As well, the lacteal, a lymphatic capillary within the villus, absorbs nutrients (dietary fats) for distribution to the body.

3. Microvilli are tiny projections located on the outer absorptive epithelial cells of the villi and are often referred to as the brush border. The microvilli assist with absorption and the microvilli's plasma membranes excrete d (mainly for protein and carbohydrate digestion).

4. Dispersed intermittently among the absorptive epithelial cells a epithelial cell called goblet cells. These cells secrete a lubricat interspersed in among the absorptive epithelial cells of the vil

crine cells (another type of epithelial cell) that belong to the enteric endocrine system and these cells produce enterogastrones (hormones) in response to the current food particles in the intestinal luminal environment.

The villus epithelium, including absorptive columnar, goblet, and enteroendocrine cells renews itself every 3-6 days. The villi cells are shed at the tip of each villus.

5. With celiac disease, autoimmune damage makes the intestinal villi dysfunctional. The absorptive cells of the damaged villi become cuboidal, sometimes squamoid, when the absorptive cells should be columnar. Basically, this means the villi loose the ability to absorb food properly [4,5,16].

The crypt (area at base of each villi) become elongated resulting in crypt hyperplasia. As well, the affected small intestine's lamina propria cellularity is increased resulting in an infiltration of lymphocytes. This indicates that the immune system is reacting to the ingested gluten and cross reacting, causing damage to intestinal cells.

6. Autoimmune damage to the villi (villus flattening) can lead to malabsorption of nutrients. This can lead to multiple nutrient deficiencies.

The extent of malabsorption is dependent on the total length of the small intestine affected. Typically, proximal small bowel damage is more severe and it tends to diminish distally. Nutrient deficiencies can result in a variety of multisystem symptoms that are described in Chapters 3-15 in this book [5,16].

The damaged villi also have difficulty producing digestive enzymes and this can lead to different types of food intolerance (i.e. lactose intolerance).

7. Adverse reactions to various food antigens in the small intestine (allergies) can also lead to villus flattening. With gluten intolerance, reactions to other food antigens (in addition to gluten) is a risk. Increased expression of zonulin (a human protein) in the intestinal tissues increases permeability allowing macromolecules (ex. food antigens, bacterial, and viral particles) exposure to the immune system. The immune systems exposure to gluten and the subsequent autoimmune reaction is thought to be responsible for the intestinal and other systemic damage seen in Celiac Disease. Unfortunately, the increased bowel permeability can also increase the risk of developing food allergies [3,15,20,21,23].

Identification of food allergies is important to help preserve the integrity of the intestinal villi. Reactions to food antigens may be responsible for continuing gastrointestinal symptoms even when you are maintaining a strict gluten-free diet [20,21].

8. There are bacteria, viruses, and parasites that may affect intestinal villi health, possibly leading to villous flattening. As well, intestinal lymphoma, certain medications, and immunodeficiency syndromes may affect villi health [5,22,24].

   Individuals with undiagnosed CD are at a higher risk for intestinal infections, lymphoma, and the use of medications which may be ordered to treat the many multisystem symptoms of undiagnosed CD.

9. Preservation of the villi epithelial cell's function and integrity is dependent on the availability of luminal and bloodstream sources of nutrients. The villi require nutrients to remain viable and functional.

   Damaged intestinal villi and a diet that is deficient in nutrients can decrease the availability of nutrients for villi health. This may lead to abnormal growth, division, and differentiation of villi cells possibly adding to the dysfunctional flattened villi [10,11,13,14].

   For example, in animal studies, prolonged vitamin A deficiency in rats led to decreased height of the intestinal villi [10], decreased cell division and differentiation were noted, and reduced goblet cells were found in the villus [10,11]. Another animal study described how vitamin A deficiency in mice combined with a rotavirus infection caused more inflammation and damage to the villus tips [12].

   A few human studies have shown that vitamin A supplementation can help to lesson diarrhea episodes with intestinal illnesses in impoverished countries where vitamin A intake is often inadequate [6-9].

   You can imagine how a vitamin A deficiency, often present in undiagnosed CD, could add to the autoimmune damage, increase malabsorption due to the negative effect on the villi, and increase the risk of intestinal infections which may further hinder the villi. Vitamin A deficiency is just one example, multiple nutrient deficiencies, often present in CD, could further decrease intestinal health.

10. Dysfunctional villi can lead to a variety of gastrointestinal symptoms. Some of the symptoms occur as a result of malabsorbed nutrients remaining in the intestine and increasing the osmotic load. Others are a result of a nutrient deficiency. Some symptoms can include diarrhea, flatulence, abdominal cramping, constipation, occult blood, steatorrhea, bloating, vomiting, and infections. See my

Gastrointestinal Symptoms chapter for more detail. As mentioned previously, the resulting nutrient deficiencies can cause many other multisystem symptoms that are discussed within Chapters 3-15 of this book.

Steps To Improve Villi Health

You can see how autoimmune damage to villi along with other factors (i.e. nutrient deficiencies, certain medications, infections, and food allergies) can collectively or individually decrease the function and integrity of small intestinal villi. With this in mind, I believe there are many steps that may help to improve intestinal villi health.

1. Consume a nutrient rich diet. This will help supply all the required nutrients for intestinal villi health. Consult a registered dietician to ensure your diet is complete.

2. Ask your MD and your dietician about a nutrient supplement.

3. Consume a strict gluten-free diet. Re-check ingredient lists on the foods, vitamins, supplements, and medications you consume to ensure that all are gluten-free.

   Products that were once gluten-free may not be now due to a change in the ingredients. It's worth viewing the label each time you buy a product. Also, check with companies to ensure that there is no cross contamination at their company due to packaging gluten and non-gluten foods on the same machine. It can be time consuming, but well worth the effort.

4. Consider asking your MD/Gastroenterologist to do blood tests to see if you still have circulating antibodies. This can help you to see if you are still exposed to gluten. Remember, that false negatives can occur with blood tests so this method isn't 100% effective.

   An upper endoscopy with biopsies can be used to assess villi health and for follow-up.

5. If symptomatic, talk to your doctor about stool tests for parasites, fungal and bacterial infections. An overstressed intestinal immune system, maladaptive intestinal environment, and damaged mucosa may predispose individuals to develop bacterial or fungal bowel infections and provide an environment for parasites to thrive.

6. Ensure adequate hydration is maintained. All human cells, including intestinal villi cells, require water for hydration. Usually, 8-10 glasses of fluids should be consumed every day. However, the recommended fluid intake can depend on your current hydration status, your age and your health history. For example, an individual with a cardiac or kidney medical history may have fluid restrictions. Check with your doctor.

7. Take precautions to avoid infections. Wash your hands, keep healthy, and avoid contact with others who have infections.

8. Check for allergies and food intolerance (i.e. lactose intolerance). Ask about a referral to an allergist or see a naturopathic doctor for blood tests. Ask your doctor about the need for digestive enzymes while your bowel is healing.

    See more about allergy testing in Chapter 16, "Diagnosis".

    See more about the need for digestive enzymes in Chapter 20, "What If the Gluten-Free diet Doesn't Work", under recommendation #5.

    Read about lectins and how lectins may affect intestinal health in Chapter 2 under "The Pathophysiology Of Non-Celiac Gluten Intolerance" and in Chapter 27, "Twelve Theories: Why has the Prevalence Of Celiac Disease Increased? under "The Lectin Theory"

9. Consult your doctor about an effective probiotic. I take probiotics regularly. Please see the discussion about this in Chapter 20, 3rd recommendation for more information and concerns with probiotics.

10. Review all medications with your MD and a Pharmacist. Ask if any affect the intestinal villi.

CHAPTER 20
What If The Gluten-Free Diet Doesn't Work?

What if you have been on the gluten-free diet for a while and it doesn't seem to be working? With some, the symptoms resolve soon after a gluten free diet is initiated. For others, it can take many months, a year, or more. Also, what if the diet was working, but now it isn't? There can be many different reasons for this. For example, with ongoing bowel symptoms, possible causes can include lactose intolerance, pancreatic insufficiency, bacterial or fungal overgrowth, parasites, accidental gluten consumption, bowel strictures, small bowel lymphoma, ulcerative jejunitis, a new food intolerance/allergy, microscopic colitis, refractory sprue, liver or gallbladder dysfunction, side effect of a drug, and vitamin/mineral deficiency or toxicity if taking high supplement doses. A lectin intolerance or the new presence of other autoimmune diseases may cause similar symptoms [1-4, 8-11,13-17,19-33].

If you are experiencing ongoing symptoms or a re-occurrence of symptoms, discuss the following possibilities with your doctor (who is hopefully knowledgeable about gluten intolerance), your gastroenterologist, and any other specialists involved in your care.

12 Recommendations To Discuss With Your Doctor, Gastroenterologist, And Other Specialists

1. With bowel involvement, ask your doctor about an upper endoscopy and colono-scopy (with inspection of the stomach, duodenum, jejunum, upper and lower ileum and colon) with biopsies. This will help rule out lymphoma, other cancers, refractory sprue, ulcerative jejunitis, microscopic colitis, or another disease process.

    There are many possible causes so try to keep that in mind emotionally when you read this first recommendation (avoid focusing on the cancer part).

2. With bowel symptoms, stool tests for parasites, fungal and bacterial infections may be helpful. An overstressed intestinal immune system, maladaptive intestinal environment, and damaged mucosa may predispose individuals to develop bacterial or fungal bowel infections or provide an environment for parasites to

thrive. Some infections (i.e. giardiasis) can cause villus flattening as well and this could affect the absorption of nutrients [10,13-15].

Keep in mind that infections (i.e. candidiasis, etc) can gain access to the blood stream (with a leaky gut) and this could lead to symptoms throughout the body. Report any symptoms to your doctor.

3. Probiotics might help to inhibit pathogens (infectious agents) and modulate the immune system. The risk for infections is high since the intestinal flora is in a state of dysbiosis (microbial imbalance) while undiagnosed with celiac disease, dermatitis herpetiformis (most have this with DH) and likely for many people with a non-celiac gluten intolerance. Therefore, it seems reasonable to suspect that probiotics would be helpful to reestablish a healthy microbial balance in the small bowel.

With this in mind, probiotics may be very helpful, but there may also be concerns. There are many mysteries with the use of probiotics. For example, with a gluten intolerance, what are the best and safest strains to use? Is there a possibility that patients with a gluten intolerance may respond to probiotics differently?

A 2008 study, "Antigenic Proteins Of Lactobacillus Acidophilus That Are Recognized By Serum IgG Antibodies In Children With Type 1 Diabetes And Coeliac Disease", highlights the possibility of an immune response. This study suggests that an immune response (mediated by IgG antibodies) could occur [34].

An additional concern, use caution with probiotics if you are immunosuppressed (i.e. with AIDS, chemotherapy, with immunosuppressive drugs) or if you are very ill or in the hospital. Probiotic microbes might cause an infection in individuals that are vulnerable [18].

Conversely, another study with in-vitro models, showed that bifidobacteria up-regulated anti-inflammatory cytokines (cytokines carry signals between cells) which may be very beneficial for celiac patients. Human clinical trials are necessary to further investigate this effect [14].

Overall, is there enough research to know how probiotics will affect individuals with CD, DH, or non-celiac gluten intolerance? Currently, I take probiotics and I have not had a reaction that I'm aware of. In fact, I feel very healthy and energetic. However, as we know with silent CD, pathological changes can be occurring within the body without any obvious symptoms.

After reviewing the literature and talking to a doctor, I am going to continue taking probiotics since this supplement seems to be improving my health. As well, I work with many patients in the hospital who have gastrointestinal infections. Therefore, probiotics are a good preventative treatment for me.

I wonder whether probiotics are a good idea for someone who is newly diagnosed. The bowel is very leaky at that time and I worry about the flora gaining access to the immune system and the systemic circulation. Theoretically, this might lead to an infection or increase the risk of an immune reaction complete with antibodies against the various flora. Conversely, probiotics may be very beneficial during this time to help correct microbial balances. As well, there is some evidence that supplementation with probiotics may help to prevent allergies, lesson allergic responses, strengthen the immune system and decrease the risk for infections [18]. With this in mind, probiotics are a very worthwhile consideration. Overall, all pros and cons associated with probiotic supplementation need to be carefully evaluated. Discuss these concerns with your doctor and to be safe, get approval before taking probiotics.

Yogurt and kefir are generally good sources of probiotics. I take a probiotic supplement. Usually, there are probiotics available at health food stores that you can check into. It is important to ensure all probiotics consumed are gluten-free.

4. Re-check ingredient lists on the foods, vitamins, supplements, and medications you consume to ensure that all are gluten-free. Products that were once gluten-free may not be now due to a change in the ingredients. Accidental ingestion of gluten could lead to ongoing symptoms. It's worth viewing the label each time you buy a product. Also, check with companies to ensure that there is no cross contamination at their company due to packaging gluten and non-gluten foods on the same machine. Contamination can also occur while growing, harvesting, transporting or preparing the food as well. These checks can be time consuming, but well worth the effort.

    Ask your doctor or gastroenterologist to do blood tests to see if you still have circulating antibodies. This can help you to see if you are still exposed to gluten. For celiac disease, a better test to check celiac related mucosal health is an endoscope with biopsies. While evaluating the results, keep in mind that there can be false negatives.

5. Ask about tests to check pancreatic, liver, and gallbladder function. As discussed in the "Gastrointestinal Symptoms" chapter, these organs aide in digestion and can

be affected. Resulting malabsorption can lead to flatulence, diarrhea, and bowel infections (as well as symptoms related to the organ affected). Tests can help to rule out these possibilities.

Keep in mind that pancreatic insufficiency can occur with gluten intolerance. One study mentioned that 30% of the gluten-free celiac patients with persistent diarrhea had pancreatic insufficiency. Fecal elastase-1 (Fe-1) levels were used to assess for pancreatic insufficiency and the results were low in 20 out of 66 patients. In this group, 19 out of 20 patients improved with pancreatic supplement-ation and the fecal elastase-1 levels started to increase demonstrating that the pancreatic insufficiency was resolving. This group was followed for 4 years and the patients discontinued the supplements once their symptoms disappeared. 11 out of 19 patients were still taking their supplements at the 4 year mark to control symptoms [13].

Talk to your doctor about taking digestive enzymes to aide in digestion. I took enzymes for the first 2-3 months to aide digestion. Collectively, inflammation in the stomach, brush border, and pancreas may affect the production of enzymes, therefore, digestive enzymes may be helpful to decrease symptoms until these areas heal.

6. With bowel symptoms, ask your doctor about testing for lactose intolerance. Lactose is found in dairy products. It is a disaccharide and requires lactase-phlorizin hydrolase (enzyme) produced within the intestines to digest it.

Loss of this brush border enzyme results in hypolactasia (low lactase production), and this can occur from the intestinal epithelial damage. Once the undigested lactose passes into the colon, it is broken down by commensal bacteria. This process produces CO_2 and hydrogen which cause abdominal discomfort, bloating, flatulence, and possibly diarrhea [4].

This may be temporary, since lactase production may resume once the bowel has healed. In others, it is a permanent condition.

7. Ask about blood tests to check for vitamin and mineral deficiencies or toxicities which could lead to a variety of symptoms throughout the body [2].

8. Consume nutritionally dense foods to help meet your nutritional needs. Avoid processed foods or foods high in processed refined sugar. Eat natural foods, hopefully, without additives if possible.

Ensure the fats you consume are healthy (include omega 3). Adequate fat intake is necessary for absorption of vitamin A, D, E, and K. Overall, you need to ensure an adequate intake of fat and water soluble vitamins, minerals, trace elements, electrolytes, proteins, fats, and carbohydrates. Ask your doctor/Gastroenterologist about a multivitamin.

Ask for a referral to a registered dietitian (who is knowledgeable about gluten intolerance and the gluten-free diet) to review your nutritional needs. Some patients find a grain-free, paleolithic, specific carbohydrate, or an elimination diet helpful (see Chapter 21), but you need to ensure you are consuming all the nutrients your body requires. A registered dietitian can provide guidance. Naturo-pathic doctors (ND) are usually more knowledgeable about these therapeutic diets than medical doctors. Inquire about your ND's knowledge. Medical doctors who specialize in gluten intolerance are an exception.

Also, with diarrhea or vomiting, ask your MD about checking your electrolyte levels since electrolytes can be lost through both emesis (vomit) and diarrhea. Your doctor may prescribe an electrolyte replacement drink and medications if you are having frequent vomiting or diarrhea.

9. Ensure adequate hydration is maintained. Usually, 8-10 glasses of fluids should be consumed every day. However, the recommended fluid intake can depend on your current hydration status, age and your health history. For example, an individual with a cardiac or kidney medical history may have fluid restrictions. Check with your MD.

   Remember, caffeinated fluids do not do a great job of hydrating you since these fluids promote diuresis and may increase peristalsis leading possibly to more diarrhea. Flushed dry skin, poor skin turgor, dry mouth and lips, coated tongue, low concentrated urine output, decreased level of orientation, irritability, or confusion are some symptoms that may indicate you are getting dehydrated. These symptoms may mean something more serious is happening as well so inform your doctor about any new symptoms.

10. Ask your doctor, specialists, and gastroenterologist about the possible presence of other autoimmune diseases that may cause the symptoms you are having. Some possibilities that may cause bowel symptoms are Graves Disease (hyperthyroid-ism-diarrhea, weight loss), Hashimoto's Disease (hypothyroidism-), Sjögren's Syndrome, Microscopic Colitis, or Addison's Disease. As well, there are many other autoimmune diseases, conditions (i.e. adrenal insufficiency, etc) and

syndromes that can cause symptoms in different areas of the body. Your doctor can investigate these possibilities.

Investigate and test for infections. Newly diagnosed patients or people with complications may be more vulnerable to infections. This can cause a variety of symptoms. Some patients who are elderly may actually become confused and have delirium while they have infections (i.e. pneumonia, urinary tract infection, etc). This requires prompt treatment.

11. Increased bowel permeability is present with gluten intolerance and can increase the risk of developing food allergies. This could lead to a variety of symptoms throughout the body [2,3,5-7,11].

    As well, food allergies can affect the health of the bowel and may cause some absorptive problems. For example, reactions to some foods (i.e. soy, dairy) could lead to villous flattening which may contribute to bowel and malabsorption symptoms [3,11]. Consider asking for a referral to an allergist or see a naturo-pathic doctor for allergy tests. See more about allergy testing in the diagnosis chapter.

    An allergy to lectins may also contribute to ongoing symptoms while on a gluten-free diet. Lectins are glycoproteins that are present in grains and some other foods such as legumes, some seeds, nightshades (i.e. potatoes and tomatoes, etc) and dairy [20-33]. Lectins are discussed in more detail in Chapter 2 under "Non-Celiac Gluten Intolerance" and also in Chapter 21 under "A Paleolithic diet".

12. Ask about checking drug levels for any medications you are taking. Review side effects with a pharmacist to see if any of the medications you take could be responsible for your symptoms. Ask the MD about checking your BUN and creat-inine levels to ensure your kidneys are functioning well. Dysfunction may lead to a drug or vitamin toxicity.

CHAPTER 21

Could A Grain-Free, Specific Carbohydrate, Paleolithic, Or Elimination Diet Be Helpful?

Some people find that a gluten-free diet doesn't take away all of their symptoms. Their medical doctor has investigated their persistent symptoms thoroughly with physical assessments and tests, but everything came back negative (nothing was found). Further investigations for allergies and other possibles causes had negative results. They were eating a nutritious strict gluten-free diet and taking all prescribed supplements. However, some symptoms still persisted.

Then, either through a suggestion from a naturopathic doctor or through their own research, they decided to try another type of therapeutic diet. Some people have tried a grain-free diet, a specific carbohydrate diet, a paleolithic diet, or an elimination diet. I have heard about many success stories with each diet. Perhaps, the success was due to a lectin intolerance, a glutamic acid or aspartic acid sensitivity (gluten, dairy, and soy), an exomorphin sensitivity (gluten and diary) or the relief may be due to allergies to other foods that happen to be absent in the chosen diet [6-8]. More research will help to unveil the reasons. For now, these people are thankful to have relief and are living symptom free.

In the following pages, I have outlined each diet with some resources to further investigate whether this diet is something you would like to consider. With these diets, a consultation with a registered dietitian is ideal to ensure you are receiving all of your daily required nutrients. Nutrient deficiencies can lead to a variety of symptoms and sometimes permanent damage. Eating a wide range of fresh, healthy, and preferably organic foods while on these diets can help with success.

Inform your medical doctor (plus other specialists) and your naturopathic doctor about your dietary changes. Naturopathic doctors (ND) are usually knowledgeable about these diets (verify that your ND is knowledgeable). Also, ensure that all other causes have been ruled out by your doctors and that you have received testing for food allergies.

A Grain-Free Diet

A grain-free diet eliminates all grains (even gluten-free grains) from your diet. I consumed a grain-free diet for a period of time, but now have progressed to a paleolithic diet. I feel much more energetic and symptom free eating this way.

My gluten-free diet took away my gastrointestinal symptoms, but I still had some asthma symptoms to deal with. I found that eliminating all grains (even gluten-free grains) improved my chronic cough and asthma. Reintroduction of any of the gluten-free grains would result in coughing and asthma symptoms. A consultation with an allergist revealed that I have a severe allergic response (IgE mediated) to grasses. Just after testing, I developed huge wheals on my arm with a rash and the roof of my mouth became very itchy. Since grains are essentially grasses, my allergist mentioned that the relief I experience on a grain-free diet is likely due to my severe allergy to grasses.

I have also encountered others who feel better eating grain-free. This could be due to allergies to some of the gluten-free grains, a reaction to something else (lectins, etc) in the gluten-free grains, or the fact that eliminating all grains decreases the risk of cross contamination issues. Some gluten-free grains can be contaminated with grains containing gluten while growing, harvesting, storing, transporting, packaging, or while being sold (i.e. in bulk bins, if the same scoops are being used for gluten and non-gluten grains).

If it is a contamination issue, then the source of contamination should be removed. Calling the companies that supply your gluten-free grains to verify that the grains are gluten-free and testing the products with an at home test kit for gluten may help to find the source. Ensuring that your grains are gluten-free may be all that is needed to feel well. You may not need to go completely grain-free.

On this diet, I ate a wide variety of fruits, vegetables, nuts, seeds (not any from grains), unprocessed natural meat, natural seafood, fish, beans, lentils, peas, fresh herbs, seaweed, and coconut. I also took a grain-free multivitamin, omega 3 supplements and probiotics.

Allergy testing may help you to clarify which gluten-free grains are specifically causing the symptoms. It may not be necessary to remove all the gluten-free grains from your diet if you are only allergic to a few. If a lectin intolerance is present, than a paleolithic diet helps to remove lectins from the diet.

A Specific Carbohydrate Diet

Elaine Gottschall B.A., M.Sc. created the specific carbohydrate diet for people with intestinal diseases. She spent years researching the effects of various sugars on the digestive tract and investigated the changes that occur in the bowel with inflammatory bowel disease. She was very interested in the effects food had on the intestinal tract and behavior. Her findings led to the creation of this diet to help restore a healthy equilibrium in the bowel [2,3].

I have her book, have read her website and tried some of her recipes when I was initially diagnosed with CD. I can understand why this diet may provide relief to individuals with ongoing symptoms. All grains are eliminated from the diet (which decreases cross contamination issues) and the carbohydrates included are all easily digested and quite healthy.

For more information, go to www.breakingtheviciouscycle.info and

www.breakingtheviciouscycle.info/beginners_guide/beginners.htm.

There is a link to many testimonials (from amazon.com readers) at the bottom of the "Information For Beginners Guide". The book can be found at www.amazon.ca, www.amazon.com, at some health food stores, and may be at various bookstores.

Inform your medical doctor (plus other specialists) and your naturopathic doctor about your dietary changes. Naturopathic doctors (ND) are usually knowledgeable about these diets (verify that your ND is knowledgeable). Also, ensure that all other causes have been ruled out by your doctors and that you have received testing for food allergies.

A Paleolithic Diet

A paleolithic diet is often referred to as a cave man/woman diet, close to what our ancestors ate when they lived a nomadic lifestyle. The diet eliminates dairy, grains, sugar (except honey), foods from the nightshade family, legumes, mined table salt, and processed refined oils (cold pressed olive oil is okay). An individual with a lectin sensitivity may benefit from this type of diet. It is low in carbohydrates, the fats included are healthy, lean meats are encouraged, and lots of non-starchy fruits and vegetables are included so there is lots of fiber [1,4,5].

Advocates of this diet feel that it increases health because it is comprised of foods that we are genetically designed to eat. As a result, the food is digested easily and advocates mention that inflammation within the body is decreased due to the removal of lectins (and possibly other harmful substances) in the diet. However, it is possible for inflammation to occur if allergies to some of the foods are present, this needs to be ruled out.

For example, I eat a paleolithic diet, however, I have to eliminate some of the foods allowed (i.e. oranges, celery, sesame seeds and bananas) due to allergies. My story, under "An Elimination Diet", explains how my transition to a paleolithic diet took place.

Information about lectins can be found in Chapter 2 under "The Pathophysiology Of Non-Celiac Gluten intolerance". A list of paleolithic diet books can be found in Chapter 30 "Support For A New Lifestyle" under "Paleolithic Books"

A dietitian can help to ensure that you are getting all of your daily nutrients. If you avoid salt, then add seaweed or another food with iodine to help ensure that you won't become deficient. Advocates of the paleolithic diet tend to discourage the use of salt. I use sea salt since I believe coastal residents would have had exposure to this natural salt.

An Elimination Diet

An elimination diet helps to identify which foods are causing a reaction and symptoms. With this diet, suspected allergenic foods are removed from the diet and reintroduced one at a time over a specified period. A dietary log helps to keep track of the foods eaten and responses. Symptoms are monitored and adjustments in diet are made. Hopefully, by the end, the offending foods will be identified and a healthy diet established.

Concerns With An Elimination Diet

For me, the elimination diet was very beneficial. I was able to identify other foods that were contributing to my symptoms and as a result, I am much healthier. However, there are a few concerns that should be considered when an individual is considering this diet.

When a reaction occurs, it can be very difficult to identify the offending part of the food. (i.e. fruit may be coated with corn wax, etc). As well, with delayed allergies, analysis of the reactions can be confusing. I must admit, the elimination diet can be a challenge. It is very important to adhere to the foods on the diet without any cheating and it is important to keep a food diary so that you can review and analyze the results.

An additional concern, weight loss often occurs while on an elimination diet. For some this may sound appealing. However, for others, weight loss could be life threatening if they are emaciated, weak, and have nutrient deficiencies.

A third concern, if someone has anaphylactic allergies, this diet should not be used without the close supervision of a medical doctor and appropriate medications (i.e. Ventolin, antihistamines, Epipen, etc) nearby. An adverse reaction at home could be life threatening. Keep in mind that the reactions can be stronger after the initial cleansing diet is done. For these reasons, it is wise to discuss this diet with your doctor and get approval before implementing it.

An allergist can test for anaphylactic allergies prior to trying this type of diet. Your doctor will likely suggest blood testing for other allergies instead of the elimination diet if you have anaphylactic allergies (due to the risks). Guidance from your allergist, naturopathic doctor, and your medical doctor is important, everyone is unique with individual needs. If your doctor recommends the elimination diet, any foods that you are allergic to should be eliminated from this type of diet and not introduced at any time.

A fourth concern, every time you have a reaction while on the elimination diet, a day or two is lost due to feeling ill. This can affect your work or your time with your family. Having the blood tests to help identify food reactions may help to avoid this loss of time.

With these concerns in mind, I proceeded with the elimination diet. A doctor suggested that I try it plus I wanted to try this method of identifying food reactions for myself. Now, it would be interesting to have blood tests done to see if the results match my findings (see my findings under "My Results").

Blood Tests For Allergies

Some doctors feel that it is easier to do the blood tests for food allergies instead of doing the elimination diet. Blood tests are not 100% accurate, however, the results can provide a base to start from. Your doctor may suggest that you use the elimination diet to confirm the results (as long as you don't have any risk of an anaphylactic response).

There are five classes of antibodies that are present in our bodies, IgA, IgD, IgE, IgG and IgM. Unfortunately, for many patients, only the IgE mediated food reactions are invest-igated by an allergist since this type of allergy is well researched and acknowledged amongst allergists.

Some other people are lucky to have the IgG mediated food reactions investigated as well. This may have been offered during a naturopathic consultation. IgG is often chosen because IgG (as subtypes IgG1, IgG2, IgG3, and IgG4) is the most abundant antibody class in the blood and it has high specificity toward antigens (i.e. allergenic foods).

Testing for IgA antibodies against foods is valuable as well. IgA antibodies protect the mucosal membranes in the respiratory tract, the gastrointestinal tract, the reproductive tract, the urological tract and can be found in the blood. IgA antibodies are the most abundant antibody class in the body and are quite efficient at binding antigens with up to four antigen binding sites (IgG only has two). With this in mind, it is reasonable to suspect that these antibodies can react to various foods, just like IgA antibodies react to gluten. There are blood tests available that can check for this type of reaction [9,10].

It is important to recognize that false negatives can occur with these blood tests, just like the gluten intolerance tests. An elimination diet is sometimes used to help identify foods that are causing a reaction or to confirm the results of the blood tests. Discuss this further with your doctor [9,10].

More research will help to reveal how IgD and IgM antibodies may be involved with food reactions. Immature B cells have IgM antibodies on their surface and once mature, these cells also carry IgD antibodies on their surface. IgM antibodies are very involved in the early stages of a reaction. In fact, IgM predominates in early reactions to perceived invaders before IgG (or other antibodies) are involved and is very efficient at activating the complement cascade (other chemicals) to help with attacking an invader. Unfortunately, with IgD, the function is less clear. IgD can activate basophils and mast cells to produce antimicrobial factors so it appears to be involved in the early stage of a reaction. Overall, more research into the function of IgM and IgD antibodies may lead to other tests that can identify early reactions to food molecules. These two antibodies may contribute more than we realize.

In my experience, the allergist often only tests for IgE mediated reactions during a consultation and offers the elimination diet to help identify other allergies. Whereas, a naturopathic doctor usually investigates the other forms of food reactions through the use of blood tests (might use an elimination diet as well). This may vary from country to country, so clarify what tests your allergist and naturopathic doctors can do for you.

With blood tests, keep in mind that you may be reacting to something not included in the tests. This could be a food dye, an additive, or an intolerance to something else in the foods (i.e. a lactose intolerance). An elimination diet along with other tests may help to investigate this possibility [9,10]. You can discuss the elimination diet with your doctor, naturopathic doctor or allergist, they should be able to provide resources and guidance for this diet.

162

Ask About Key Words To Look For In Ingredients

Once your allergies are diagnosed, be aware of key words to look for on ingredient lists while shopping. Sometimes, this extra information may be overlooked by your allergist. Ask for a complete list of ingredients that can be derived from the foods you are allergic to so that you can successfully avoid that food. As well, an allergy medical alert bracelet may be a worthwhile consideration in case of future emergencies.

The following story may illustrate why a complete list of key words from your allergist, naturopathic doctor or registered dietitian is important for success. My husband, two of my daughters, and I have a corn allergy. With a corn allergy, you need to be aware that ingredients such as dextrose, glucose, fructose, citric acid, maltodextrin, zein, and vitamin C (many more keywords as well) can be derived from corn. The list of possible ingredients derived from corn is actually more extensive than with gluten. Even intravenous infusions in the hospital can contain corn (in the dextrose), it can coat table salt (to stabilize the iodine) and can be used in low fat milks (1%, 2%, and skim) to carry the fat soluble vitamins A and D (it won't say corn on the label, just vitamin A and D added). As well, the vegetable oil used in many products is often from corn and there can be small amounts of cornstarch in many products (sometimes undeclared) such as icing sugar. Much to my dismay, the wax on some fruit can also contain corn.

Many people just think of corn kernels, popcorn, cornstarch, corn syrup, corn oil and corn flour when they identify foods they need to avoid with a corn allergy. Unfortunately, the list is much more extensive. If my family and I only avoided the obvious sources of corn, then we likely wouldn't feel well because we would still be getting some derivatives of corn. Knowing my complete list of ingredients to avoid helps me to take knowledgeable steps to improve our health.

When I purchase a product, I always call the company and clarify what each ingredient is made from so that we can avoid all corn derivatives. The extra time spent checking can be well worth it. For example, when my daughter was young, I thought she had a dairy allergy because she would get a rash and a stomach ache when she drank milk. Then, I called the company and discovered that there was corn oil in her 2% milk. I realized that she could still drink milk, I just needed to buy homogenized milk. Allergy testing helped to confirm that she didn't have a milk allergy. Corn allergies can be very difficult because corn isn't one of the allergens that has to be declared on labels so it is important to call the company to verify it is corn free.

Talk to your allergist and/or naturopathic doctor about key words you need to be aware of. As you can see with the example above, it is worthwhile.

My Experience

I had a consultation with an allergist to test for IgE reactions to foods and pollens. The allergist did a skin scratch test. With this test, 40 droplets (containing the allergenic part of each food and pollen) were put on my two forearms. Then a needle scratched my skin just under each droplet. After some time, if the skin became red under the droplet with a raised area (called a wheal), then the test was considered positive.

My test results revealed that I have a severe allergic response (IgE mediated) to grasses. The area on my arm around the grasses site had an extensive rash and my arm was swollen. Since grains are essentially grasses, my allergist mentioned that the relief I experience on a grain-free diet (mentioned previously) is likely due to my severe allergy to grasses.

I also had small wheals on my skin from shrimp, corn, wheat, peanuts, tomato, sesame seed, celery, dairy, oranges, and bananas. Once the test was done, the roof of my mouth became very itchy and I had some mild asthmatic symptoms. These food allergies appeared to trigger my asthma symptoms. My throat did not swell at all.

Following this, I tried an elimination diet with my allergist's approval. I hoped that the elimination diet would help to identify other foods that may be causing a reaction. At this point, I could have chosen to go to a naturopathic doctor for further testing. However, I decided to try the diet to see what kind of results I could get with it.

I didn't take any anti-histamines, aspirin, Advil type products or my nasal spray (Flonase) while on this diet because these medications might dampen or mask a reaction. If your doctor has ordered any of these medications or other medications and vitamins (with additives, food dyes, or other potential allergens) to be taken regularly, then perhaps the blood tests from the naturopathic doctor would be a better choice than the elimination diet to identify the offending foods and additives.

I had medications at home to treat a reaction, if necessary. However, I didn't need to use any medication.

Peppermint and spearmint might make a reaction worse so I avoided these two foods as well. I also avoided preservatives and dyes in the elimination diet foods since a reactions to these two things might cause confusion with the results.

I outlined the elimination diet I tried in the following pages. I modified the diet, eliminating gluten (due to celiac disease) and GF grain (because of my severe IgE reaction to grasses). I also eliminated the foods that tested positive in my IgE related skin prick test at

164

the allergist (see previously) and foods that I never eat. Other people who try this diet could adjust it so that the foods they know they react to are taken out. As well, I added probiotics and vitamins in at the end since I normally take both.

The cleansing diet, consisting of hypoallergenic foods, lasted for 6 days. My lungs felt clear and I didn't have any asthma symptoms. However, I did have itchy skin a couple of times with a small rash on my face that lasted a couple of hours. I also noticed that the roof of my mouth was frequently itchy. I suspected that potatoes might be the culprit since I was eating a lot of potatoes and it seemed to occur after I consumed this food. I removed potatoes from my diet. During this time, I lost a pound a day.

After 6 days, I started to introduce other foods in to my diet. A new food was introduced every three days. Again, I didn't eat any of the foods I tested positive to at the allergist. I also eliminated all gluten-free grains due to my severe grass allergy. My allergist urged me to try quinoa and amaranth, but these grains caused symptoms as well (heavy feeling in my stomach and nausea). The other foods I reacted to while implementing the elimination diet included the legume family (not surprising with my peanut allergy), potatoes, and apples. As previously mentioned, this diet helped me to see that I seem to thrive on a paleolithic styled diet.

This experience raised a concern: Some people may go to the allergist, get diagnosed with a wheat allergy (IgE mediated), but not get the full diagnosis of having a gluten intolerance issue. Once they start to eat wheat free they may feel better. but not entirely, since they are still getting rye and barley, and contaminated oats. It would be difficult to test them since much of the gluten would be taken out of the diet with eating wheat free (may cause false negatives).

With this in mind, I think everyone with allergies should be screened for a gluten intolerance to decrease this risk.

As mentioned previously, I have an IgE mediated antibody reaction to wheat. Individuals with a gluten intolerance usually have an IgA or IgG antibody reaction to gluten unless they have an IgE mediated allergy too (which I have).

My Modified Elimination Diet

For 6 days, I only ate foods included in the cleansing diet:

- Unprocessed natural turkey and lamb (with no additives)
- Well cooked potatoes (without skin). I reacted to the potatoes.

- Canned or cooked plums, prunes, nectarines, apricots, cherries, peaches and yams (should be no sugar and no gluten). Can be canned in pear juice, but should be free of other additives
- Fresh or cooked spinach. Can be canned, but ensure it is gluten-free and free of additives
- Fresh lettuce
- Olive oil (I used extra virgin, cold pressed)
- Canned or fresh cranberry and blueberry juice (free of additives, labels should only say cranberries and blueberries)
- Salt (I used sea salt with no additives, sometimes table salt can be coated with dextrose from corn to stabilize the iodine)
- Plain water (no coffee or tea)
- No spices

During the 6 days I monitored myself for any reactions and wrote down any symptoms in my food log. It is possible to react to something in the basic foods during this period. I reacted to the potatoes. Symptoms can occur in almost every system of the body and can be just as elusive and vague as the gluten intolerance symptoms. For example, some people may only experience a feeling of exhaustion or a heavy feeling in their stomach, others may have more obvious symptoms such as heartburn, itching, diarrhea, headache, or stomach upset, etc (many other symptoms too).

After the initial 6 days, I was ready to introduce other foods (see below). It was important for me to eat as much of the food being introduced/tested as I could to see if there would be a reaction. Once a reaction occurred, I would stop eating the food that triggered a reaction and consider myself allergic/intolerant to that food group. Following a reaction, I would return to the basic cleansing diet plus the foods that I already tried with no reactions. I would stay on that diet for 5-6 days to cleanse my body, then introduce the next food group. My allergist only recommended waiting until the symptoms disappeared before introducing the next food group, but I waited 5-6 days just to be sure that the previous reaction didn't interfere with a potential future one.

Dairy

Then after 6 days, dairy products can be introduced for 3 days, including foods such as butter, white cheeses, plain yogurt, and milk. Watch for and avoid any additives (i.e. gluten, corn derivatives such as dextrose, glucose, fructose, etc) or dyes and be aware that sour cream can contain corn and so can many types of milk (1%, 2%, and skim milk). I would avoid anything with other ingredients or corn because it can make it more difficult to figure out the culprit with a reaction. With no reactions, someone on this diet can proceed to the next food group.

I didn't include dairy because I know I am allergic to it.

Gluten-Free Grains

If no reaction to the above foods, gluten-free grains can be introduced for 3 days. Ensure all are gluten-free with no cross contamination or other additives.

I didn't include gluten-free grains because of my severe grass allergy and allergic reaction that I experienced during the consultation. Previous to my allergy testing, I had tried all the different gluten-free grains and noticed that I coughed after I ingested them and sometimes I would have asthma symptoms as well.

Legume and Peas

If no reaction to the above foods, then the legume pea family can be introduced for 3 days. Foods can include peanuts, soya bean, kidney beans, navy beans, Lima beans and green peas. After my 5 day cleansing diet, I started with this group (since I know I react to the other two). I didn't try peanuts since I know I have an allergy to this. I kept track of any reactions on the dietary log.

For people with a peanut allergy, talk to your allergist, doctor and registered dietitian for approval before introducing legumes and peas. Of course, the peanuts would be strictly avoided with a peanut allergy.

I reacted to legumes and peas so I waited 5 days before I introduced the next food.

Other Foods

Then, I introduced beef. With no reaction, I introduced chicken, then pork, then egg (each with 3 days in between). I only introduced the next food if no reaction occurred with the previous one. Otherwise, I would wait 5 days to clear the reaction.

Then with no reaction, I was able to introduce the following foods, each 3 days apart. I ate as much as I could of that food during the 3 days. Again, I only introduced the next food if no reaction occurred with the previous one. Following a reaction, I would return to the basic diet plus the foods that I already tried with no reactions. I would stay on that diet for 5 days to cleanse my body, then introduce the next food group. For this phase of the diet, I wrote down all of the foods that I commonly eat. I didn't include the foods that I am allergic to (according to the allergy tests). All fruits, vegetables and nuts were eaten raw for the 3 day test. I cooked the squash, zucchini, parsnips, onions, leeks, and asparagus since I would normally eat these foods cooked.

Foods (introduced 1 at a time, each 3 days apart)

Apple	Strawberry	Raspberry
Pears	Potato	Cherries
Apricots	Nectarines	Peaches
Plums	Prunes	Cod
Halibut	Salmon	Sole
Trout	Tuna	Whitefish
Coconut	Maple Syrup	Honey
Almonds	Brazil nuts	Cashew nuts
Pecans	Hazelnuts	Walnuts
Sunflower seeds	Grapes	Lemons
Grapefruit	Carrots	Parsnip
Onion	Leek	Asparagus
Scallops	Crab	Lobster
Radish	Cauliflower	Broccoli
Cantaloupe	Watermelon	Honeydew melon
Cucumber	Squash	Zucchini
Mustard	Garlic	Rosemary
Sage	Oregano	Marjoram
Parsley	Sugar	Tea
Probiotics	Vitamins	

Once I completed the elimination diet, I kept note of any other new foods introduced over the next few months and logged any reactions.

Keep your family doctor informed about new or ongoing symptoms. Your doctor may choose to do other tests to rule out other causes. A registered dietitian (who specializes in allergies) can guide you through this process with an elimination diet and can help to ensure you get all of your daily nutrients.

In my skin test, I tested mildly positive to foods in many different food groups (foods within each group are related to each other). For example, I tested positive to shrimp which is in the shellfish family. If this happens to you, clarify with your allergist whether you should avoid the whole food group completely or try some of the other foods in the food group (that you didn't test positive to) while doing your elimination diet. Your allergist will have to advise you whether this is safe.

The previous elimination diet is the one I tried (I modified it to suit my needs), check with your allergist or naturopathic doctor for one that is right for you since they may have a different recommendation.

> *Caution: Starting the diet without consulting an allergist or a doctor could place you at risk for life threatening allergic reactions, weight loss, and nutrient deficiencies which could be life threatening, especially if you are ill, emaciated, or recovering from illness. I am just including my experience with an elimination diet as an example to demonstrate what an elimination diet is like. Please do not follow my elimination diet unless your allergist or naturopathic doctor (and medical doctor) advises that you follow it. Your doctors will likely modify it to suit your needs or may supply his/her own elimination diet.*

My Results

While I was progressing through the diet, it became increasingly more evident that I was reacting to the foods that are taboo on a Paleolithic diet plus a few extra. It is reasonable to suspect that lectins or some other component of the reactive foods were causing my symptoms or perhaps just allergenic responses were responsible. Likely, a combination of these factors contributed to this outcome. What ever the cause, I am currently consuming a paleolithic diet, am symptom free, and am thankful for my good health.

Allergy Bracelet

Consider the use of an medial alert allergy bracelet. This is usually a metal bracelet that has your allergies engraved into it. Wear it all all times in case of an emergency. It will provide a valuable source of information for the doctors and nurses if you are admitted to the hospital and for some reason you are unable to talk to share your history.

The Food Diary

Below is a chart that I created and used while on the elimination diet. It was helpful to record the foods I was introducing and to analyze any reactions that occurred. This chart can be taken with you to your allergist and/or your doctor.

Date	Food Introduced	Reactions?	Plan of Action

CHAPTER 22
Charts To Track Progress

In this chapter, a test chart is included to track progress. I suggest that you also keep a file with a photocopy of all of your test results. This may be of value if you need to go to the ER or if you see a different doctor while on vacation. You can take this record and your file with you to show to the new doctor.

A second chart is provided to keep track of all the tasks you would like to complete. I included some of the tasks I completed while starting my new gluten-free lifestyle.

Test Chart To Track Progress

Normal test results can vary from lab to lab and in different countries (ex. some are metric and some are not). Log the normal range found on your lab result sheet, then your results.

Type Of Test	Normal Range (may vary in different countries)	Date and result	Date and result	Date and result	Date and result	Date and result
White Blood Cells						
Red Blood cells						
Hemoglobin						
Ferriton (Iron)						
Blood Sugar						
Thyroid Test						
ALP (liver)						

Type Of Test	Normal Range (may vary in different countries)	Date and result	Date and result	Date and result	Date and result	Date and result
AST (liver)						
ALT (liver)						
Bilirubin (liver)						
Vitamin A						
Vitamin D						
Vitamin E						
Vitamin K						
Vitamin B-1						
Vitamin B-6						
Vitamin B-12						
Folic Acid (Folate)						

Type Of Test	Normal Range (may vary in different countries)	Date and result	Date and result	Date and result	Date and result	Date and result
Other B Vitamins						
Calcium						
Magnesium						
Phosphorus						
Copper						
Zinc						
Total Protein						
Albumin						
BUN (Kidney)						
Creatinine (Kidney)						
Electrolytes						

Type Of Test	Normal Range (may vary in different countries)	Date and result	Date and result	Date and result	Date and result	Date and result	Date and result
Bone Density Test							
Stool Tests For Parasites, Bacteria, And Fungii							
Lactose Intolerance Test							
D-Xylose (Absorption Test)							
Cholesterol (can elevate once GF and absorbing food)							
Height And Weight	Normal range will vary with age						
Gluten Intolerance Blood Tests							
Endoscope							

Chart Of Tasks

You can write down tasks to accomplish. I included some examples.

Goals And Tasks	Description	Date Completed
Dietitian	Ask your doctor about a referral to a registered dietitian who is knowledgeable about the gluten-free diet. Take blood test results to the dietitian.	
Other Tests	Ask your doctor about a referral for a bone density test, lactose intolerance test and other tests	
Follow-up Scope	With celiac disease (and many with DH), ask your doctor about a follow-up endoscopy to check intestinal healing. It is important to know whether the intestine has healed completely.	
Schedule Follow-up	Schedule follow-up appointments with your doctor, naturopathic doctor, specialists, and dietitian to monitor your healing and progress. Follow-up tests and blood tests may need to be ordered. Children need growth and development monitored.	
Blood Tests	Ask your doctor about ordering recommended blood tests (see previous chart for blood test results and about supplements for any deficiencies. Ask doctor about follow-up antibody tests to ensure antibody levels are normalizing.	

Goals And Tasks	Description	Date Completed
Allergy Testing	Ask your doctor about a referral to an allergist or see a naturopathic doctor for allergy testing. Ask about testing for different types of food intolerance.	
Test Relatives	Talk to the doctor about testing your children for DH, CD, and a non-celiac gluten Intolerance. Inform relatives about their increased risk and the diagnostic tests that are available to check for a gluten intolerance.	
Probiotics	Talk to your doctor and gastroenterologist about using probiotics.	
Support Group	Join a support group and check out gluten-free forums online. Ask about local GF restaurants and bakeries	
Disaster Kits	Create a GF disaster kit for your home and your vehicles	
GF School	1. Stock your children's backpack with non-perishable GF treats (ask school if this is okay). 2. Create a GF disaster kit to keep at the school for your kids. 3. Put labeled GF treats in the freezer at school for your kids (let the teachers know). 4. Talk to teacher, principle, and other parents.	

Goals And Tasks	Description	Date Completed
Recipes	Look for books at the library, used book stores, or your favorite local store. Also available on Amazon.ca and Amazon.com. Check out blogs with recipes	
Exercise Program	Ask your doctor if there are any limits with exercising first, then choose an exercise program you enjoy.	
Medications And Vitamins	Check with the pharmacist and companies to ensure medications and vitamins are gluten-free. Ask your doctor about the need for nutrient supplements.	
Immunize	Ensure immunizations are up to date. Consider flu and pneumonia vaccines if immunosuppressed or if you have conditions that affect the immune system (check with your doctor). If immunized against hepatitis B, ensure antibody levels are sufficient to protect against the disease (ask your doctor).	
Digestive Enzymes	Ask your doctor whether digestive enzymes are needed? Check for the presence of pancreatic insufficiency (Test Fecal elastase-1 (Fe-1) levels).	
Task:		
Task:		

CHAPTER 23
Two Alternative Approaches To Relieve Allergies

The human body is amazing. It is so complex with many perplexing mysteries that are yet to be solved. I keep an open mind to alternative approaches because I believe that anything is possible. I also carefully analyze the possible benefits and associated risks before I try something new. I am not going to try something that may put me at risk. With this in mind, I would like to introduce you to two alternative approaches that may be helpful to manage and relieve allergies.

One approach attempts to relieve allergic reactions by healing the bowel and creating a favorable environment for healthy intestinal flora (beneficial bacteria in the bowel). This approach makes sense considering that the increased intestinal permeability likely led to the reactions in the first place. Taking steps to heal the bowel and decrease intestinal permeability would logically help to prevent future reactions to other foods and may eventually provide relief with current food reactions.

The other approach requires an open mind and the ability to think outside the box. It involves the use of energy medicine to relieve allergies. I know it is difficult to believe, but I have talked to several people who have benefited from its use.

In the following pages, I'll outline each approach. This information will help you to be aware of all of your options. Then, you can discuss these approaches with doctors who are knowledgeable and decide whether either of these approaches are right for you.

Healing The Bowel Approach

With this approach, a combination of treatments and recommendations help to promote a healthy intestinal environment. Therapy can include the use of digestive enzymes, healthy fats, a healthy diet (lots of raw foods and lots of fiber), food combining, immune system support, vitamin therapy, emotional support, prebiotics, probiotics, and steps to create a healthy acid-base balance. During this time, professional care is provided by a doctor and the patient avoids the foods that they react to [1].

The hope with this approach is that inflammation will decrease, immune reactions to foods will lesson (or diminish) and the body will reach a state of equilibrium and optimum health. The belief is that the patient may be able to consume some of the foods they were reacting to after a period of time has passed [1]. A doctor should monitor you very closely to provide guidance and I suggest re-testing (for allergies) to see if you are still allergic to the foods before anything is reintroduced. In fact, reintroduction of foods will be contrain-dicated if possible reactions are life threatening (i.e. anaphylactic allergies). Get approval from your doctor before reintroducing foods.

I bought a book, "Allergies, A Disease In Disguise", that provides a great resource for this type of approach. It was written by Carolee Bateson-Koch. She is a doctor of chiropractic and naturopathy. She is very focused on treating allergies with diet modification and natural therapies.

Bateson-Koch, DC, ND. Allergies, Disease In Disguise. How To Heal Your Allergic Condition Permanently And Naturally. Alive Books. 1994.

Energy Medicine Approach

Energy medicine has been utilized for health and wellness for centuries. The belief with this type of approach is that imbalances in the energy fields of the body can lead to patho-logical changes, diseases, allergic conditions, and other types of illness. With treatment, the belief is that the energy field can be rebalanced and sometimes the negative changes can be reversed. You may recognize some of the common names for different types of energy medicine such as acupuncture, Ayurveda, traditional Chinese medicine {use prana and qi (CHEE)}, magnetic field therapy, yoga, Therapeutic Touch, Reiki, or reflexology.

One type, Nambudripad's Allergy Elimination Technique, NAET, (and other variations of this method) is specifically designed to treat allergies. I have met some people over the last few months who have had tremendous success with this technique so I thought that it would be worth mentioning in this book.

More research needs to be done to explore this method of allergy relief. Close supervision and guidance should be provided by a doctor and I suggest re-testing (for allergies) to see if you are still allergic to the foods before anything is reintroduced. Reintroduction of foods will be contraindicated if possible reactions are life threatening (i.e. anaphylactic allergies). Get approval from your doctor before reintroducing foods.

The NAET approach was created by Dr. Devi S. Nambudripad, MD, DC, Lac, PhD (Acu). If interested, you can visit her website at www.naet.com and evaluate whether this is a method of interest to you. She has a list of practitioners on her site and several books [2].

I have included a few case examples that highlight how some people have benefited. At the end, I have included my thoughts about this unusual practice.

Case 1: I spent a lot of time in the spring, summer and fall in the hospital because of my asthma. I needed assistance in breathing that a normal puffer could not handle. I knew that I was allergic to cats, but I wasn't diagnosed with any other allergies (I may have had some). After two sessions of removal, I can now can play golf without any hesitancy, haven't been hospitalized, nor even used a puffer since. I can be around a cat without worry.

Case 2: My son was allergic to seafood and dairy. After a series of NAET treatments, I had him retested for allergies and the allergies appear to be gone. He can now eat these foods.

Case 3: I had an allergic reaction when I ate anything with garlic in it - nausea, stomach cramps, etc. Then I heard about a holistic treatment called energy medicine for this. One whole session was devoted to removal of only garlic. After the removal, I had garlic bread, garlic seafood and had no symptoms, whatsoever. This has continued to be the case after 3 years. Other sensitivities were discovered and removed at a subsequent session.

Case 4: My husband had an allergy to celery. The naturopathic doctor tried NAET and it took his allergy away. He can eat celery with no problems now.

Case 5: After testing, I discovered that I had allergies to turkey, cucumber, and olive oil. I think these allergies are gone now after the energy treatment because I don't seem to react to these foods.

My Thoughts

I'm not sure why these people are experiencing relief with energy medicine. Perhaps, some of the people avoided the problematic foods for so long that their body isn't as reactive. This could lead to the perception that the allergy was removed by the practitioner's energy methods. Secondly, the practitioner may have promoted some or all of the therapies mentioned in the "Healing The Bowel Approach".This may have helped to diminish reactions to food leading the patient to believe it was energy medicine. Thirdly, the power of thought and beliefs can influence outcomes. If the patient believes that the treatment will remove their allergies, then perhaps, something happens physiologically to create a shift in the way their body reacts to foods. Another consideration: NAET may really work either in isolation or in combination with the theories mentioned above. Future research will help to unveil the reasons.

I haven't tried a series of NAET treatments to see if this approach works. If I try it in the future, I'll do a blog post explaining my experience and the outcome.

I do have a concern that a practitioner might claim to be able to remove a gluten intolerance. Personally, I would never believe this type of claim. Reintroducing gluten would be very risky and could lead to permanent damage (i.e. cancer, nervous system damage, etc) and other potential complications. Retesting for a gluten intolerance (after energy treatments) would not be accurate since a GF diet along with many other issues (see diagnosis chapter) can lead to false negative test results. Therefore, you can't rely on retesting to confirm whether it worked or not.

As well, I would never reintroduce gluten following treatments with energy medicine because gluten is difficult for humans to digest and undigested gluten can lead to a permeable bowel. This leaky gut effect along with immune reactions and inflammation can cause many health problems. With this in mind, I'm gluten-free for life:)

CHAPTER 24

Food Can Heal Or Make You Ill: Could Other Autoimmune Diseases Be Triggered By Immune Reactions To Food?

Autoimmune Reactions In Gluten Intolerance

Celiac disease, dermatitis herpetiformis, and some forms of non-celiac gluten intolerance (i.e. gluten ataxia) are considered autoimmune diseases since antibodies can be created against the affected person's bodily tissues. Initially, antibodies are created against gluten and then the body cross reacts producing antibodies against endomysial tissue in the bowel, against the enzymes transglutaminase 2, transglutaminase 3 or transglutaminase 6 or against other organs, nerves, and tissues. The reactions can be IgA or IgG antibody mediated reactions [12,13].

The treatment, a strict gluten-free diet for life, is recommended to halt the inflammatory reactions and promote recovery. For some, this works. For others, they need to investigate allergies and modify their diet further to achieve an optimum state of health. For more reactive types, like me, the diet needs to be limited to a grain-free, paleolithic or specific carbohydrate styled diet before the patient feels completely well. Every individual is unique with specific needs.

Can Immune Reactions To Food Trigger The Symptoms Evident In Other Autoimmune Diseases?

If initial reactions to food can cause autoimmune reactions in the three forms of gluten intolerance, why couldn't this chain of reactions occur with other autoimmune diseases? The trigger could be gluten, lectins, corn, dairy, a food additive or another food allergen/antigen. Various antibodies (IgA, IgE, IgD, IgG, IgM) could be involved, either in isolation in combination.

Case Example: Crohn's Disease

I have a close relative with Crohn's disease. This is another autoimmune disease that affects the bowel. Upon diagnosis, he was offered a drug to suppress his immune system and help decrease the inflammation. When he asked about diet, the gastroenterologist told him that diet modification would not help him because Crohn's disease didn't appear to be related to diet. I was quite surprised by this guidance because, for me, it seemed logical to suspect that Crohn's disease could be associated with something in the diet. After all, what is the bowel most exposed to? Food!

Luckily, my relative, a professional engineer, was used to questioning new information and agreed that a change in diet may be needed. He went on the specific carbohydrate diet and was off his medication within 5 months. Further investigation revealed that he reacts to corn and corn derivatives (high fructose corn syrup, dextrose, glucose/fructose, citric acid, etc). Corn is in most grocery store products so this was quite a challenge to remove from his diet. He also has an allergy to almonds, broccoli, cauliflower, chocolate, and legumes. Diet modification has helped him to heal himself. If he accidentally consumes corn or the other foods he is allergic to, then the symptoms promptly return. Currently, he is very healthy with no symptoms. With his last follow-up scope, the gastroenterologist was amazed at the healthy appearance of his bowel.

This story highlights the fact that autoimmune reactions in Crohn's disease (and possibly other diseases) may be triggered by something in the diet. I also met another individual with Crohn's disease who had the same results. This strengthens the possibility that diet modification may relieve symptoms in individuals with Crohn's disease.

Dr. Loren Cordain's Research

A researcher, Dr. Loren Cordain, PhD, (from Colorado State University, USA) discussed the use of a Palaeolithic diet for Multiple Sclerosis in a 2007 video, "Potential Therapeutic Characteristics of Pre-agricultural Diets In The Prevention And Treatment Of Multiple Sclerosis", www.wildhorse.insinc.com/directms03oct2007/. Dr. Cordain shared how 4 individuals with multiple sclerosis benefited from this diet (halted symptoms) and believes this diet may benefit others with various autoimmune diseases as well. The video is located on Dr. Ashton Embry's (Ph.D) website at Direct-MS [www.direct-ms.org/].

A paleolithic diet removes lectins from the diet. Lectins are in all grains, the nightshade foods, some seeds, legumes and dairy. According to studies, lectin does appear to have

186

neurological effects once it gains access to the systemic circulation (through a leaky gut) [1,2,4-11].

Dr. Alessio Fasano's Research

In individuals with a gluten intolerance, gluten consumption can lead to increased expression of zonulin (a human protein) in the intestinal tissues. This increases intestinal permeability allowing macromolecules (ex. food antigens, bacterial, and viral particles) exposure to the immune system. The immune systems exposure to gluten and the subsequent reaction is thought to be responsible for the intestinal and other systemic damage seen with a gluten intolerance [14,15].

The increased bowel permeability can also increase the risk of developing food allergies. Dr. Alessio Fasano and his research team feel that the increased intestinal permeability (due to zonulin) is part of the underlying pathogenesis involved in CD and possibly many other autoimmune diseases. With this in mind, testing for a gluten intolerance along with food allergy tests would be a worthwhile consideration for people with autoimmune diseases.

Dr. Alessio Fasano is a researcher from The University Of Maryland Center For Celiac Research in Baltimore, MD, US.

Conclusions

I believe that our overall health is very strongly associated to the health of our bowels and the food that we ingest. Testing for a gluten intolerance, nutrient deficiencies, and allergies (IgE, IgA, IgG mediated) along with an elimination diet (to confirm the results, if needed) could help to identify the triggers in an autoimmune disease. If a gluten-free diet doesn't work, then the recommendations in Chapter 20, "What If The Gluten-Free Diet Doesn't Work" may be helpful. Some people find relief with a grain-free, specific carbohydrate, or paleolithic diet (Chapter 21). A naturopathic doctor or a doctor who specializes in gluten intolerance would likely be the best resource to help rule out these possibilities. A registered dietitian (who understands gluten intolerance) can help to ensure that you are consuming all of your required nutrients.

A therapeutic healthy diet along with prebiotics, probiotics, digestive enzymes (if needed), vitamin therapy, food combining, immune system support, and emotional support may help to promote a healthy intestinal environment and recovery. Some alternative medicine techniques (i.e. Reiki, therapeutic touch) may also help.

More research is needed to investigate possible links between food antigens and other autoimmune diseases. A therapeutic diet would be an attractive alternative to the use of medications (with possible side effects) and other possibly invasive procedures. Further research and increased awareness can help medical professionals and patients put the pieces of the puzzle together.

Probiotics promote the development of regulatory T cells in the immune system. This may help to decrease auto-immune related damage since regulatory T cells control immune responses and help to protect our tissues from immune damage [16].

The recommendations in the chapters listed below may be helpful for people suffering from an autoimmune disease.

- *Chapter 16 Diagnosis*

- *Chapter 19 Celiac Disease: Helping The Villi Heal. Even if you don't have intestinal damage, the recommendations in this chapter may help you to maintain a healthy intestinal environment.*

- *Chapter 20 What if the Gluten-Free Diet doesn't Work.*

- *Chapter 21 Could A Grain-Free, Specific Carbohydrate, Paleolithic, Or Elimination Diet be Helpful?*

- *Chapter 23 Two Alternative Approaches To Relieve Allergies*

Food For Thought: Would A Healthy Gluten-Free Diet During Childhood Along with Probiotics Decrease The High Prevalence Of Other Food Allergies?

Food Allergies Are More Common

Food allergies appeared to be fairly rare when I was in elementary school. However, the presence of various food allergies is very common now. What caused this change? Perhaps the symptoms were just under recognized and under diagnosed. This might explain some allergies that presented with vague symptoms, but what about the increased prevalence of anaphylactic allergies? I wonder whether the increased prevalence and density of gluten in the modern diet has increased gut permeability and increased the risk and prevalence of other food allergies. This theory seems reasonable when you examine the pathophysiology of celiac disease, dermatitis herpetiformis, and non-celiac gluten intolerance.

Theoretically, an overload of gluten in our society's modern diet, could overstimulate the intestinal gates to open, exaggerate the production of zonulin, further opening the gates and allow multiple food macromolecules to gain exposure to the immune system. In the end, the immune system would be just doing its job, reacting to large food molecules that shouldn't be there.

Altered intestinal flora, increased use of certain medications, lectins, and high intake of refined carbohydrates may also affect intestinal permeability.

The Hygiene Hypothesis

Some researchers have thought that the increased prevalence of food allergies could be related to the Hygiene Hypotheses. They have proposed that our current living environments in developed countries are too clean and this may be contributing to the rise in allergies. These researchers suspect that our immune systems have become misguided (now that there are less parasites and germs to react to) and are mistakenly reacting to food antigens and other environmental triggers (i.e. foods, pollen) that are generally considered harmless and not real invaders [13,14,18].

To support this, studies have shown that food allergies seem to be less prevalent in under-developed countries. Theoretically, the people living in these situations may be exposed to more germs and some researchers have thought that this may keep the immune system busy so it is less likely to react to harmless foods, pollens, etc [10-14,18].

Gluten And Altered Intestinal Flora Theory

Intestinal flora that are in a state of imbalance may also increase intestinal permeability. We naturally have helpful intestinal flora present in our intestine that have a role keeping the presence and growth of bad intestinal bacteria or fungi under control. Any environmental influence that alters our good flora versus bad flora balance, could put the gastrointestinal system at risk for infections and altered intestinal permeability. As discussed under pathophysiology, reactions to gluten can lead to increased intestinal permeability (a leaky gut). This can lead to immune responses to foods and increase our risk of getting a gluten intolerance or food allergies [1-4,9,17].

There are a number of other environmental influences that could threaten the integrity of the bowel, upset the healthy microbial balance and increase the risk of a leaky gut. For one, antibiotic use has increased significantly in developed countries and this may upset the natural balance of flora in our intestines. The high use of antibiotics medically and in the food supply of developed countries supports the hygiene theory (less germs to keep immune system busy), but it can also lead to a leaky gut and possibly increase the effect gluten can have on the permeability of the small intestine [10,12,14].

As well, people in developed countries generally ingest more refined carbohydrates and sugar (cane sugar and high fructose corn syrups) which may also promote the growth of pathogenic bacteria or fungi in the small bowel. This may potentiate the effect of antibiotics and gluten on the intestine's microbial balance further affecting bowel permeability. Certain medications (such as NSAIDS) are also used more in developed countries and this can cause intestinal inflammation and increase permeability. All of these factors combined with an overload of gluten (and lectins) may cause a leaky gut leading to an immune reaction with food molecules.

Some studies and researchers have suggested that individuals with low levels of intestinal probiotic microbes have a higher incidence of allergies [16,20,21,22]. Other studies have demonstrated allergic reactions may be alleviated with the use of probiotic supplements

[16,23,24,25]. These findings appear to strengthen the "Gluten And Altered Intestinal Flora Theory". However, more research is needed to investigate whether the research results are due to the leaky gut effect or whether the probiotics affect the function of the immune system (possibly affect the regulatory T cells that control reactions and protect our tissues) in a way that decreases allergic reactions [16].

Conclusions

I think that the higher risk for imbalanced intestinal flora and a leaky gut in developed countries may be primarily responsible for the increase in allergies. Researchers need to look closer at how gluten and other factors in our diet (i.e. medications, lectins, refined carbohydrates and sugar) may be contributing to a leaky gut and the increased prevalence of allergies. As well, more research is needed to further investigate how imbalanced intestinal flora can affect our immune system and how intestinal flora can affect allergic reactions.

A healthy gluten-free diet (with only healthy food choices and low or no added sugar) plus probiotics, from birth onward, could be the perfect primary prevention to the development of food allergies. For others, a paleolithic diet may be needed to decrease the risk of increased bowel permeability due to a lectin intolerance.

Less use of medications that can increase bowel permeability, healthier diets, and the removal of antibiotics from our food supply (with raising different animals) may also be helpful to maintain a healthy microbial balance in our intestine and lesson the risk of food allergies.

Note: Please read about concerns with probiotics Chapter 20, recommendation #3.

CHAPTER 26
Is A Gluten-Free Or A Grain-Free Diet Healthier For Dogs And Cats?

Is a gluten-free or a grain-free diet healthier for dogs and cats? It seems reasonable to suspect that these animals would be healthier if they ate a natural diet, close to what their canine ancestors ate. Dogs and cats have canine teeth (to assist with consuming meat), historically preferred meat and likely their ancestors ingested very little grains. Some digested grains might have been ingested from the stomachs and bowels of the herbivores they ate. These grains would have been altered and broken down by the digestion process in the herbivore and are therefore different than the undigested grains currently added to cat and dog food. The digested grains may have been tolerated better by these animals historically or perhaps they still did react to the digested grains to some degree.

In humans, we know that gluten containing grains can be difficult to digest and can cause increased bowel permeability possibly leading to an immune reaction. I suspect that dog and cat food with gluten containing grains could be difficult to digest as well. Overall, I believe dog and cat food with added grains is a change from the diet that their ancestors ate and could cause an immune reaction. Zookeepers have long recognized that each of their animals should eat a diet that is similar to their ancestor's diet. As well, the animals are healthier if they eat the same food that they ingested in their original habitat. A change in diet could make the zoo animals sick. Theoretically, the same ideology could be applicable to dogs and cats.

Gluten and/or dairy can cause a variety of multisystem related symptoms in humans. Hypothetically, an immune reaction could cause similar symptoms in dogs and cats. There are articles that identify that dogs can have food allergies and sensitivities. One discussed a family of Irish setters with gluten sensitive enteropathy (like celiac disease) and one found heightened immune activity in the intestinal mucosa of dogs with enteropathies [1-8].

If your dog or cat has health problems that you think may be related to gluten, talk to your veterinarian about trying a gluten-free (or grain-free) and dairy-free diet for a few months to see if an improvement occurs. The potential increased quality of life and savings in veterinarian bills might be well worth the change. I found that the grain-free diet was actually cheaper than the previous formula I was using for my dog.

Our dog, an Australian Sheppard (Aussie), consumes a grain-free diet. This change was inspired by our gluten-free lifestyle. Since we eat gluten-free, it seemed like a good idea to make our dog's diet grain-free to decrease our potential exposure to gluten. This change had a few pleasant side effects. Prior to eating grain-free, our Aussie had a little arthritis in her one hip, excess gas at times, occasional looser stools, and would vomit small amounts of whitish emesis or her dog food at least once a week. Once grain-free, her coat became shinier, and the gas, vomiting, loose stools and arthritis resolved. I was quite happy to see this improvement and to me it made sense. Dogs have canine teeth for a reason. After all, have you ever seen a dog hungrily chewing on a bushel of wheat (or any other grain)?

According to John B. Symes, D.V.M., wheat, dairy, and soy contain high levels of glutamic acid and aspartic acid. These two non-essential amino acids can over activate the receptors of the nerve cells and lead to excitotoxicity in animals. His research suggests that this can lead to nerve and brain impairments which are evident in many neurodegenerative diseases. His website can be found at dogtorj.com.

Theoretically, it may be possible for dogs and cats to have a lectin intolerance, an exomorphin (gluten and dairy) intolerance, food allergies, or a food intolerance (due to lack of digestive enzymes).

Please review all your dog and cat's health problems with a veterinarian before changing their diet. Your veterinarian can recommend a good gluten-free or grain-free brand of food available in your area. If a gluten-free or grain-free diet does not remove your dog or cat's symptoms, then ask your veterinarian about whether other food allergies may be the cause.

Other people's Experiences

Case 1: Three years ago, my 12 year old Australian Shepard''s health started deteriorating. He began choking on his water and began having accidents (urinating) in the house. He became very weak and had difficulty walking.

I read a blog post about gluten intolerance and I decided to put him on a gluten-free diet. Within a week, I started to notice improvements. By the time a month passed, he was significantly stronger and all of his symptoms were almost gone. Now 3 years have passed. He is so energetic and isn't having any more problems.

Case 2: I totally agree that a Dogs over all health is absolutely a reflection to what they ingest. In my own experience with my two large breeds, they both have an intolerance to turkey, which causes them to have very strong odored loose stool with mucus in it, to the point of not being able to wait to get outside to relieve themselves. Believe me when you have two dogs that way 100 pounds and over, you learn very quickly what not to feed them.

Our one dog I found through process of elimination and some research, has a corn allergy. Which unfortunately is found in so many dog foods because it is a cost effective filler. When we first got him he was about a year old, and was living at a shelter, where the choices of kibble were not high quality and/or not from the same supplier. They were just grateful for the foods they were able to receive. When I first got him, his ears were filled with a soft thick black substance, that had a terrible sour yeast like odor to it. His ears were inflamed and very sore. Eventually, once we were able to figure out his main intolerance was corn we were able to clear his ears up permanently.

I have noticed in other dogs as well, that a grain and corn free diet makes a tremendous difference in coat appearance, normal bowel health, less mucus in eyes, and ears that are free off inflammation and yeast. That is just to name a few benefits. Therefore it only makes sense that if so many systems in your dogs body are functioning healthier, than they are going to be a much happier and more energetic canine.

Case 3: *I have 3 dogs. I am gluten-free so I decided to put all of them on a grain-free diet. I took all grains out, not just gluten because dogs don't normally eat grains. This diet cleared up the one dog's ear infection, my other dogs skin condition and improved all of their energy levels.*

Case 4: *My cat was a very fussy eater, slept too much, frequently vomited (sometimes hairballs) and had a skin condition. My veterinarian put her on a grain-free diet and all the symptoms cleared up. What an easy solution and easier than dealing with ongoing vet bills.*

CHAPTER 27

Twelve Theories: Why Has The Prevalence Of Celiac Disease (And Possibly Non-Celiac Gluten intolerance) Increased?

According to a study, the prevalence of celiac disease (CD) has increased dramatically over the last 50 years. This study examined the sera (collected between 1948-1954) of 9,133 healthy individuals from an Warren Air Force Base, USA, and tested it for tissue transglutaminase antibodies and the samples with abnormal results were also tested for endomysial antibodies. Then 12,768 people, matched for age and gender, were selected from Minnesota, USA, to undergo the same testing. The results were surprising, the researchers found that prevalence of celiac disease has increased significantly in the last 50 years (4-4.5 fold) [2].

This study misses all the people with a non-celiac gluten intolerance (and some with DH) since it only tests the sera for celiac disease. I would suspect that the prevalence of dermatitis herpetiformis (DH) and non-celiac gluten intolerance has increased as well. A future study looking for the presence of IgA and IgG antigliadin antibodies, along with anti-transglutaminase 2, anti-transglutaminase 3, and anti-transglutaminase 6 antibodies in the sera 50 years ago versus now might help to reveal whether the prevalence of gluten intolerance (CD, DH, and non-celiac) has increased over the last 50 years.

What has caused an increase in the prevalence of CD? Many theories have emerged, but nothing has been exclusively proven. In the following pages are some examples of some some theories that may explain, combined or singularly, the increased prevalence. The development of celiac disease is thought to be related to genetic, environmental (i.e. gluten, stress, infection, etc), and immune system factors. The theories discussed in the following pages are associated with one or more of these contributing factors. Some of the theories are currently being considered by researchers, others are just hypothetical possibilities.

Theory 1 - High Density Of Gluten In Food Theory

The first theory makes the most sense to me. Bio-engineers have genetically modified wheat to produce a high gluten load since it is valued for baking. Therefore, our foods have a much higher gluten load now than they did 50 years ago. If gluten relaxes the gates in our small intestine and allows gluten to interact with the immune system, then you can imagine the effect that a higher dose of gluten would have on our bowel permeability and on our immune systems, especially if introduced from an early age in infant formulas and baby foods [23,46-51].

This gluten overload would likely stimulate a reaction in a higher percentage of people due to the "overdose effect" and may be responsible for the increased prevalence of CD. As well, bread is processed differently now than it was 50 years ago so this may also contribute in some way.

Theory 2 - The Hygiene Hypothesis

The second theory is the "Hygiene Hypothesis". This theory proposes that our current living environments are too clean and this may be contributing to the rise in allergies and autoimmune diseases. Some researchers suspect that our immune systems have become misguided (now that there are less parasites and germs to react to) and are now reacting to food antigens and other environmental triggers (i.e. foods, pollen) that are generally considered harmless and not real invaders [16,18,19].

One study highlighted how this theory may be involved in CD. Ten CD patients were intentionally infected with human hookworms to investigate the effect on the immune system and intestinal health. Once infected, the patient's were given bread containing gluten to eat. The patients with the worms had less inflammation with less damage to the intestine. Much more research is needed before this treatment is safely available [16]. As well, the study only mentioned that there was less inflammation and damage, the damage was still there which leads me to believe the associated risks with consuming gluten would still be high.

Another consideration: The immune system is stressed when you are fighting off a virus, parasite (i.e. worms), bacteria, or food antigens. Protective mechanisms in the immune system can dampen the response if the immune system is continuously reacting. Therefore, if infected with one of these invaders (i.e. parasite), the response to secondary invaders (i.e gluten consumption) may not be as strong. Perhaps the immune response is weaker due to protective mechanisms or immune stressors (i.e. the worms) and, as a result, the immune response is weaker (it is fighting two perceived invaders instead of one) [52]. With this in mind, I personally am not about to expose myself to germs and worms quite yet. More research will help to clarify whether the worms are triggering protective mechanisms, stressing the immune system and making its responses weaker or whether the worms are helping to keep the immune system focused on the role it was created to do.

Overall, it is an interesting theory and should be investigated further, but I do have some concerns with the belief that our immune system is abnormal and requires treatment (see Chapter 28).

Theory 3 - Imbalanced Intestinal Flora Theory

The altered intestinal flora theory looks at how the intestinal environment may be different now, than it was 50 years ago. We naturally have helpful intestinal flora present in our intestine that have a role keeping the presence and growth of bad intestinal bacteria or fungi under control. Any environmental influence that alters our good flora versus bad flora balance, could put the gastrointestinal system at risk for infections and altered intestinal permeability. This can significantly increase the risk for a gluten intolerance.

As discussed under pathophysiology, the ingestion of gluten can lead to increased intestinal permeability (a leaky gut), immune responses, inflammation and intestinal damage [15,24-27]. This can lead to microbial imbalances in the intestine that further increase the leaky gut effect. The overload of gluten in our society's current foods could potentiate this outcome and increase the prevalence of CD. Overall, this theory, along with theory 1 could significantly increase the risk of CD, DH, or a non-celiac gluten intolerance.

There are other factors that can cause intestinal microbial imbalances as well. Unfortunately, the helpful flora may be negatively affected by traces of antibiotics in our foods, in our water supply (potentially, if people are pouring left over antibiotics down the drain and contaminating the water supply), and in our medications since oral antibiotics have been used prolifically over the last 50 years. Could this increase in humanities exposure to antibiotics have altered our intestinal flora in a way that promotes digestive problems, promotes intestinal permeability, and increases the risk of an immune reaction to gluten [75]?

Other factors may potentiate this effect by promoting the growth of bad bacteria or fungus. For one, we eat a lot less fermented foods now than we did 50 years ago. These foods would have naturally introduced beneficial bacteria to our intestines [75]. Secondly, high levels of various types of sugar (corn sugar such as dextrose, glucose/fructose, high fructose corn syrup or cane sugar, etc) are prevalent in our modern diet and this likely promotes the growth of pathogenic bacteria or fungi, further hindering digestion and possibly increasing bowel permeability. Combined, all of these influencing factors may have negatively changed our intestinal flora over the last 50 years.

Imbalanced intestinal flora can lead to an overgrowth of Candida Albicans (yeast) in the bowel. One study suggested that the biochemical structure of yeast is similar to gluten. If molecular mimicry occurred (see next theory), then the immune system would react to the yeast, but would also cross react to gluten leading to a gluten intolerance. As previously discussed, the likelihood of our intestinal flora being imbalanced is high. Therefore, the risk for a yeast infection and a cross reaction with gluten may also be high. [75]. With this in mind, imbalanced intestinal flora along with yeast overgrowth could contribute to the increased prevalence of CD.

According to Dr. Alessio Fasano, an individual's intestinal microbes can change during a lifetime, so it reasonable to suspect that over a 50 year period (within a person's lifetime), the previously mentioned influencing factors could lead to a difference in the balance of our intestinal microbes. Dr. Fasano also mentioned that this change could influence the onset of celiac disease symptoms [15,27].

Can microbial imbalances affect genetic expression? This is an interesting thought. Microbes could influence the expression of genes that are expressed within each person. This can happen if the microbial imbalance causes a leaky gut and this allows an inter-action between the immune system and gluten. This reaction can promote uploading or a heightened expression of the susceptibility genes on the antigen presenting cells (part of the immune system). We know this occurs with CD and it could possibly occur with non-celiac gluten intolerance [72].

For example, imagine an asymptomatic (with no symptoms) individual who is genetically susceptible for CD, but doesn't have any diagnostic signs of CD. Now, imagine this person with silent celiac genes is ill with a bacterial infection and has to take a course of antibi-otics. Their intestinal flora would be altered, intestinal permeability may increase leading to a leaky gut and possibly an immune response. This, in theory, may trigger a higher percentage of susceptibility genes to be expressed in the population that carry these genes [1,15,72].

In summary, the variety of factors, mentioned previously, could have negatively impacted our beneficial flora over the last 50 years and this could have increased the prevalence of CD.

Are probiotics a possible solution? Probiotics are promoted as a way to increase intestinal health for many with various gastrointestinal conditions. Could the use of probiotics and prebiotics help decrease the risk of developing CD, DH, or a non-celiac gluten intolerance [15,27,75]? As well, could less antibiotics, less sugar, and an increased consumption of fermented foods help preserve the natural balance in our intestinal flora and ultimately keep the genetic expression of the genes involved in CD, DH, or non-celiac gluten intolerance silent? This is an interesting thought. However, undigested gluten's could still affect the permeability of the bowel in the absence of the above factors so gluten consumption may still pose a risk.

Overall, this is an interesting theory with lots of promise, I'm excited to see more research in this area.

Theory 4 - The Molecular Mimicry Theory

A fourth theory involves molecular mimicry. For this theory to be successful, the person needs to be exposed to a microbial or viral infection and, given the right conditions immunologically, the immune system reacts to the infection, but it also cross reacts with self antigens (cells of your body) or food molecules that have some similar amino acid sequences. For an autoimmune reaction to be successful, the individual's major histocompatibility complex (part of the immune system) must have the ability to present a self antigen peptide (part of your body) and the B (antibodies) and T cells must have receptors that recognize self antigens (part of your body) [22].

Usually, our immune system has built in safeguards to help prevent this type of cross reaction. Some researchers believe that these safeguards can fail and this may lead to immune reactions to something physiological (self antigen with an autoimmune disease) or environmental (allergy to food, pollen, etc) that we shouldn't be reacting to [22].

With CD, we know that the immune system reacts to gluten and cross reacts with self antigens (parts of our bowel and other areas in our body). Possibly, the reaction to gluten was triggered by an earlier reaction to a virus or some other perceived invader. This could cause an immune related cross reaction with gluten if the amino acid sequences were similar between gluten and the virus. Then, the reaction to gluten and/or the virus (or other invader) could cause a cross reaction (autoimmune) with self antigens (parts of the body) [21,25,73].

Could a new type of virus or bacterial be causing a cross reaction and be the underlying culprit behind the increased prevalence of celiac disease? Paul W. Ewald, author of

"Plague Time, The New Germ Theory Of Disease" would likely agree that germs might be involved. In his book, he describes how germs have triggered other diseases and cancers. Could a new type or increased prevalence of a germ (i.e. Klebsiella present in babies with colic) be increasing the prevalence of Celiac Disease [12,13] and possibly non-celiac gluten intolerance through molecular mimicry? In one study, researchers noticed that babies with colic also had the bacterium Klebsiella with gut inflammation evident. The researchers were suspecting that the bacteria caused the gut inflammation and this may increase the babies infected to gastrointestinal conditions later in life, such as celiac disease or irritable bowel [12].

As well, the anti-tissue transglutaminase antibody in CD tends to react to rotavirus leading researchers to wonder whether rotovirus may have caused a cross reaction causing an immune response to gluten [20].

Mycotoxins could be involved as well. Could a mycotoxin (a fungal metabolite) in our foods contribute to the increased prevalence of celiac disease? There are several mycotoxins that could alter intestinal homeostasis, this could lead to increased gut permeability and an immune reaction to gluten. Another possibility, the ingestion of a mycotoxin could ignite a reaction between the immune system and gluten and this could progress to an auto-immune reaction [9].

Contrary to the previous thoughts, could an underlying gluten intolerance have increased the risk for getting Klebsiella or another viral or bacterial infection? Once infected, the antibodies reacting to gluten might cross react against the bacteria or virus responsible for the infection. This may give the illusion that a virus or bacteria may be responsible for triggering the onset of CD. Overall, this raises a question, which came first, the gluten intolerance or the infection? Future research will hopefully clarify this mystery.

Theory 5 - The Genetic Theory

Could there be genetic reasons for the increased prevalence? Perhaps, the percentage of people with celiac genes is greater now than 50 years ago.

Additionally, as discussed under "The Imbalanced Intestinal Flora Theory" genetic expression can be influenced by environmental factors. Perhaps, the high gluten load in our modern day foods, increased use of antibiotics, or other factors are increasing intestinal permeability, causing an immune reaction, and activating celiac susceptibility genes [72]. This may lead to an increased prevalence of celiac disease.

Theory 6 - The Zonulin Theory

A sixth theory, perhaps something else, in addition to gluten, is stimulating the overproduction of zonulin. As discussed previously, an increased expression of zonulin is a problem because this human protein stimulates the tight intercellular junctions in the small intestine to open allowing the undigested gluten to enter and interact with the immune system. The immune system can then react to this invader and mount an attack [8,14]. Therefore, anything affecting zonulin production (i.e. medications, pesticides, food additives, something else in grain such as lectins), could, in theory, increase the risk of CD, DH, or a non-celiac gluten intolerance.

Just a thought: zonulin is the precursor to Haptoglobin 2 that is present in 80% of humans. Haptoglobin binds to hemoglobin in our blood and it is associated with inflammatory diseases, such as atherosclerosis, autoimmune diseases, or infections. Humans have evolved to have Haptoglobin 2 and we are unique. Apes, chimpanzees, and monkeys do not have Haptoglobin 2 or autoimmune diseases (very rarely) [3,15]. They typically don't eat grains either so perhaps that is why they haven't evolved to have Haptoglobin 2 or a prevalence of autoimmune diseases. Interesting food for thought.

Theory 7 - The Leaky Gut Theory

Perhaps, something else, in addition to gluten and intestinal microbial imbalances, is increasing the permeability of the bowel. This could include increased use of medications (i.e. NSAIDS), undetected parasites, gastrointestinal infections, high levels of caffeine intake, high intake of refined carbohydrates or the high level of stress that is common in our modern society [21,24,25,28]. Collectively or in isolation, perhaps these factors contribute to increased intestinal permeability, eventually leading to celiac disease or a gluten intolerance.

As well, our grains have been genetically modified over the last 50 years to include many different varieties. Perhaps something else (other than gluten) in these grains is contributing to a leaky gut effect and ultimately an increased prevalence of celiac disease.

Theory 8 - Wheat Germ Agglutinin (Lectin) Theory

Lectins are glycoproteins that are present in grains (even gluten-free grains) and some other foods such as legumes, seeds, nightshades (i.e. potatoes, tomatoes, etc) and dairy. Like gluten, lectins are difficult to digest and undigested lectins in the gut could lead to increased bowel permeability (leaky gut) [6,29,32,34,53,55,57,61,62,65,77].

In two studies, IgA and IgG antibodies against wheat germ agglutinin (WGA) were elevated in people with celiac disease. These particular antibodies were only directed against WGA, not gluten indicating that the immune system views it as a separate antigen (invader) [4,5].

Theoretically, lectins may increase the risk for a gluten intolerance due to the effects on bowel permeability. As mentioned under theory 1, grains have been genetically modified to contain more proteins (such as gluten and possibly lectins). Unfortunately, this may increase the density of lectins in our current foods. Lectins may increase the risk of celiac disease by altering the intestinal mucosal membrane (brush border) ultimately affecting the villi and crypts. This adverse effect is due to decreased production of intestinal epithelial cells along with the lectin induced damage to the small intestine [6,29,32,34,53,55,57,61,62,65,77].

Does this sound familiar? It certainly seems to parallel the damage that gluten can cause in the bowel. Increased prevalence of lectins in our foods could contribute to the increased prevalence of celiac disease since it may increase bowel permeability increasing the risk of an immune reaction to both ingested gluten and lectins [4,5,36].

Note: Lectins are a problem if increased bowel permeability occurs and the lectins encounter the immune system or the circulation. Due to gluten and lectin's combined effect on bowel permeability, this seems likely.

Theory 9 - The Vitamin D Deficiency Theory

Vitamin D deficiency has been on the rise and is associated with a number of autoimmune diseases. Perhaps, people spend more time inside and use more sunscreen when they are outdoors than they did 50 years ago. Combined, this would decrease our skin's production of vitamin D. This, theoretically, might somehow contribute to the increased prevalence of celiac disease.

I personally don't think our lifestyle is solely responsible for the low vitamin D. It is reasonable to suspect that many with autoimmune diseases may not be absorbing vitamin D very well from their foods, due to patchy intestinal damage associated with celiac disease or they may have flattened villi due to other food allergies. Another thought, could the use of medications to treat some autoimmune diseases decrease the absorption of vitamin D as well?

Theory 10 - The Pesticide, Herbicide And Gut Theory

Could the modern day pesticides and herbicides, used on grain crops, be increasing bowel permeability and stimulating the overproduction of zonulin? This would open the intestinal gates, allowing gluten to interact with the immune system.

I think future studies should investigate this possibility. Medications can have side effects and some can affect bowel permeability, so why couldn't pesticides and herbicides have similar effects?

Theory 11 - The Early Exposure To Gluten Theory

Does early exposure to gluten in infancy increase the risk of developing CD? In an article, by Dr. Fasano, he mentioned a study that suggests delaying gluten ingestion until after the first year of life to help decrease the risk. A later introduction appears to reduce the risk of developing celiac disease. The high density of gluten in our foods (some infant formulas and baby foods) may be overwhelming and very difficult for an infant's small intestinal enzymes to digest. This, in theory, could lead to increased bowel permeability and an immune response, ultimately ending with a celiac diagnosis, dermatitis herpetiformis [15], or a non-celiac gluten intolerance.

The preliminary results of this study (at University Of Maryland) didn't show whether CD might develop later in the infants who had delayed gluten introduction. Once gluten has been introduced for many years, perhaps the outcome wouldn't be any different, just delayed until later in life [15]. In other words, delaying the gluten could just delay the inevitable. Only time and more research (including the final results of this long-term study) will reveal the true outcome.

In another study, breast feeding during the introduction of gluten combined with increasing the length of breastfeeding appeared to reduce the risk of developing celiac disease. This study doesn't clarify whether this just delays the risk or whether it offers long-term protection. More studies are needed [17].

Theory 12 - The Labor And Gut Theory

In one study, researchers looked at data collected from 1,950 children affected by colitis, celiac disease, and other bowel diseases. The rate of cesarean and vaginal birth was evaluated and compared to children who didn't suffer from any bowel diseases. They found that children appeared to have a much higher risk of developing celiac disease when they were born through a C-section [10]. This risk may be due to decreased exposure to microorganisms in the vaginal tract. Perhaps, the vaginal canal provides microorganisms that colonize babies gastrointestinal tracts during a vaginal delivery and this helps to provide a balanced healthy gastrointestinal immune system. According to this "hygiene hypothesis" type theory, a Cesarian birth might deny exposure to these helpful microorganisms. Could an increase in cesarean sections increase the prevalence of celiac disease?

I'm not completely convinced. Perhaps this finding is due to the fact that women with undiagnosed celiac disease have a higher risk of complications with pregnancies and labor. Could the high rate of cesarean births be due to the mothers (possibly undiagnosed Celiacs) having complications and, therefore, requiring a C-section to safely deliver their babies? Since most Celiacs remain undiagnosed, this seems like a real possibility. However, no conclusions can be made at this point. More research is needed to help clarify how cesarean sections may increase the risk.

More Research Needed

To summarize, all 12 theories may contribute (either singularly, but more likely combined) to the increased prevalence of CD. I believe that an overload of gluten and lectins in our modern foods, imbalanced intestinal flora, over stimulation of zonulin, and increased gut permeability are the leading causes of CD, DH, and non-celiac gluten intolerance. Certainly, molecular mimicry could contribute as well. Research is needed to investigate each possibility and, hopefully, this will shed more light onto the risks associated with each contributing factor and may lead to some preventative guidelines.

Chapter 28

More Thoughts About Gluten Intolerance: Is Our Immune System Really Abnormal?

For years, I learned that celiac disease is an abnormal autoimmune reaction to gluten. I was led to believe that my body had somehow failed me and my immune system was dysfunctional. My natural inclination to question everything has led me to a different view.

Thousands of years ago, we did not eat grains. We ate foods that were naturally available to us such as fruits, vegetables, sea vegetables, nuts, seeds, meat, fish, and seafood [3-6]. Our ancestors didn't have to grind these foods into a flour or process these foods in any way to digest them. It was a natural process and these foods were easily digested. Current research validates how healthy these foods are for us.

Then humans started using grains as a source of food. This new food source seemed very appealing to alleviate famine and to allow the nomadic nature of humans to change to a more stationary lifestyle [3-7]. Towns were created and this agricultural way of life seemed less stressful. You can see how the benefits associated with the addition of grains seemed appealing.

However, with all change comes a period of adaptation. In our evolutionary history (prior to grains), we had consumed foods that were easy to digest. Now, humans were asking their bodies to adapt to a new food and to digest something that the intestine hadn't been exposed to before [1,2]. This was a huge request because our bodies had evolved for millions of years to have the gastric, intestinal brush border and pancreatic enzymes necessary to digest fruits, vegetables, sea vegetables, nuts, seeds, meat, fish, and seafood, not grass. As a result, this unrealistic expectation led to a cascade of immune reactions and gluten intolerance symptoms.

When I reviewed the dietary history of humanity, it became fairly obvious to me that our immune systems may not be abnormal at all. We may just be reacting to foods we were never genetically designed to eat. Our immune systems may be reacting normally to an invader that was never meant to be ingested. I understand that our immune system does cross react which is evident with the production of auto-antibodies. However, this cross reaction wouldn't have occurred if humanity hadn't introduced gluten into our diet.

Others who don't appear to have gluten intolerance may have evolved and adapted over the last 10,000 years so that they can tolerate gluten with a lower risk of a leaky gut and a reaction. However, even this is questionable since many people with an undiagnosed gluten intolerance have very little or no symptoms, yet their risk for complications still exists. Perhaps these other, apparently, asymptomatic people do have symptoms of gluten intolerance that manifests with a vague presentation. Also, as discussed in the patho-physiology chapter, some studies suggest that humans do not have all of the enzymes required to digest gluten and as a result a leaky gut and an innate immune reaction can occur. Only future research into the full spectrum of gluten intolerance will uncover to what extend everyone reacts.

For now, I believe that if grains containing gluten didn't exist, then celiac disease, dermatitis herpetiformis and non-celiac gluten intolerance wouldn't exist. In summary, my immune system would likely be considered normal if humans hadn't introduced grains over 10,000 years ago. I believe my immune system reacts to gluten because it is a foreign antigen/toxin that I am not designed to eat. Yes, there is an autoimmune component with anti-endomysial antibodies and anti-tissue transglutaminase antibodies flagging self antigens (i.e. tissue and an enzyme in my bowel) for destruction, but this cross-reaction wouldn't have occurred if gluten was never introduced onto my dinner plate.

CHAPTER 29
About The Author: My Struggle With Undiagnosed Celiac Disease

As a toddler, I was frequently in and out of our local hospital with pneumonia and tonsillitis. Infections and antibiotics were a way of life for me.

As time passed, I developed into a tall, but thin child. My low weight didn't make sense because I ate copious amounts of food. During family gatherings, my relatives would frequently comment about my appetite and my aunts marveled at my slim size. Everyone assumed that my slim build was due to my active lifestyle, growth spurts, and perhaps a high metabolism. No one suspected that it was due to a malabsorption issue, likely because I didn't have any gastrointestinal symptoms and I was tall. We now know that many people with celiac disease do not have gastrointestinal symptoms and many are tall, despite the malabsorption problems. Not everyone with celiac disease has short stature.

In addition to the low weight, I would occasionally get pressure and burning in my chest that was diagnosed as growing pains. Now, I know that this was likely indigestion, a symptom of CD. I also remember having problems with forgetfulness and sometimes it was difficult to think (I call this foggy brain).

With puberty, came anemia, canker sores, restless legs, leg cramps, brittle nails, low blood pressure, more foggy headed days, ovarian cysts, indigestion and I frequently felt an unusual heavy feeling in my abdomen after eating bread or pasta. The symptoms would exacerbate with any physiological or psychological stress. My mother experienced some of the same symptoms for years so I didn't think it was that unusual. Our doctor prescribed iron pills for our anemia with no further investigations. I now have labeled this, "The Band Aide Treatment", since it just addresses the symptoms without diagnosing the cause.

As more time passed, I went to university, graduated with honors (a real struggle on my foggy head days), and naturally started to avoid some of the foods (bread, pasta) that sat heavy in my stomach and depleted my energy. This helped me to feel better and I didn't question it further since I assumed that bread and pasta were very filling foods that made most people feel full and tired.

I married and shortly after I became pregnant with our first child. I had anemia and palpitations during the pregnancy. My daughter was born 3 weeks early due to my water breaking and, luckily, she appeared to be a healthy baby with no apparent health problems. My health problems continued. Three weeks postpartum, I started having loose stools multiple times a day and this lasted a few weeks. All tests were negative (a celiac screen was not included).

With my second pregnancy, I was hospitalized and put on bed rest, due to premature interuterine contractions and pain. I also had anemia with this pregnancy and delivered 2 weeks early. My second baby appeared to be healthy. My ill health continued, three weeks postpartum, the loose stools started again and I lost all my pregnancy weight. I was checked for parasites, had a colonoscopy, and investigations stopped there since the loose stools stopped after a few weeks. An upper endoscopy would have diagnosed celiac disease but it was not offered, instead the doctor diagnosed me with hormonal irritable bowel syndrome.

With my third pregnancy, I had inter-uterine fetal growth restriction and had to decrease my activity. I remember adding lots of pasta and bread into my diet to help increase weight (exactly the opposite of what I needed since the pasta and bread had a high gluten content). My third child was born 1 and 1/2 weeks early at 6 pounds, 6 ounces. Three weeks postpartum, the loose stools returned. Again, I was checked for parasites and had a colonoscopy. Since my results were negative, I was told that I conclusively had irritable bowel syndrome. With ongoing intermittent diarrhea, I was loosing nutrients. It was difficult to keep up my breast milk supply, I had to stop breast feeding my third child after six weeks due to poor quality and production. Due to diarrhea and malabsorption, I likely had multiple nutrient deficiencies

This time, my symptoms didn't subside, only more were added. Muscle weakness, arthritis symptoms, weight loss, various nervous system symptoms, frequent lung infections, fatigue and skin rashes were more warning signs that I desperately needed help. During this time, I also had 3 little girls, ages 10 months, 2 years, and 4 years. It was a real struggle trying to be an energetic creative mother for my children. I remember my mom flew out to visit and she was in tears when she saw me. She said that I looked like I had terminal cancer. In many ways, she was right, my body was deteriorating, but not from cancer. Gluten toxicity was affecting every part of my body leading to inflammation and damage. During this period, I lost quality time with my family, my friends, and time at my work.

After a long undiagnosed journey with many symptoms, I managed to finally link my ill health to celiac disease. A gastroenterologist confirmed a celiac diagnosis and I have been living gluten-free for the last 6 years. Once diagnosed, I had my siblings, parents, and children screened. My mother and daughter also had positive results. My mother had canker sores, restless legs, leg cramps, brittle nails, and anemia. My daughter only presented with occasional stomach aches and pale skin. Finally, we were all able to heal.

My Mission To Increase Awareness

Once I was diagnosed, I learned that only 3-5% of people with CD are diagnosed. This, along with my personal experience, inspired me to fulfill a mission to do my part to increase awareness and diagnosis. Working with a variety of patients at the hospital has allowed me to identify potential Celiacs in the hospital population. Many undiagnosed Celiacs have frequent doctors visits and are admitted to the hospital with a variety of diagnoses. I have requested Celiac screening for many patients.

Once my youngest entered grade 1, I knew I could begin writing a blog about celiac disease and gluten intolerance. In addition to my blog, I also began increasing awareness as Celiac Nurse on Facebook, and CeliacNurse1 on Twitter.

As time passed, I began to seek other ways to use my 21 years of nursing (including 5 years of gastroenterology) and 6 years of living successfully with celiac disease to help others. Currently, I am a Celiac Nurse and Gluten Intolerance Consultant at Stuart Healthcare Solutions (my company) in British Columbia, Canada. With this position, I am able to provide support services to assist with diagnosis, education, health assessments, a new lifestyle and problem solving when complication arise. This professional focus has become my passion. Helping others navigate the maze associated with gluten toxicity has become a way of life.

I am an optimist and I believe that change is possible. Imagine, a future with everyone diagnosed, doctors and nurses who are knowledgeable about the full spectrum of gluten intolerance, and all the restaurants, companies, and grocery stores competently selling GF products and meals. This is what I visualize as I start each day. A better future for myself, my children, my future grandchildren, and others who are adversely affected by this little protein called gluten.

> Shelly Stuart, R.N., B.Sc.N.
>
> Celiac Nurse And Gluten Intolerance Consultant
>
> Stuart Healthcare Solutions, BC, Canada

Blogs: www.celiacnurse.com and www.paleolithicrn.blogspot.com

Twitter: "CeliacNurse1", "PaleolithicRN", and "GlutenToxicity"

Facebook: "Celiac Nurse" and an author page, "Gluten Toxicity"

Member of the Canadian Celiac Association

Member of Sigma Theta Tau International

CHAPTER 30
Support For A New Lifestyle

I would like to dedicate this chapter to all of the heroic souls who are advocating for those who are suffering from gluten intolerance. Collectively, the people in the following pages work tirelessly to promote awareness, diagnosis, and provide tips and recipes to help increase success with the GF lifestyle. Thank you everyone for all of your generous contributions. Together, we can increase the rate of diagnoses and improve people's quality of life.

Support Groups

Canadian Celiac Association [www.celiac.ca]

Living Gluten-Free Community in Vancouver [lgfc.ca/]

Gluten Intolerance Group Of North America (GIG) [www.gluten.net]

National Foundation For Celiac Awareness US [www.celiaccentral.org]

American Celiac Disease Alliance US [www.americanceliac.org]

Celiac Kids [www.celiackids.org]

Celiac Sprue Association US [www.csaceliacs.org]

National Foundation for Celiac Awareness US [www.celiaccentral.org]

Celiac Disease Foundation US [www.celiac.org]

Raising Our Celiac Kids (ROCK) [www.celiackids.com]

Australia [www.coeliacsociety.com.au]

Ireland [www.coeliac.ie]

UK [www.coeliac.co.uk]

Do you live near or travel to New York City in the USA? There is a large group called "The New York City Celiac Disease Meet-up Group". Erin Smith (the lead organizer) asked if I could include this social support group in my book. (This group is not aligned with any national organization, it is an independent group). Website: www.meetup.com/celiac. I haven't personally attended, but if I'm in NY sometime I'll give it a try.

There may be other support groups available in your area.

Celiac Disease Centers (US)

1. Celiac Disease Center at Columbia University [www.celiacdiseasecenter.org]

    Dr. Peter Green works at this center.

2. The University of Chicago Celiac Disease Center [www.celiacdisease.net]

3. The University of Maryland Center for Celiac Research [www.celiaccenter.org]

    Dr. Alessio Fasano works at this center.

4. WM K. Warren Medical Research Center For Celiac Disease

    [www.celiaccenter.ucsd.edu]

5. The Beth Israel Deaconess Medical Center:

    www.bidmc.org/CentersandDepartments/Departments/DigestiveDiseaseCenter/Ce
    liacCenter.aspx

6. Stanford Hospital Celiac Sprue Clinic:

    www.stanfordhospital.org/clinicsmedServices/clinics/gastroenterology/celiacSprue.
    html

These clinics are all located in the USA. Ask your doctor and your local celiac association for celiac disease centers located in your area.

Gluten Intolerance Group (GIG) Of North America

Information and support can be found at www.gluten.net for people affected by a gluten intolerance. Their website has many resources including:

Educational Materials: www.gluten.net/publications.php

Gluten-Free Restaurants: www.glutenfreerestaurants.org/find.php

GF Magazines

Living Without Magazine: www.livingwithout.com

Gluten-Free Living Magazine: www.Gfliving.com

Delight Gluten-Free Magazine: www.delightgfmagazine.com

Easy Eats www.glutenfreemag.com

Online GF Forums/Social Networks

www.celiac.com/gluten-free

www.glutenfreefaces.com

www.grandmasgfbakingncooking.ning.com/forum

www.forums.glutenfree.com

www.the-gluten-free-chef.com/gluten-free-forum.html

www.forums.delphiforums.com/celiac

Travel And Dining

www.triumphdining.com

www.theceliacscene.com

www.glutenfreetravelsite.com

www.glutenfreeonthego.com

www.glutenfreerestaurants.org

www.glutenfreemaps.com

www.glutenfreepassport.com

www.celiachandbook.com

www.glutenfreeregistry.com

www.bobandruths.com

www.wetravelglutenfree.com

www.celiacsite.com (Under"Travel" has cruise info, travel tips, etc)

www.celiactravel.com (GF restaurant cards and much more)

www.glutenfreerestaurants.org/find.php

Food Allergy Magazines

Allergic Living Magazine: www.allergicliving.com

Living Without Magazine: www.livingwithout.com

Gluten-Free Doctors With Blogs

These doctors share many helpful tips on their blogs. I believe that their efforts have significantly improved the health of people, globally, who have been suffering from undiagnosed celiac disease, dermatitis herpetiformis, and non-celiac gluten intolerance. They are truly heroes and heroines in this race to end the suffering and to save lives.

1. Dr. Stephen Wangen is a licensed and board certified physician located in Seattle, Washington State, USA. Dr. Wangen founded the Irritable Bowel Syndrome Treatment Center and the Center For Food Allergies. He is also the research director of the Innate Health Foundation.

   Books: Author of "The Irritable Bowel Syndrome Solution" and "Healthier without Wheat, A New Understanding of Wheat Allergies, Celiac Disease, and Non-Celiac Gluten Intolerance".

   Blog: www.ibstreatmentcenter.blogspot.com
   Website: www.ibstreatmentcenter.com
   Website: www.HealthierWithoutWheat.com
   Website: www.centerforfoodallergies.com
   Website: www.innatehealthfoundation.org

   Phone: 1-206-264-1111 or 1-888-546-6283

2. Dr. Rodney Ford (pediatrician, gastroenterologist, allergist) in Christchurch, New Zealand. He has an e-clinic for result interpretation and diagnostic help.

   Books: He is the author of "The Gluten Syndrome" and many other books that can be found at his website.
   Website: www.drrodneyford.com
   Blog: www.celiac.com/blogs/4/Dr-Rodney-Fords-Blog.html
   Blog: www.gluten-freeplanet.blogspot.com

3. Dr. Scot Micheal Lewey (Gastroenterologist) in Colorado Springs, Colorado State, US.

   Website: www.gacsonline.com/physicians-nps/dr-lewey

   Dr. Lewey's Blog: www.thefooddoc.com/blogpage.html

4. Drs. Vikki and Richard Petersen. D.C., C.C.N.

216

Founders of HealthNOW Medical Center in Sunnyvale, California

Phone: 1-408-733-0400

Book: Authors of "The Gluten Effect"
Website: www.healthnowmedical.com
Blog: www.glutendoctors.blogspot.com
Youtube: www.youtube.com/healthnowmedical

5. Dr. Jean Layton, ND, in Bellingham, Washington State, US.
   Website: www.laytonhealthclinic.com/pages/jean.html
   Blog: www.gfdoctorrecipes.com

GF Bloggers

These heroic people are tirelessly trying to increase awareness. They share stories of inspiration, tips, product reviews, and recipes from their personal lives. I have met many of these lovely bloggers on Facebook and Twitter.

GF Bloggers In BC, Canada (where I live)

www.celiacnurse.com (my blog)

www.glutenfreenotebook.com

www.glutenfree-vancouver.blogspot.com

www.glutenfreeguineapig72.blogspot.com

Global GF Bloggers

www.glutenfreediet.ca/blog

www.gfgoodness.com

www.elanaspantry.com

www.glutenfreeworks.com

www.gfreelife.com

www.blog.guaranteedgf.com

www.thesavvyceliac.com

www.gluten-freeliving.blogspot.com

www.celiac.com (has a gluten-free mall and many bloggers on one site)

www.glutenfreefitness.com

www.glutenfreegirl.blogspot.com

www.glutenfreegoddess.blogspot.com (vegan, gluten-free, dairy-free)

www.dishtoweldiaries.com

www.wellbladder.com

www.glutenfreehomemaker.com

www.glutenfreehelp.info

www.glutenfreern.com

www.glutenfreemike.com

www.celiacbites.com

www.surefoodsliving.com

www.theceliacmaniac.com

www.glutenfreetriathlete.com/blog

www.celiacsite.com

www.glutenfreeda.blogspot.com (also www.glutenfreeda.com)

www.adventuresofaglutenfreemom.com

www.glutenfreefun.blogspot.com

www.mondaysceliac.com

www.celiacsite.com

www.noglutennoproblem.blogspot.com

www.simplysugarandglutenfree.com

www.glutenfreeday.com

www.theglutenfile.com

www.grandmasgfbakingncooking.ning.com

www.glutenfreemom.typepad.com

www.glutenfreeonashoestring.com

www.glutenfreeislife.com

www.glutenfreephilly.blogspot.com

www.glutenfreeoptimist.blogspot.com

www.atxglutenfree.wordpress.com

www.bonbongazette.com

www.befreeforme.com/blog

www.celiacstips.com

www.go-with-your-gut.com/blog/

www.glutenfreeda.blogspot.com

www.celiacadvocate.com

www.celiacchicks.com

www.beyondricecakes.com

www.glutenfreejenna.com

www.sacgfgirl.blogspot.com

www.celiaceats.blogspot.com

www.celiacfacts.wordpress.com

www.creativecookinggf.wordpress.com

www.glutenfreebetsy.com

www.glutenfreeeasily.com

www.gfingf.blogspot.com

www.glutenfree-journey.blogspot.com

www.glutenfreeraleigh.blogspot.com

www.glutenwatchers.com

www.freerangecookies.com

www.goodwithoutgluten.blogspot.com

www.glutenwatchers.com

www.heythattastesgood.com

www.blog.kitchentherapy.us

www.tatefamilyblog.com

www.thewholegang.org

www.celiacfacts.wordpress.com

www.stephsceliacdisease.blogspot.com

www.gflinks.com

www.celiackids.com

www.glutenfreebloggers.com (community of bloggers)

www.glutenfreemommy.com

www.gluten-free-around-the-world.com/gluten-free-blog.html

www.glutenfreeforgood.com

www.gingerlemongirl.blogspot.com

www.glutenfree.wordpress.com

www.glutenfreejungle.com

www.glutenfreehub.com

www.simplysugarandglutenfree.com

www.glutenfreehippie.com

www.gluten-free-blog.com

www.legardenbakery.com/blog

www.nourishingmeals.com

www.glutenfreelifestylecoach.com/category/blog/

www.isabelskitchencorner.wordpress.com

www.the-gluten-free-chef.com/gluten-free-blog.html

www.megsfoodreality.blogspot.com

www.thehealthyapple.com

www.glutenfreeeasily.com

www.glutenfreeislife.com

www.customchoicecereal.com/blog

www.theglutenfreespouse.blogspot.com

www.glutenfibrofree.com

www.mydarlinglemonthyme.blogspot.com

www.glutenfreeli.com

www.glutenfreebirmingham.com

www.celtic-celiac.blogspot.com

www.free-from.com/blog

www.celiacinthecity.wordpress.com

www.whatthefood.blogspot.com

www.glutenfreeproductreviews.blogspot.com

www.glutenfreetwentysomething.com

www.abakinglife.blogspot.com

www.gfsocialmedia.blogspot.com

www.glutenfreeguerrillas.healthunlocked.com

www.glutenfreeguerrillas.tumblr.com

www.glutenfreerecipebox.com

This list of bloggers is provided as a helpful resource, not an endorsement. I haven't been able to review all of the content of each blog due to continual new content and revisions of content. This is just a helpful list. You can use this book as a guide when you are reviewing content on various blogs.

Support For GF Bloggers

www.glutenfreebloggers.com

www.problogger.net

GF Radio

www.glutenfreeonlineradio.com

Gluten-Free TV

Gfree TV: www.gfree.tv

Gluten Free Life TV: www.glutenfreelife.tv

Celiac Chicks TV: www.celiacchicks.com/2010/06/glutenfree-tv.html

Paleolithic Blogs

PaleolithicRN blog at www.paleolithicrn.blogspot.com. Also on Twitter as "PaleolithicRN" (my blog and Twitter account)

Mark's Daily Apple blog at www.marksdailyapple.com

The Paleo Diet blog at www.thepaleodiet.blogspot.com

Robb Wolf's blog at www.robbwolf.com/blog/

Further Reading

GF Cook Books

Silvana Nardone (Foreword by Rachael Ray). **Cooking for Isaiah: Gluten-Free & Dairy-Free Recipes for Easy Delicious Meals**. Readers Digest, August 26, 2010.

Elana Amsterdam. **The Gluten-Free Almond Flour Cookbook**. Celestial Arts; 1 Original edition, July 28, 2009.

Elana Amsterdam. **Gluten Free Cupcakes: 50 Irresistible Recipes Made With Almond And Coconut Flour.** Celestial Arts, April 26, 2011.

Richard J. Coppedge JR., C.M.B. **Gluten-Free Baking With The Culinary Institute Of America.** The Culinary Institute Of America, 2008.

Shauna James Ahern and Daniel Ahern. **Gluten Free Girl And The Chef.** Wiley, Aug 30 2010.

Bette Hagman. **Cooks Fast And Healthy.** Henry Holt And Company LLC. 2000.

Bette Hagman, **The Gluten free Gourmet.** Henry Holt And Company LLC, 2000.

Donna Washburn And Heather Butt. **125 Gluten-Free Recipes.** Robert Rose 2003

Lisa A. Lundy. **The Super Allergy Girl Gluten-Free, Casein- Free, Nut-Free Allergy And Celiac Cook Book.** The Rooster Crows, 2007. I haven't read this book yet, it looks like a good resource for recipes

Nicola Graimes. **The Gluten, Wheat, And Dairy Free Cookbook.** Parragon Publishing, 2004. I haven't read this book yet, but it looks great.

Shirley Plant. **Finally Food I Can Eat.** (has recipes free of wheat, yeast, eggs, dairy, gluten, soy, corn, nuts, and sugar). General Store Publishing House. November 25, 2007. I haven't read this book yet, but it looks like it would be very helpful for people with allergies.

Celiac Disease Books

Peter HR Green And Rory Jones. **Celiac Disease A Hidden Epidemic.** Harper Collins, 2006. (a newer Edition is out)

Cleo Libonati. **Recognizing Celiac Disease.** Gluten Free Works Publishing, 2007.

Gluten Intolerance Books

James Braly, MD, and Ron Hoggan, MA. **Dangerous Grains.** Penguin Group, Inc., 2002.

Dr. Stephen Wangen. **Healthier Without Wheat.** Innate Health Publishing, 2009.

Dr. Rodney Ford. **The Gluten Syndrome.** RRS Global Ltd, 2008.

Shari Lieberman, PhD, CNS, FACN. **The Gluten Connection,** Rodale, 2007.

Paleolithic Books

This is a list of books that discuss lectins and the paleolithic diet. I haven't read all of them, but decided to list them anyway so that you are aware of the books that are available.

Loren Cordain. The Paleo Diet: **Lose Weight and Get Healthy by Eating the Food You Were Designed to Eat.** Wiley (December 20, 2002).

Loren Cordain. **The Paleo Diet For Athletes: A Nutritional Formula For Peak Athletic Performance**. Rodale Books; 1 edition, October 13, 2005.

Robb Wolf. **The Paleo Solution: The Original Human Diet.** Victory Belt Publishing, September 14, 2010.

Mark Sisson. **The Primal Blueprint: Reprogram Your Genes For Effortless Weightloss, Vibrant Health, And Boundless Energy.** Primal Nutrition, Inc.; 1ST edition, June 1, 2009.

Mark Sisson and Jennifer Meier. **The Primal Blueprint Cookbook: Primal, Low Carb, Paleo, Grain-Free, Dairy-Free, And Gluten-Free.**

A. Pusztai. **Plant Lectins**. Cambridge University Press, 1991.

Allergy Books

Carolee Bateson-Koch DC ND. **Allergies, Disease In Disguise. How To Heal Your Allergic Condition Permanently And Naturally.** Alive Books, 1994.

Dr. James Braly And Patrick Holford. **Hidden Food Allergies: The Essential Guide To Uncovering Hidden Food Allergies And Achieving Permanent Relief.** Basic Health Publications; 1ST edition (September 14, 2006).

Other Health Books

Gary Huffnagle, PhD. **The Probiotics Revolution**. Bantam Books, 2007.

Elaine Gottschall B.A., MSc. **Breaking The Vicious Cycle**. 1994.

Michael Pollan. **The Omnivore's Dilemma**. Penguin Books, 2008.

Wendy Cohen, RN. **The Better Bladder Book**. Hunter House, Oct 21, 2010.

Larry Trivieri, JR., and John W. Anderson. **Alternative Medicine, The Definitive Guide.** Inno Vision Health Media, 2002.

Deepak Chopra. **Ageless Body, Timeless Mind**. Three Rivers Press, 2010.

Bibliography

Introduction

1. Feldman Mark, MD, Friedman Lawrence S, MD, Sleisenger, Marvin H, MD, *Gastrointestinal and Liver Disease Pathophysiology/Diagnosis/Management,* 7th Edition, Volume11, 2002,Saunders

2. Green PH, Cellier C (October 2007). Medical progress: Celiac Disease. *N. Engl. J. Med.* 357 (17): 1731–43.

3. West J, Logan RF, Hill PG, et al. Seroprevalence, correlates, and characteristics of undetected coeliac disease in England. *Gut* 2003;52:960–5.

4. Green PHR et al. Economic benefits of Diagnosis. *Journal of Insurance Medicine*, 2008;40:218-228

5. Albert A. Kyle, Edward L. Kaplan, Dwight R. Johnson, William Page, Frederick Erdtmann, Tricia L. Brantner, W. Ray Kim, Tara K. Phelps, Brian D. Lahr, Alan R. Zinsmeister, Joseph Melton III, Joseph A. Murray. Increased Prevalence and Mortality in Undiagnosed Celiac Disease. *Gastroenterology*, Volume 137, Issue 1 , Pages 88-93, July 2009.

6. Johnston SD, Watson RGP, McMillan SA, Sloan J, Love AHG. Prevalence of coeliac disease in Northern Ireland. *Lancet* 1997; 350:1370.

7. www.celiacdisease.net

8. Hin H, Bird G, Fisher P, Mahy N, Jewell D. Coeliac disease in primary care, case finding study. *Br Med J* 1999; 318:164–7.

9. Paul J. Ciclitira, Mathew W. Johnson, David H. Dewar and H. Julia Ellis. The Pathogenesis Of Coeliac Disease. *Molecular Aspects of Medicine* Volume 26, Issue 6, December 2005, Pages 421-458.

10. MI Torres, MA Lopez Casado, A Rios. New Aspects In Celiac Disease. *World Journal Gastroenterol.*, 2007, February 28; 13 (8): 1156-1161.

Chapter 1

1. Shewry PR, Halford NG. Cereal seed storage proteins: structures, properties and role in grain utilization. *J Exp Bot* 2002;53:947-58. PMID__ 11912237.

2. Carolyn D. Berdanier, Johanna Dwyer, and Elaine B. Feldman. Handbook Of Nutrition And Food, Second Edition, 2007.

3. Shane M. Devlin, MD, FRCPC Christopher N. Andrews, MD, FRCPC Paul L. Beck, MD, PHD, FRCPC. Celiac Disease. *Canadian Family Physician*, CME update for family physicians. May, 2004.

4. Children's Digestive Health And Nutrition Foundation
    http://www.cdhnf.org/wmspage.cfm?parm1=40

5. Mahida YR. Immunological Aspects of Gastroenterology. Kluwer Academic Publishers 2001.

6. David A Nelson, JR., MD., MS., University of Arkanas for Medical Sciences, Little Rock, Arkansas. Gluten-Sensitive Enteropathy (Celiac Disease): More Common Than You Think. *American Family Physician*, December 15, 2002.

7. Feldman Mark, MD, Friedman Lawrence S, MD, Sleisenger, Marvin H, MD, Gastrointestinal and Liver Disease Pathophysiology/Diagnosis/Management 7th Edition, Volume11, 2002,Saunders

8. Barrett KE. Gastrointestinal Physiology. Lange Medical Books/McGraw-Hill 2006.

9. Kagnoff MF. AGA Institute Medical Position Statement on the Diagnosis and Management of CD. *Gastroenterology*, Official Journal of the American Gastroenterological Association (AGA). December 2006.

10. Farhadi A, Banan A, Fields J, Keshavarzian A. Intestinal barrier: an interface between health and disease. *Journal of Gastroenterology And Hepatology*. 2003; 18:479-497.

11. Liu Z, Li N, Neu J. Tight junctions, leaky intestines, and pediatric diseases. *Acta Paediatrica*, 2005; 94:386-393.

12. Clemente MG, De Virgiliis S, Kang JS, et el.Early effects of gliadin on enterocyte, intracellular signalling involved in intestinal barrier function *Gut*, Feb. 2003; 52 (2):218-23.

13. Lammers KM, Lu R, Brownley J, *et al* (July 2008). "Gliadin induces an increase in intestinal permeability and zonulin release by binding to the chemokine receptor CXCR3". *Gastroenterology* 135 (1): 194–204

14. Hausch F, Shan L, Santiago NA, Gray GM, Khosla C. Intestinal digestive resistance of immunodominant gliadin peptides. *Am J Physiol Gastrointest Liver Physiol*. 2002;283(4):G996–G1003.

15. Green, PH. The many faces of celiac disease: clinical presentation of celiac disease in the adult population. *Gastroenterology.* 2005;128:S74-78.

16. Brandimarte G, Tursi A, Giorgetti GM. Changing trends in clinical form of celiac disease. Which is now the main form of celiac disease in clinical practice? *Minerva Gastroenterol Dietol.* 2002;48:121-30.

17. Celiac Disease. Health Canada

    http://www.hc-sc.gc.ca/fn-an/securit/allerg/cel-coe/index-eng.php

18. Alessio Fasano and Carlo Catassi. Current approaches to diagnosis and treatment of celiac disease: an evolving spectrum. *Gastroenterology* 2001:120636-651.

19. Triticeae glutens www.wikipedia.org

20. Gluten www.wikipedia.org

21. Amendola, J., Rees, N., & Lundberg, D. E. (2002). *Understanding Baking*

22.

23. Talley NJ, Valdovinos M, Petterson TM, Carpenter HA, Melton LJ 3rd. Epidemiology of celiac sprue: a community-based study. *Am J Gastroenterol.* 1994 Jun;89(6):843-6.

24. Talley NJ, Valdovinos M, Petterson TM, Carpenter HA, Melton LJ 3rd. Epidemiology of celiac sprue: a community-based study. *Am J Gastroenterol.* 1995 Jan;90(1):163-4.

25. Oliveira RP, Sdepanian VL, Barreto JA, Cortez AJ, Carvalho FO, Bordin JO, de Camargo Soares MA, da Silva Patrício FR, Kawakami E, de Morais MB, Fagundes-Neto U. High prevalence of celiac disease in Brazilian blood donor volunteers based on screening by IgA antitissue transglutaminase antibody. Eur J Gastroenterol Hepatol. 2007 Jan;19(1):43-9.

26. Gee-Herter-Heubner Disease [www.wrongdiagnosis.com]

27. www.celiacdisease.net

28. Neela Sundar, Rosemary Crimmins, and Gillian L Swift . Clinical presentation and incidence of complications in patients with coeliac disease diagnosed by relative screening. Postgrad Med J. 2007 April; 83(978): 273–276.

29. Hadjivassiliou M, Maki M, Saunders DS, Williamson CA, Grunewald RA, Woodroof NM, Korponay-Szabo IR. Autoantibody Targeting of Brain and Intestinal Transglutaminase in Gluten Ataxia. *Neurology* 2006 Feb.14;66(3):373-7.

30. Health Canada's Position on the Introduction of Oats to the Diet of Individuals Diagnosed with Celiac Disease (CD). "Celiac disease and the safety of oats.

http://www.hc-sc.gc.ca/fn-an/securit/allerg/cel-coe/oats_cd-avoine-eng.php

31. Evolutionary Aspects of Nutrition and Health: Diet, Exercise, Genetics and Chronic Disease. World Review of Nutrition and Dietetics, vol. 84. Edited by A. P. Simopoulos. Basel: Karger. 1999. Pp. 145. Book review: SE Humphries. *Annals of Human Genetics* Volume 63, Issue 4, pages 377–381, July 1999

32. Marks J, Shusters S, Watson AJ. Small Bowel Changes In Dermatitis Herpetiformis. Lancet, 1966;ii:1280-1282.

33. Dermatitis Herpetiformis www.nlm.nih.gov/medlineplus/ency/article/001480.htm

34. www.celiac.ca Accessed September 2010.

35. K. Fälth-Magnusson, K.-E. Magnusson . Elevated levels of serum antibodies to the lectin wheat germ agglutinin in celiac children lend support to the gluten-lectin theory of celiac disease. Pediatric Allergy and Immunology. Volume 6, Issue 2, pages 98–102, May 1995.

Chapter 2

1. Shane M. Devlin, MD, FRCPC Christopher N. Andrews, MD, FRCPC Paul L. Beck, MD, PHD, FRCPC. Celiac Disease. *Canadian Family Physician*, CME update for family physicians. May, 2004.

2. Peter Parham. The Immune System. Garland Science; 3 edition (January 19, 2009)

3. Russell P. Hall, Thomas J. Lawley and Stephen I. Katz. Dermatitis Herpetiformis. *Springer Seminars In Immunopathology,* Volume 4, Number 1, March 1981.

4. Sardy M, Karpati S, Merkl B, Paulsson M, Smyth N.Epidermal transglutaminase (TGase 3) is the autoantigen of dermatitis herpetiformis. *J Exp Med*.Mar 18 2002;195(6):747-57.

5. Hull CM, Liddle M, Hansen N, et al. Elevation of IgA anti-epidermal transglutaminase antibodies in dermatitis herpetiformis. *Br J Dermatol*. Jul 2008;159(1):120-4.

6. Marietta EV, Camilleri MJ, Castro LA, Krause PK, Pittelkow MR, Murray JA. Transglutaminase autoantibodies in dermatitis herpetiformis and celiac sprue. *J Invest Dermatol*. Feb 2008;128(2):332-5.

7. Bardella MT, Fredella C, Saladino V, et al. Gluten intolerance: gender- and age-related differences in symptoms. *Scand J Gastroenterol*. Jan 2005;40(1):15-9.

8.   LM Solid, J Kolberg, H Scott, J Ek, O Fausa, P Brandtzaeg. Antibodies to wheat germ agglutinin in coeliac disease. *Clin Exp Immunol.* 1986 January; 63(1): 95–100.

9.   K. Fälth-Magnusson, K.-E. Magnusson . Elevated levels of serum antibodies to the lectin wheat germ agglutinin in celiac children lend support to the gluten-lectin theory of celiac disease. *Pediatric Allergy and Immunology.* Volume 6, Issue 2, pages 98–102, May 1995.

10.   Brunngraber EC. Possible role of glycoproteins in neurol function. *Perspectives in Biology And Medicine*, 12, pg. 467-70, 1969.

11.   Clevers HC, de Bresser A, Kleinveld H, Gmelig-Meyling FH, and Ballieux RE. Wheat germ agglutinin activates human T lymphocytes by stimulation of phosphoinositide hydrolysis. *The Journal of Immunology*, 136, pg. 3180-3, 1986.

12.   De George JJ and Carbonetto S. Wheat germ agglutinin inhibits nerve fiber growth and concanavalin A stimulates nerve fiber initiation in culture of dorsal root ganaglia neurons. *Developmental Brain Research* 28, 169-75, 1986.

13.   Cuatrecasas P and Tell GPE. Insulin-like activity of concanavalin A and wheat germ agglutinin: direct interactions with insulin receptors. *Proceedings Of The National Academy of Sciences.* USA 70, 485-9, 1973.

14.   Casalounge C, Pont Lezica RC. Potato lectin: a cell wall glycoprotein. *Plant Cell Physiology*, 26, pg. 1533-9, 1985.

15.   Ceri H, Falkenberg-Anderson K, Fang R, Costerton JW, howard R and Barnwell JG. Bacteria-lectin interactions in phytohemagglutinin-induced bacterial overgrowth of the small intestine. *Canadian Journal Of Microbiology* 34, 1003-8, 1988.

16.   Carpender G, Cohen S. Influence of lectins on the binding of 125-1 labelled EGF to human fibroblasts. *Biochemical And Biophysical Research Communications* 79, pg. 545-52, 1977.

17.   JH Ovelgonne, JFJG Koninkxa, A Pusztaib, S bardoczb, W Koka, SWB Ewenc, HGCJM Hendriksa, JE van Dijka. Decreased levels of heat shock proteins in gut epithelial cells after exposure to plant lectins. *Gut.* 2000 May;46(5):679-87.

18.   Pusztia A, F Greer and G Grant. Specific uptake of dietary lectins into the systemic circulation of rats, *Biochem Soc. Trans.*, 17: 481-482, 1989.

19.   Pusztai A. Dietary lectins are metabolic signals for the gut and modulate immune and hormonal functions. *Eur. J. Clin. Nutr*, 47: 691-699, 1993.

20. Vasconcelos IM and JT Oliveira. Antinutritional Properties Of Plant Lectins. *Toxicon*, 44: 385-403, 2004.

21. Fabian RH, Coulter JD. Transneuronal transport of lectins. *Brain Research* 344, 41-48, 1985.

22. Wheat germ agglutinin induces NADPH-oxidase activity in human neutrophils by interaction with mobilizable receptors. *Infection and Immunity.* 1999 Jul;67(7):3461-8.

23. Kidney bean (phaseolus vulgaris) lectin induced lesions in rat small intestine. 2 ultrastructural studies. *The Journal Of Comparitive Pathology* 92, 357-73, 1982.

24. Zang J, D Li, X Piao and X Tang. Effects Of Soybean Agglutinin On Body Composition And Organ Weights In Rats. *Arch Anim Nutr.*, 60: 245-253, 2006.

25. Brady PG, AM Vannier and JG Banwell. Identification of dietary lectin, wheat germ agglutinin, in human intestinal contents. *Gastroenterology*, 75: 236., 1978.

26. Freed DLJ. Dietary lectins and the anti-nutritive effects of gut allergy. In: Protein Transmission Through Living Membranes. *Elsevier/North Holland Biomedical Press,* pages: 411-422, 1979.

27. Bulajic M, CuperlovicM, Movsesinjan IM, Borojevil D. Interaction of dietary lectin (phytohemagglutinin) with the mucosa of rat digestive tract. *Immunofluorescence Studies. Periodicum Biologorum*, 38, 331-76, 1986.

28. Gloria V. Guzyeyeva. Lectin Glycosylation As A Marker of Thin Gut inflammation. *The FASEB Journal.* 2008;22:898.3

29. D Bernardo, J A Garrote, L Fernandez-Salazar, S Riestra, E Arranz. Is gliadin really safe for non-coeliac individuals? Production of interleukin 15 in biopsy culture from non-coeliac individuals challenged with gliadin peptides *Gut* 2007;56:889-890

30. A. Pusztai, S. W. B. Ewen, G. Grant, D. S. Brown, J. C. Stewart, W. J. Peumans, E. J. M. Van Damme and S. Bardocz Antinutritive effects of wheat-germ agglutinin and other N-acetylglucosamine-specific lectins. *The British Journal of Nutrition* 1993 Jul;70(1):313-21.

31. Borges LF, Sidman RL.Axonal transport of lectins in the peripheral nervous system. *Journal Of Neuroscience*, 2, pg. 647-53, 1982.

32. Tchernychev B, Wilchek M.. Natural human antibodies to dietary lectins. *FEBS Lett.* 1996 Nov 18;397(2-3):139-42.

33. Broadwell RD, Balin BJ, Salcman M.. Transcytotic pathway for blood-borne protein through the blood-brain barrier. *Proceedings from the National Academy of Sciences* U S A. 1988 Jan;85(2):632-6.

34. Begbic R, King TP. The interaction of dietary lectin with porcine small intestine and production of lectin-specific antibodies. In Lectins Biology, Biochemistry, *Clinical Biochemistry* (Bog-Hansen TC, Breborovicz J eds). Vol 4, pages 15-27. Walter de Gruyter, Berlin and New York, 1985.

35. Damak S, Mosinger B, Margolskee RF. Transsynaptic transport of wheat germ agglutinin expressed in a subset of type II taste cells of transgenic mice. *BMC Neuroscience*. 2008 Oct 2;9:96.

36. Dolapchieva S. Distribution of concanavalin A and wheat germ agglutinin binding sites in the rat peripheral nerve fibres revealed by lectin/glycoprotein-gold histo-chemistry. *The Histo Chem Journal.* 1996 Jan;28(1):7-12.

37. Boldt DH, Banwell JG. Binding of isolectins from red kidney bean (phaseolus vulgaris) to purified rat brush border membranes, *Biochimia et Biophysica Acta* 843, 230-7, 1985.

38. Hashimoto S, Hagino A. Wheat germ agglutinin, concanavalin A, and lens culinalis agglutinin block the inhibitory effect of nerve growth factor on cell-free phosphorylation of Nsp100 in PC12h cells. *Cell Struct and Function* 1989 Feb;14(1):87-93.

39. Liu WK, Sze SC, Ho JC, Liu BP, Yu MC. Wheat germ lectin induces G2/M arrest in mouse L929 fibroblasts. *J Cell Biochem*. 2004 Apr 15;91(6):1159-73

40. Bonavida B, Katz J. Studies on the induction and expression of T-cell mediated immunity. xv. Role of non-MHC papain-sensitive target structures and Lyt-2 antigens in allogenic and xenogeic lectin dependent cellular cytotoxicity (LDCC). *The Journal Of Immunology,* 135, 1616-23, 1985.

41. Yevdokimova NY, Yefimov AS. Effects of wheat germ agglutinin and concanavalin A on the accumulation of glycosaminoglycans in pericellular matrix of human dermal fibroblasts. A comparison with insulin. *Acta Biochim Pol.* 2001;48(2):563-72.

42. Sasano H, Rojas M, Silverberg SG. Analysis of lectin binding in benign and malignant thyroid nodules. *Arch Pathol Lab Med.* 1989 Feb;113(2):186-9.

43. Lebret M, Rendu F. Further characterization of wheat germ agglutinin interaction with human platelets: exposure of fibrinogen receptors. *Thromb Haemost.* 1986 Dec 15;56(3):323-7.

44. Ohmori T, Yatomi Y, Wu Y, Osada M, Satoh K, Ozaki Y. Wheat germ agglutin-in-induced platelet activation via platelet endothelial cell adhesion molecule-1: involvement of rapid phospholipase C gamma 2 activation by Src family kinases. *Biochemistry*. 2001 Oct 30;40(43):12992-3001

45. David L J Freed, Allergist. Do dietary lectins cause disease? The evidence is suggestive—and raises interesting possibilities for treatment. *BMJ*. 1999 April 17; 318(7190): 1023–1024.

46. JH Ovelgonne, JFJG Koninkxa, A Pusztaib, S bardoczb, W Koka, SWB Ewenc, HGCJM Hendriksa, JE van Dijka. Decreased levels of heat shock proteins in gut epithelial cells after exposure to plant lectins. *Gut*. 2000 May;46(5):679-87.

47. D Bernardo, J A Garrote, L Fernandez-Salazar, S Riestra, E Arranz. Is gliadin really safe for non-coeliac individuals? Production of interleukin 15 in biopsy culture from non-coeliac individuals challenged with gliadin peptides Gut 2007;56:889-890

48. David A Nelson, JR., MD., MS., University of Arkanas for Medical Sciences, Little Rock, Arkansas. Gluten-Sensitive Enteropathy (Celiac Disease): More Common Than You Think. *American Family Physician*, December 15, 2002.

49. Feldman Mark, MD, Friedman Lawrence S, MD, Sleisenger, Marvin H, MD, Gastrointestinal and Liver Disease Pathophysiology/Diagnosis/Management 7th Edition, Volume 11, 2002, Saunders

50. Hadjivassiliou M, Aeschlimann P, Strigun A, Sanders DS, Woodroofe N, Aeschlimann D. Autoantibodies in gluten ataxia recognize a novel neuronal trans-glutaminase. *Ann Neurol* 2008 Sep;64(3):332-43.

51. Lammers KM, Lu R, Brownley J, *et al* (July 2008). "Gliadin induces an increase in intestinal permeability and zonulin release by binding to the chemokine receptor CXCR3". *Gastroenterology* 135 (1): 194–204

52. Hausch F, Shan L, Santiago NA, Gray GM, Khosla C. Intestinal digestive resistance of immunodominant gliadin peptides. *Am J Physiol Gastrointest Liver Physiol*. 2002;283(4):G996–G1003.

53. Shan L, Qiao SW, Arentz-Hansen H, *et al* (2005). Identification and Analysis of Multivalent Proteolytically Resistant Peptides from Gluten: Implications for Celiac Sprue. *J. Proteome Res*. 4 (5): 1732–41.

54. Bodinier M, Legoux MA, Pineau F, *et al*. (May 2007). "Intestinal translocation capabilities of wheat allergens using the Caco-2 cell line". *J. Agric. Food Chem*. 55 (11): 4576–83.

55. Thomas KE, Sapone A, Fasano A, Vogel SN (February 2006). "Gliadin stimulation of murine macrophage inflammatory gene expression and intestinal permeability are MyD88-dependent: role of the innate immune response in Celiac disease". *J. Immunol.* 176 (4): 2512–21.

56. Clemente MG, De Virgiliis S, Kang JS, et el.Early effects of gliadin on enterocyte, intracellular signalling involved in intestinal barrier function *Gut,* Feb. 2003; 52 (2):218-23.

57. G. Fluge, H. Olesen, M. Gilljam, P. Meyer, T. Pressler, O. Storrösten, F. Karpati, L. Hjelte. Co-morbidity of cystic fibrosis and celiac disease in Scandinavian cystic fibrosis patients. Journal of Cystic Fibrosis, Volume 8, Issue 3, Pages 198-202.

58. Mario Curione, Maria Barbato, Pietro Cugini, Silvia Amato, Silvia Da Ros, Simonetta Di Bona. Association of cardiomyopathy and celiac disease: an almost diffuse but still less know entity. *Arch Med Sci* 2008; 4, 2: 103–107.

59. Hadjivassiliou M, Aeschlimann P, Strigun A, Sanders DS, Woodroofe N, Aeschlimann D. Autoantibodies in gluten ataxia recognize a novel neuronal trans-glutaminase. *Ann Neurol* 2008 Sep;64(3):332-43.

60. Lammers KM, Lu R, Brownley J, *et al.* (March 2008). "Gliadin Induces an Increase in Intestinal Permeability and Zonulin Release by Binding to the Chemokine Receptor CXCR3". *Gastroenterology* 135 (1): 194–204,2008.

61. Green, PH. The many faces of celiac disease: clinical presentation of celiac disease in the adult population. *Gastroenterology.* 2005;128:S74-78.

62. Brandimarte G, Tursi A, Giorgetti GM. Changing trends in clinical form of celiac disease. Which is now the main form of celiac disease in clinical practice? *Minerva Gastroenterol Dietol.* 2002;48:121-30.

63. Alessio Fasano and Carlo Catassi. Current approaches to diagnosis and treatment of celiac disease: an evolving spectrum. *Gastroenterology* 2001:120636-651.

64. Alessio Fasano, M.D. Physiological, Pathological, and Therapeutic Implications of Zonulin-Mediated Intestinal Barrier Modulation. *American Journal of Pathology,* 2008;173:1243-1252.

65. Hadjivassiliou M, Sanders DS, Grünewald RA, Woodroofe N, Boscolo S, Aeschlimann D. Gluten sensitivity: from gut to brain. *Lancet Neurol.* 2010 Mar;9(3):318-30.

66. Willy J. Peumans, Hetty M. Stinissen, and Albert R. Carlier. Isolation and partial characterization of wheat-germ-agglutinin-like lectins from rye (Secale cereale)

and barley (Hordeum vulgare) embryos. *Biochem J.* 1982 April 1; 203(1): 239–243.

67. Constanze Ebert, Barbara Nebe, Hermann Walzel, Heike Weber and Ludwig Jonas. Inhibitory effect of the lectin wheat germ agglutinin (WGA) on the proliferation of AR42J Cells. *Acta Histochemica* Volume 111, Issue 4, July 2009, Pages 336-343.

68. A. Pusztai. Plant Lectins. Cambridge university Press, 1991.

69. Bender AE, Reaidi GB, Toxicity of kidney beans (Phaseolus vulgaris) with particular reference to lectins. *The Journal of Plant Foods* 4, 15-22, 1982.

70. Barrett DJ, Edwards JR, Pietrantuono BA, Ayoub EM. Inhibition of human lymphocyte activation by wheat germ agglutinin: a model for saccharide specific suppressor factors. *Cellular Immunology,* 81, 287-97, 1983.

71. *Gastroenterology.* 2007 Oct;133(4):1175-87. Epub 2007 Aug 14.

72. Di Sabatino A, Pickard KM, Gordon JN, Salvati V, Mazzarella G, Beattie RM, Vossenkaemper A, Rovedatti L, Leakey NA, Croft NM, Troncone R, Corazza GR, Stagg AJ, Monteleone G, MacDonald TT. Evidence for the role of interferon-alfa production by dendritic cells in the Th1 response in celiac disease. *Gastroenterology.* 2007 Oct;133(4):1175-87. Epub 2007 Aug 14.

73. Hadjivassiliou M, Maki M, Saunders DS, Williamson CA, Grunewald RA, Woodroof NM, Korponay-Szabo IR. Autoantibody Targeting of Brain and Intestinal Transglutaminase in Gluten Ataxia. *Neurology* 2006 Feb.14;66(3):373-7.

74. Bottaro G, Failla P, Rotolo N, Azzaro F, Spina M, Castiglione N, Patané R. [The predictive value of antigliadin antibodies (AGA) in the diagnosis of non-celiac gastrointestinal disease in children]. *Minerva Pediatr.* 1993 Mar;45(3):93-8.

75. Hadjivassiliou M, Grünwald R, Sharrack B, Sanders D, Lobo A, Williamson C, Woodroofe N, Wood N, Davies-Jones A. Gluten Ataxia in Perspective: Epidemiology, Genetic susceptibility, And Clinical Characteristics. *Brain* 2003 Mar;126(pt 3): 685-91.

76. Hadjivassiliou M, Sanders DS, Grünewald RA, Woodroofe N, Boscolo S, Aeschlimann D. Gluten sensitivity: from gut to brain. *Lancet* Neurol. 2010 Mar;9(3):318-30.

77. M. Hadjivassiliou, MD, M. Mäki, MD, D. S. Sanders, MD, C. A. Williamson, PhD, R. A. Grünewald, DPhil, N. M. Woodroofe, MD and I. R. Korponay-Szabó, MD. Autoantibody targeting of brain and intestinal transglutaminase in gluten ataxia. *NEUROLOGY* 2006;66:373-377.

78. Floreani A, Chiaramonte M, Venturini R, Plebani M, Martin A, Giacomini A, Naccarato R. Antigliadin antibody classes in chronic liver disease. Ital J Gastroenterol. 1992 Oct;24(8):457-60.

79. Reichelt KL, Jensen D. IgA antibodies against gliadin and gluten in multiple sclerosis. *Acta Neurol Scand*. 2004 Oct;110(4):239-41.

80. Akçay MN, Akçay G. The presence of the antigliadin antibodies in autoimmune thyroid diseases. *Hepatogastroenterology*. 2003 Dec;50 Suppl 2:cclxxix-cclxxx.

81. Paimela L, Kurki P, Leirisalo-Repo M, Piirainen H. Gliadin immune reactivity in patients with rheumatoid arthritis. *Clin Exp Rheumatol*. 1995 Sep-Oct;13(5):603-7.

82. Fukudome S, Yoshikawa M. Opiod Peptides Derived from Wheat Gluten: Their Isolation And Characterization. *Febs Letts*. 1992. January 13 ;296(1) : 107-11.

83. C Zioudrou, R A Streaty and W A Klee . Opioid peptides derived from food proteins. The exorphins. *The Journal Of Biological Chemistry*, April 10, 1979. 254: 2446-2449

84. A. Pusztai. Plant Lectins. Cambridge University Press, 1991.

85. Shattock P, Whiteley P. (2002) "Biochemical aspects in autism spectrum disorders: updating the opioid-excess theory and presenting new opportunities for biomedical intervention" "Autism Research Unit, University of Sunderland, UK.

86. Carolee Bateson-Koch DC ND. Allergies: A Disease In Disguise. Alive books, 1994.

87. Jönsson T, Ahrén B, Pacini G, Sundler F, Wierup N, Steen S, Sjöberg T, Ugander M, Frostegård J, Göransson L, Lindeberg S. A Paleolithic diet confers higher insulin sensitivity, lower C-reactive protein and lower blood pressure than a cereal-based diet in domestic pigs. Nutr Metab (Lond). 2006 Nov 2;3:39.

88. Drago, Sandro; El Asmar, Ramzi; Di Pierro, Mariarosaria; Grazia Clemente, Maria; Sapone, Amit Tripathi Anna; Thakar, Manjusha·; Iacono, Giuseppe; Carroccio, Antonio; D'Agate, Cinzia; Not, Tarcisio; Zampini, Lucia; Catassi, Carlo; Fasano, Alessio·Gliadin, zonulin and gut permeability: Effects on celiac and non-celiac intestinal mucosa and intestinal cell lines. Scandinavian Journal of Gastroenterology, Volume 41, Number 4, March 2006 , pp. 408-419(12).

Chapter 3

1.   Hausch F, Shan L, Santiago NA, Gray GM, Khosla C. Intestinal digestive resistance of immunodominant gliadin peptides. *Am J Physiol Gastrointest Liver Physiol*. 2002;283(4):G996–G1003.

2.   Shan L, Qiao SW, Arentz-Hansen H, *et al* (2005). Identification and Analysis of Multivalent Proteolytically Resistant Peptides from Gluten: Implications for Celiac Sprue. *J. Proteome Res*. 4 (5): 1732–41.

3.   Shane M. Devlin, MD, FRCPC Christopher N. Andrews, MD, FRCPC Paul L. Beck, MD, PHD, FRCPC. Celiac Disease. *Canadian Family Physician*, CME update for family physicians. May, 2004.

4.   David A Nelson, JR., MD., MS., University of Arkanas for Medical Sciences, Little Rock, Arkansas. Gluten-Sensitive Enteropathy (Celiac Disease): More Common Than You Think. *American Family Physician*, December 15, 2002.

5.   Feldman Mark, MD, Friedman Lawrence S, MD, Sleisenger, Marvin H, MD, Gastrointestinal and Liver Disease Pathophysiology/Diagnosis/Management 7th Edition, Volume11, 2002,Saunders

6.   Hadjivassilou M and Grünwald RA, Davies-Jones GAB. Gluten Sensitivity As a Neurological Illness. *Journal of Neurology*, Neurosurgery, and Psychiatry 2002;72:560-563

7.   Lejarraga H, et el. Normal Growth Velocity Before Diagnosis Of Celiac Disease. *J Pediatr Gastrenterol Nutr* 2000;30:552-556

8.   Pruessner Harold T, MD. Detecting Celiac Disease In Your Patients. *American Family Physician*. March 1st, 1998.

9.   Green, PH. The many faces of celiac disease: clinical presentation of celiac disease in the adult population. *Gastroenterology*. 2005;128:S74-78.

10.   Brandimarte G, Tursi A, Giorgetti GM. Changing trends in clinical form of celiac disease. Which is now the main form of celiac disease in clinical practice? *Minerva Gastroenterol Dietol*. 2002;48:121-30.

11.   Celiac Disease. Health Canada.

      http://www.hc-sc.gc.ca/fn-an/securit/allerg/cel-coe/index-eng.php

12.   Alessio Fasano and Carlo Catassi. Current approaches to diagnosis and treatment of celiac disease: an evolving spectrum. *Gastroenterology* 2001:120636-651.

13. Alessio Fasano, M.D. Physiological, Pathological, and Therapeutic Implications of Zonulin-Mediated Intestinal Barrier Modulation. *American Journal of Pathology,* 2008;173:1243-1252.

14. Mäki M, Mustalahti K, Kokkonen J, Kulmala P, Haapalahti M, Karttunen T, Ilonen J, Laurila K, Dahlbom I, Hansson T, Höpfl P, Knip M.. Prevalence of Celiac disease among children in Finland. *N Engl J Med.* 2003 Jun 19;348(25):2517-24.

15. Catassi C, Rätsch IM, Gandolfi L, Pratesi R, Fabiani E, El Asmar R, Frijia M, Bearzi I, Vizzoni L. Why is coeliac disease endemic in the people of the Sahara? Lancet. 1999 Aug 21;354(9179):647-8.

16. V. Kumar, M. Jarzabek-Chorzelska, J. Sulej, Krystyna Karnewska, T. Farrell, and S. Jablonska Celiac Disease and Immunoglobulin A Deficiency: How Effective Are the Serological Methods of Diagnosis? *Clinical and Diagnostic Laboratory Immunology, November* 2002, p. 1295-1300, Vol. 9, No. 6

17. Talley NJ, Valdovinos M, Petterson TM, Carpenter HA, Melton LJ 3rd. Epidemiology Of Celiac Sprue: A Community Based Study. *Am J Gasterenterol* 1994 Jun;89(6):843-6.

18. www.celiac.ca

19. www.celiac.org.uk

20. www.patient.co.uk/doctor/Dermatitis-Herpetiformis.htm

Chapter 4

1. Shane M. Devlin, MD, FRCPC Christopher N. Andrews, MD, FRCPC Paul L. Beck, MD, PHD, FRCPC. Celiac Disease. *Canadian Family Physician,* CME update for family physicians. May, 2004.

2. Mahida YR. Immunological Aspects of Gastroenterology. *Kluwer Academic Publishers* 2001.

3. Hadjivassilou M and Grünwald RA, Davies-Jones GAB. Gluten Sensitivity As a Neurological Illness. *Journal of Neurology, Neurosurgery, and Psychiatry* 2002;72:560-563

4. David A Nelson, JR., MD., MS., University of Arkanas for Medical Sciences, Little Rock, Arkansas. Gluten-Sensitive Enteropathy (Celiac Disease): More Common Than You Think. *American Family Physician*, December 15, 2002.

5. Rhodes RA, Tai HH, Chey WY. Impairment of Secretin Release in Celiac Sprue. *Am J Dig Dis* 23:833, 1978.

6.   Maton PN, Seldon AC, Fitzpatrick ML, et al. Defective Gallbladder Emptying And Cholecystokinin Release In Celiac Disease. Reversal by Gluten-free Diet. *Gastroenterology* 88:391, 1985.

7.   Vuoristo M, MiettinenTA. The Role Of Fat And Bile Acid Malabsorption in Diarrhoea Of Coeliac Disease. *Scand J Gastroenterol* 22:289, 1987.

8.   Egan-Mitchell Bridget, McNicholl Brian. Constipation in Childhood Coeliac Disease. *Archives of Disease in Childhood*. 1972;47,238

9.   Tursi, Antonio MD. Gastrointestinal Motility Disturbances in Celiac Disease. *Journal of Clinical Gastroenterology*: September 2004 – Volume 38 – Issue 8 – pp 642-645

10.   Gabrio Bassotti, Giuseppe Castellucci, Cesare Betti, Carla Fusaro, Maria Lucia Cavalletti, Alberto Bertotto, Fabrizio Spinozzi, Antonio Morelli and Maria Antonietta Pelli. Abnormal gastrointestinal motility in patients with celiac sprue. *Journal Digestive Diseases and Sciences*. Volume39, Number 9/September 1994.

11.   Feldman Mark, MD, Friedman Lawrence S, MD, Sleisenger, Marvin H, MD, Gastrointestinal and Liver Disease Pathophysiology/Diagnosis/Management 7th Edition, Volume11, 2002,Saunders

12.   Touloukian RJ, and Spencer RP, Ileal blood flow preceding compensatory intestinal hypertrophy. *Annals of Surgery*. vol. 175(3);Mar 1972.

13.   Pratesi R, Gandolfi L, Friedman H, Farage L, de Castro CA, Catassi C. Serum IgA Antibodies From Patients With Coeliac Disease React Strongly With Human Brain Blood Vessel Structures. *Scand J Gastroenterol* 1998;33:817-21.

14.   Aine L, Maki M, Collin P, et al. Dental Enamel Defects In Celiac Disease. *J Oral Pathol Med* 19:241, 1990.

15.   Tursi A,Brandimarte G, Giorgetti G. High Prevalence of Small Intestinal Bacterial Overgrowth in Celiac Patients With Persistance of Gastrointestinal Symptoms After Gluten Withdrawl. *Am J Gastroenterol* 98(4):839-43

16.   Kagnoff MF. AGA Institute Medical Position Statement on the Diagnosis and Management of CD. *Gastroenterology,* Official Journal of the American Gastroen- terological Association (AGA). November 2006.

17.   Marc-Emmanuel Dumas, Richard H. Barton, Ayo Toye, Olivier Cloarec, Christine Blancher, Alice Rothwell, Jane Fearnside, Roger Tatoud, Véronique Blanc, John C. Lindon, Steve C. Mitchell, Elaine Holmes, Mark I. McCarthy, James Scott, Dominique Gauguier, and Jeremy K. Nicholson Metabolic profiling reveals a

contribution of gut microbiota to fatty liver phenotype in insulin-resistant mice. *Proc Natl Acad Sci* U S A. 2006 August 15; 103(33): 12511–12516.

18. Fraquelli M, Colli A, Colucci A, Bardella MT,Trovato C, Pometta R, Pagliarulo M, Conte D. Accuracy of Ultrasonography in Predicting Celiac Disease. *Arch Intern Med*. 2004;164(2):169-74.

19. Marciani L, Coleman NS, Dunlop SP, Singh G, Marsden CA, Holmes GK, Spiller RC, Gowland PA. Gallbladder Contraction, Gastric Emptying And Antral Motility: Single Visit Assessment of Upper GI Function In Untreated celiac Disease Using Echo Planar MRI. *J Magn Reson Imaging*. 2005;22(5):634-8.

20. Deprez P, Sempoux C, Van Beers BE, Jouret A, Robert A, Rahier J, Geubel A, Pauwels S, Mainguet P. Persistant Decreased Plasma Cholecystokinin levels in Celiac patients Under Gluten Free Diet: Respective Roles of Histological Changes and Nutrient Hydrolysis. *Regul Pept*. 2002;110(1):55-63.

21. Rehfeld JF. Clinical Endocrinology and Metabolism. Cholecystokinin. *Best Prac Res Clin Endocrinol Metab*. 2004;18(4):569-86.

22. Carroccio A, Iacono G, Montalto G, Cavataio F, Marco C Di, Balsamo V, Notar-bartolo A. Exocrine Pancreatic Function in Children With Coeliac Disease Before and After a Gluten-free Diet. *Gut*. Vol 32(7): 796-799, Jul 1991.

23. Iovino Paola, Ciacci Carolina, Sabbatini Francesco, Mota Acioli Dinete, D'Argenio Giuseppe, Mazzacca Gabriele. Esophageal Impairment In Adult Celiac Disease With steatorrhea. *The American Journal of Gastroenterology*. (1998)93,1243-1249.

24. Szodoray P, Barta Z, Lakos, Szakall S, Zeher M. Coeliac Disease In Sjogren's Syndrome-A Study of 111 Hungarian Patients. *Rheumatol Int* 2004 Sep;24(5):278-82. Epub 2003 Sep 17.

25. Matz Jenilee. The Link Between Type 1 Diabetes and Celiac Disease.
http://www.myoptumhealth.com

26. Evans KE, Leeds JS, Morley S, Saunders DS. Pancreatic Insufficiency in Adult Celiac Disease: Do Patients Require Long-Term Enzyme Supplementation? *Dig Dis Sci*. 2010, May11.

27. Clinical guideline: Guidelines For The Diagnosis And Treatment Of Children: Recommendations of The North American Society For Gastroenterology, Hepatology, And Nutrition. *Journal of Pediatric Gastroenterology And Nutrition* 40: 1-9. January 2005 Lippincott Williams and Wilkins, Phildelphia.

28. Green, PH. The many faces of celiac disease: clinical presentation of celiac disease in the adult population. *Gastroenterology.* 2005;128:S74-78.

29. Brandimarte G, Tursi A, Giorgetti GM. Changing trends in clinical form of celiac disease. Which is now the main form of celiac disease in clinical practice? *Minerva Gastroenterol Dietol.* 2002;48:121-30.

30. Alessio Fasano and Carlo Catassi. Current approaches to diagnosis and treatment of celiac disease: an evolving spectrum. *Gastroenterology* 2001:120636-651.

31. Halabi IM.. Coeliac disease presenting as acute pancreatitis in a 3-year-old. *Ann Trop Paediatr.* 2010;30(3):255-7.

32. Patel RS, Johlin FC Jr, Murray JA. Celiac disease and recurrent pancreatitis. *Gastrointest Endosc.* 1999 Dec;50(6):823-7.

33. Hadjivassiliou M, Aeschlimann P, Strigun A, Sanders DS, Woodroofe N, Aeschlimann D. Autoantibodies in gluten ataxia recognize a novel neuronal trans-glutaminase. *Ann Neurol.* 2008 Sep;64(3):332-43.

34. Tatsukawa H, Fukaya Y, Frampton G, Martinez-Fuentes A, Suzuki K, Kuo TF, Nagatsuma K, Shimokado K, Okuno M, Wu J, Iismaa S, Matsuura T, Tsukamoto H, Zern MA, Graham RM, Kojima S. Role of transglutaminase 2 in liver injury via cross linking and silencing of transcription factor Sp1. *Gastroenterology.* 2009 May;136(5):1783-95.e10. Epub 2009 Jan 14.

35. Rehfeld JF. Clinical Endocrinology and Metabolism. Cholecystokinin. Best pract Res Clin Endocrinol Metab. 2004, 18 (4) :569-86.

36. Francesca Bernassola, Massimo Federici, Marco Corazzari, Alessandro Terrinoni, Marta L. Hribal, Vincenzo De Laurenzi, Marco Ranalli, Ornella Massa, Giorgio Sesti, Irwin Mclean, Gennaro Citro, Fabrizio Barbetti, and Gerry Melino. Role of transglutaminase 2 in glucose tolerance: knockout mice studies and a putative mutation in a MODY patient. The FASEB Journal. 2002;16:1371-1378.

37. Hadjivassiliou M, Maki M, Saunders DS, Williamson CA, Grunewald RA, Woodroof NM, Korponay-Szabo IR. Autoantibody Targeting of Brain and Intestinal Transglutaminase in Gluten Ataxia. *Neurology* 2006 Feb.14;66(3):373-7.

38. Marciani L, Coleman NS, Dunlop SP, Singh G, Marsden CA, Holmes GK, Spiller RC, Gowland PA. Gallbladder contraction, gastric emptying and antral motility: single visit assessment of upper GI function in untreated celiac disease using echo-planar MRI. J Magn Reson Imaging. 2005;22 (5) :634-8.

39. Fraquelli M, Colli A, Colucci A, Bardella MT, Trovato C; Pometta R, Pagliarulo M, Conte D. Accuracy of ultrasonography in predicting celiac disease. Arch Intern Med 2004; 164 (2) :169-74.

40. Kate E Evans, John S leeds, Stephen Morley, David S Sanders. Pancreatic Insufficiency In Adult Celiac Disease: Do Patients Require Long-Term Enzyme Supplementation? *Digestive Diseases and Sciences,* Springer netherlands, May 11, 2010.

41. Deprez P; Sempoux C, Van Beers BE, Jouret A, Robert A, Rahier J Geubel A, Pauwels S, Mainguet P. Persistent decreased plasma cholecystokinin in celiac patients on gluten-free diet: the respective roles of histological changes and nutrient hydrolysis. Regul PEPT. 2002, 110 (1) :55-63.

42. Drut R, Drut RM. Lymphocytic gastritis in pediatric celiac disease -- immunohistochemical study of the intraepithelial lymphocytic component. *Med Sci Monit.* 2004 Jan;10(1):CR38-42.

43. K M Feeley, M A Heneghan, F M Stevens, and C F McCarthy. Lymphocytic gastritis and coeliac disease: evidence of a positive association. *J Clin Pathol.* 1998 March; 51(3): 207–210.

44. Scot Lewey. Gallbladder Problems Common In Celiac Disease May Be Missed By Doctors Because Of Normal Tests. www.ezinearticles.com

Chapter 5

1. Gibney MJ, Vorster HH, Kok FJ. Introduction to Human Nutrition. Blackwell Publishing 2002.

2. Zamani F, Mohamadnejad M, Shakeri R, Amiri A, Najafi S, Alimohamadi SM, Tavangar SM, Ghavamzadeh A, Malekzadeh R. Gluten sensitive enteropathy in patients with iron deficiency anemia of unknown origin. Gastrointestinal and Liver Disease Research Center, Iran University of Medical Sciences, Tehran, Iran. *World J Gastroenterol* 2008 December;14(48):7381-7385

3. Gibney MJ, Marinos E, Olle L, Dowsett J. Clinical Nutrition. Blackwell Publishing 2005.

4. Djuric Z, Zivic S, Katic V. Celiac disease with diffuse cutaneous vitamin K-deficiency bleeding. *Adv Ther.* 2007 Nov-Dec;24(6):1286-9.

5. Chen CS, Cumbler EU, Triebling AT. Coagulopathy due to celiac disease presenting as intramuscular hemorrhage. *J Gen Intern Med.* 2007 Nov;22(11):1608-12. Epub 2007 Sep 1.

6. Pruessner Harold T, MD. Detecting Celiac Disease In Your Patients. *American Family Physician*. March 1st, 1998.

7. Feldman Mark, MD, Friedman Lawrence S, MD, Sleisenger, Marvin H, MD, Gastrointestinal and Liver Disease Pathophysiology/Diagnosis/Management 7th Edition, Volume11, 2002,Saunders

8. Lichtman Marshall A, William Joseph Williams, Beutler Ernest, Kaushansky Kenneth, Kipps Thomas J, Seligsohn Uri, Prchal Joseph. Williams Hematology. McGraw-Hill Professional 7th Edition, Oct. 14th 2005.

9. Walker Allan, Duggan Christopher, Watkins John. Nutrition In Pediatrics:Basic Science And Clinical Applications, Third Edition, 2003. Chapter 49: Harmatz Paul MD, Butensky Ellen RN, MSN, Lubin Bertram MD. Nutritional Anemias. 2003.

10. Graham David R, Bellingham Alistair J, Alstead Elspeth, Krasner Neville, Martindale John. Coeliac Disease Presenting As Acute Bleeding Disorders. *Postgraduate Medical Journal* (March, 1982) 58, 178-179.

11. Alessio Fasano, M.D. Physiological, Pathological, and Therapeutic Implications of Zonulin-Mediated Intestinal Barrier Modulation. *American Journal of Pathology,* 2008;173:1243-1252.

12. Canadian Celiac Association Health Survey (2007) http://tinyurl.com/n3fbj7 Also in *Digestive Diseases And Sciences* April 2007:52(4):1087-1095.

13. Mahida YR. Immunological Aspects of Gastroenterology. Kluwer Academic Publishers 2001.77. David A Nelson, JR., MD., MS., University of Arkanas for Medical Sciences, Little Rock, Arkansas. Gluten-Sensitive Enteropathy (Celiac Disease): More Common Than You Think. *American Family Physician,* December 15, 2002.

14. Devlin Shane MD, Andrews Christopher MD, beck Paul MD, Celiac Disease. *CME Update* May 2004.

15. Kagnoff MF. AGA Institute Medical Position Statement on the Diagnosis and Management of CD. Gastroenterology, *Official Journal of the American Gastroenterological Association* (AGA). December 2006.

16. Friedman Scott L, McQuaid Kenneth R, Grendell James H. Current Diagnosis And Treatment In Gastroenterology. McGraw-Hill, 2003.

17. Frye, Richard E, MD, PhD. and Jabbour, Serge A, MD. Pyridoxine Deficiency. Dec. 18, 2008, emedicine.medscape.com

18. Halfdanarson Thorvardur R. MD; Kumar Neeraj MD; Hogan William J. MBBCh; Murray Joseph A. MD. Copper Deficiency In Celiac Disease. *Journal of Clinical Gastroenterology.* February 2009, Volume 43:issue 2, pp162-164.

19. Goyens Philippe, Brasseur Daniel, Cadranel Samy. Copper Deficiency In Infants With Active Celiac Disease. *Journal of Pediatric Gastroenterology And Nutrition.* 4(4):677-680, August 1985.

20. Foy H, Kondi A: Hypochromic Anemias Of The Tropics Associated With Pyridoxine and Nicotine Acid Deficiencies. *Blood* 13:1054, 1999.

21. Shamir R, Levine A, Yalon-Hacohen M, Shapiro R, Zahavi I, Rosenbach Y, Lerner A, Dinari G. Faecal occult blood in children with coeliac disease. *Eur J Pediatr.* 2000 Nov;159(11):832-4.

22. Glanze Walter D, Anderson Kenneth N, Anderson Lois E, Urdang Laurance, Swallow Helen Harding. Mosby's Medical And Nursing Dictionary. The C.V. Mosby Company, 1986.

23. Nelson David A, JR.,MD., MS. University of Arkansas for Medical Sciences, Little Rock, Arkansas. Gluten-Sensitive Enteropathy (Celiac Disease): More Common Than You Think. *American Family Physician,* December 15, 2002.

24. Allee, Mark R, MD. and Baker, Mary Zoe, MD. Riboflavin Deficiency. emedicine.medscape.com May 18, 2009.

25. Lane Montague, Alfrey JR. Clarence P. The Anemia of Human Riboflavin Deficiency. Blood 1965, Vol. 25, No. 4, pp. 432-442. 1965 American Society of Hematology, Inc. Authors from Departments of Pharmacology And Medicine, Baylor University College of Medicine, and The Department of Medicine and Radioisotope Service, Veterans Administration Hospital, Houston, Texas.

26. Lane M, Alfrey CP: The Anemia of Human Riboflavin Deficiency. *Blood* 22:811, 1963.

27. Snyderman SE, Holt LE Jr, Carretero R, Jacobs KG: Pyridoxine Deficiency In The Human Infant. *Am J Clin Nutr* 1:200, 1953.

28. Snyderman Selma E M.D., Emmett Holt JR. L. M.D., Carretero Rosario M.D., and Jacobs Kathryn M.D. Pyridoxine Deficiency In The Human Infant. *American Journal of Clinical Nutrition,* Vol 1, 200-207, Copyright © 1953 by The American Society for Clinical Nutrition, Inc. Authors from the Department of Pediatrics, New York University College of Medicine.

29. Foy H, Kondi A: Hypochromic Anemias Of The Tropics Associated With Pyridoxine and Nicotine Acid Deficiencies. *Blood* 13:1054, 1999.

30. Semba RD, Bloem MW. The Anemia Of Vitamin A Deficiency: Epidemiology And Pathogenesis. *Eur J Clin Nutr.* 2002 Apr;56(4):271-81

31. William ML, Shoot RJ, O'Neil PL, et al. Role Of Dietary Iron And Fat On Vitamin E Deficiency Anemia Of Infancy. *N Engl J Med* 1975; 292:887-90.

32. Oski FA. Anemia In Infancy: Iron Deficiency and Vitamin E Deficiency. Pediatrics In Review. 1980;1:247-253. doi:10.1542/10.1542/pir.1-8-247. 1980, *American Academy of Pediatrics.*

33. Wilfond Benjamin S, Farrell Phillip M, Laxova Anita, Mischler Elaine. Severe Hemolytic Anemia Associated With Vitamin E Deficiency In Infants With Cystic Fibrosis. *Clinical Pediatrics,* Vol 33, N. 1, 2-7 (1994). DOI: 10.1177/000992289403300101. Departments Of Pediatrics And Nutritional Sciences, University of Wisconsin-Madison, Madison, Wisconsin.

34. Stokes PL, Melikian V, Leeming RL, et el: Folate Metabolism In Scurvey. *Am J Clin Nutr.* 28:126, 1975.

35. Masugi J, MD; Amano M, MD; and Fukuda T, MD. Copper Deficiency Anemia and Prolonged Enteral Feeding. *Annals of Internal Medicine.* 1 September 1994 | Volume 121 Issue 5 | Page 386.

36. Dunlop William M., M.D.; James G. Watson , III, M.D., F.A.C.P.; and Hume David M. , M.D., F.A.C.S. Anemia and Neutropenia Caused by Copper Deficiency. *Annals of Internal Medicine.* 1 April 1974 | Volume 80 Issue 4 | Pages 470-476.

37. Jain Sushil K, MSc,PhD, and Williams Daryl M, MD. Copper Deficiency Anemia. *Am J Clin Nutr* 1988;48:637-40. 1988 American Society for Clinical Nutrition.

38. Sood S. K., Deo M. G., and Ramalingaswami V. Anemia in Experimental Protein Deficiency in the Rhesus Monkey with Special Reference to Iron Metabolism. Blood, 1965, Vol. 26, No. 4, pp. 421-432. © 1965 American Society of Hematology, Inc.

39. Beard John L, Huebers Helmut A, Finch Clement A. Protein Depletion and Iron Deficiency in Rats. *The Journal of Nutrition.* 1984, American Institute of Nutrition.

40. Delmonte L, Aschenasy A, Eyquern A: Studies On The Hemolytic Nature of Protein-Deficiency Anemia In The Rat. *Blood* 24:49, 1964.

41. Crowley Leonard V. An Introduction To Human Disease: Pathology And Pathophysiology Correlations, 2004. Jones and Bartlett Publishing Co; 6th Edition.

42.   Pusztai, S. W. B. Ewen, G. Grant, D. S. Brown, J. C. Stewart, W. J. Peumans, E. J. M. Van Damme and S. Bardocz Antinutritive effects of wheat-germ agglutinin and other N-acetylglucosamine-specific lectins. *The British Journal of Nutrition* 1993 Jul;70(1):313-21.

43.   Scott H. Sicherer, M.D. Manifestations Of Food Allergies: Evaluation And management. *American Family Physician*, 1999.

44.   D. D. Metcalfe, Hugh Sampson, and Ronald Simon. Food Allergy: Adverse reactions to food and food additives. Wiley-Blackwell; 3 edition (Jun 16 2003)

45.   Hadjivassiliou M, Maki M, Saunders DS, Williamson CA, Grunewald RA, Woodroof NM, Korponay-Szabo IR. Autoantibody Targeting of Brain and Intestinal Transglutaminase in Gluten Ataxia. *Neurology* 2006 Feb.14;66(3):373-7.

Chapter 6

1.   Semba Richard D. Handbook Of Nutrition And Ophthalmology. Humana Press, 2007.

2.   Miller Neil R., Walsh Frank Burton, Biousse Valérie, Hoyt William Fletcher. Walsh And Hoyt's Clinical Neuro-Ophthalmology. Lippincott Williams And Wilkins, 2004.

3.   Gibney MJ, Vorster HH, Kok FJ. Introduction to Human Nutrition. Blackwell Publishing 2002.

4.   Gibney MJ, Marinos E, Olle L, Dowsett J. Clinical Nutrition. Blackwell Publishing 2005.

5.   http://www.webmd.com/eye-health/night-vision-problems-halos-blurred-vision-night-blindness

6.   Antinoro Linda. Sharpen All Five Of Your Senses By Eating Better, Smarter. *Environmental Nutrition.* May 1st, 2003.

7.   Iron deficiency could Affect Hearing And Vision. *Decision News Media* SAS, May 7th, 2001.

8.   Clark K, Sowers MR, Wallace RB, Jannausch ML, Lemke J, Anderson CV. Age-Related Hearing Loss And Bone Mass In A Population Of Rural Woman aged 60-85 yrs. *Ann Epidemiol* 1995;5:8-14.

9.   Gates G., Cobb J., D'Agostino R., Wolf P. The Relation Of Hearing In The Elderly To The Presence Of Cardiovascular Disease And Cardiovascular Risk Factors. *Arch Otolaryngol Head Neck Surg.*1993;119:156-161.

10. Makishima K. Anterior Sclerosis As A Cause Of Presbycusis. *Otolaryngology,* 1978;86:322-326.

11. Seidman MD, Khan MJ, Dolan DF, Quirk WS. Age-Related Differences In Cochlear Microcirculation And Auditory Brain Stem Response. *Arch Otolaryngol Head Neck Surg* 1996;122:1221-1226.

12. Willot JF. Aging And The Inner Ear Of Animals. In: Aging And The Auditory System. Singular Publishing Group, Inc., San Diago, CA 1991:18-55.

13. Bales Connie W., Ritchie Christine S. Handbook Of Clinical Nutrition And Aging. Humana Press, 2003.

14. Nexo E, Hansen M, Rasmussen K, Lindgren A, Gräsbeck R. How To Diagnose Cobalamin Deficiency. *Scand J Clin Lab Invest* 1994;54:61-76.

15. Hector M, Burton JR. What Are The Psychiatric Manifestations Of B-12 Deficiency? J *Am Geriatr Soc* 1988;36:1105-1112.

16. Porter KH. Age-Related Hearing Loss And Nutrition In Older Women. Dissertation. University of Georgia, 1999.

17. Healton EB, Savage MD, Brust JCM, Garrett TJ, Lindenbaum MD. Neurologic Aspects Of Cobalamin Deficiency. *Medicine* 1991;70:229-245.

18. Krumholz A, Weiss HD, Goldstein PJ, Harris KC. Evoked Responses In Vitamin B-12 Deficiency. *Ann Neurol* 1981;9:407-409.

19. Fine EJ, Hallett M. Neurophysiological Study Of Subacute Combined Degeneration. *J Neurol Sci* 1980;45:331-336.

20. Fine EJ, Soria E, Paroski MW, Petryk D, Thomasula L. The Neurophysiological Profile Of Vitamin B-12 Deficiency. Muscle Nerve 1990;13:158-164.

21. Houston DK, Johnson MA, Nozza RJ, Gunter EW, Shea KJ, Cutler GM, Edmonds TJ. Age-Related Hearing Loss, Vitamins B-12 And Folate In Elderly Women. *Am J Clin Nutr* 1999;69:564-571.

22. Shemesh Z, Attias J, Ornan M, Shapira N, Shahar A. Vitamin B-12 Deficiency In Patient's With Chronic Tinnitis And Noise Induced Hearing Loss. *AM J Otolaryngol* 1993;2:94-99.

23. Berner B, Odem L, Parving A. Age-Related Hearing Impairment And B Vitamin Status. *Acta Otolaryngol* 2000;120:633-637.

24. Roman GC, An Epidemic In Cuba Of Optic Neuropathy, Sensorineural Deafness, Peripheral sensory neuropathy And Dorsallateral Myeloneuropathy. *J Neurol Sci* 1994;127:11-28.

25. DeNoon Daniel J. Folic Acid may Slow Hearing loss. 2007 WebMD. www.webmd.com

26. Horner K. Review: Morphological Changes Associated With Endolymphatic Hydrops. *Scanning Microsc* 1993;7:223-238.

27. Sewell WF. Neurotransmitters And Synaptic Transmission. In: The Cochlea. Dallos P, Popper AN, Fay RR (eds). Springer-verlag, New York, 1996 pp501-533.

28. Sørensen, MS. Temporal Bone Dynamics, The Hard Way. *Acta Otolaryngol* 1994;512:6-22.

29. Sørensen MS, Bretlau P, Jorgensen B. Quantum Type Bone Remodelling In The Human Otic Capsule. *Acta Otolaryngol* 1992A;496:4-10.

30. Sørensen MS, Bretlau P, Jorgensen B. Bone Remodelling In The Human Otic Capsule. *Acta Otolaryngol* 1992B;496:11-19.

31. Sørensen MS, Bretlau P, Jorgensen B. Fatigue Microdamage In Perilabyrinthine Bone. *Acta Otolaryngol* 1992C;496:20-27.

32. Wangemann P, Schacht J. Homeostatic Mechanisms In: The Cochlea. Dallos P, Popper AN, Fay RR (eds). Springer-verlag, New York, 1996, 130-185.

33. Women With Hearing Loss May Benefit By Boning Up On Calcium. *Environmental Nutr.* Oct. 1998. P,8.

34. Hearing Loss And Nutrition. Timely Topics From The Department Of Human Nutrition. http://www.oznet.ksu.edu/dp_fnut/_timely/hearingloss.htm

35. Li Y, et el. The Effect Of Iron Deficiency Anemia On The Auditory Brainstem Response In Infant. *Nat Med J China* 1994;74:392.

36. Roncagliolo M, Garrido M, Walter T, Peirano P, Lozoff TB. Evidence Of Altered Central Nervous System developments In Infants With Iron Deficiency Anemia At 6 mos: Delayed Maturation Of Auditory Brainstem Responses. *Am J Clin Nutr* 1998;68:683-690.

37. Sun AH, Wang ZM, Xiao SZ, Li ZI, Zheng Z, Li JY. Sudden Sensorineural Hearing Loss Induced By Experiemental Iron Deficiency In Rats. *ORL* 1992A;54:246-250.

38. Agamanolis DP, Chester EM, Victor M, Kark JA, Hines JD, Harris JW. Neuropathology Of Experimental B-12 Deficiency In Monkeys. *Neurology* 1976;26:905-914.

39. Covell WP. Pathological Changes In The Peripheral Auditory Mechanism Due To Avitaminosis (A, B complex,C, D, and E). *Laryngoscope* 1940;2:632-647.

40. Dakshinamurti K, Singer WD, Paterson JA. Effect Of Pyridoxine Deficiency In The Neuronally Mature Rat. *Int J Vit Nutr Res* 1987;57:161-167.

41. Schaeffer MC. Attenuation Of Acoustic And Tactile Startle Responses of Vitamin B-6 deficient Rats. *Physiol Behav* 1987;40:473-478.

42. Stephens MC, Havlicek V, Dashinamurti K. Pyridoxine Deficiency And Development of The Central Nervous System In The Rat. *J Neurochem* 1971;18:2407-2416.

43. Buckmaster PS, Holliday TA, Bai SC, Rogers QR. Brainstem Auditory Evoked Potential Interwave Intervals Are Prolonged In Vitamin B-6 Deficient Cats. *J Nutr* 1993;123:20-26.

44. Seidman MD. Effects of Dietary Restriction And Antioxidants On Presbyacusis. *Laryngoscope* 2000;110:727-738.

45. Ikeda K, Kusakari J, Kobayashi T, Saito Y. The Effect Of Vitamin D Deficiency On The Cochlear Potential and The Perilymphatic Ionized Calcium Concentration of Rats. *Acta Otolaryngol* (Stockh) 1987A;435S:64-72.

46. Idrizbegovic E, Willot JF, Bogdanovic N, Canlon B. Aging And The Total Number Of calbindin D-28K And The Parvalbumin Immunopositive Neurons In The Dorsal Cochlear Nucleus Of CBA/CaJ Mice. In: Abstracts Of The ARO Midwinter Meeting 1999 p258. (abstract)

http://www.aro.org/archives/1999/258.html

47. De Chicchis AR. Vitamin D Deficiency And Auditory Function Of Genetically Disordered Mice. University Of Georgia, USA, 2004.

http://www.reeis.usda.gov/web/crisprojectpages/189531.html

48. Teranishi M, Nakashima T, Wakabayashi T. Effects Of Alpha-Tocopherol On Cisplatin-Induced Ototoxicity In Guini Pigs. *Hear Res* 2001;151:61-70.

49. Prohaska JR, Hoffman RG. Auditory Startle Response Is Diminished In Rats After Recovery From Perinatal Copper Deficiency. *J Nutr* 1996;126:618-627.

50. Sun AH, Xiao SZ, Li BS, Zhao JL, Wang TY, Zhang YS. Iron Deficiency And Hearing Loss. Experimental Study In Growing Rats. *Otorhinolaryngology* And Related Spec 1987A;49:118-122.

51. Sun AH, Xiao SZ, Zheng Z, Li BS, Chao J, Wang TY. A Scanning Electron Microscopic Study Of Cochlear Changes In Iron Deficient Rats. *Acta Otolaryngol* (Stockholm) 1987B;104:211-216.

52. Sun AH, Li JY, Xiao SZ, Li ZJ, Wang TY. Changes In The Cochlear Ion Enzymes And Adenosine Triphosphatase In Experimental Iron Deficiency. *Ann Otol Rhinol Laryngol* 1990;99:988-992.

53. Sun AH, Wang ZM, Xiao SZ, Li ZJ, Ding JC et el. Idiopathic Sudden Hearing Loss And Disturbance Of Iron Metabolism. *ORL* 1992B;54:66-70.

54. Cevette MJ, Franz KB, Brey RH, Robinette MS. Influence of Dietary Magnesium On The Amplitude Of Wave V Of The Auditory Brain Stem Response. *Otolaryngol Head Neck Surg* 1989;101:537-541.

55. Ising H, Handrock M, Gunther T, Fischer R, Dombrowski M. Increased Noise Trauma In Guinea Pigs Through Magnesium Deficiency. *Arch Otorhinolaryngol* 1982;236:139-146.

56. Joachims Z, Babisch W, Ising H. Dependence of Noise Induced Hearing Loss Upon Perilymph Magnesium Concentration. *J Acoust Soc Am* 1983;74:104-108.

57. Gunther T, Rebentisch E, Vormann J. Enhanced Ototoxicity Of Salicylate By Magnesium Deficiency. *Magnesium Bulletin* 1989;11:15-18.

58. Eberhardt MJ, Halas ES. Developmental Delays In Offspring Of Rats Undernourished or Zinc Deprived During Lactation. *Physiol Behav* 1987;41:309-341.

59. Herbert V, Das KC. Folic Acid And Vitamin B-12. In: Modern Nutrition In Health And Disease. Shils ME, Olsen JA, Shike M (eds). Lea And Fabiger, Philadelphia, PA,1994, pp 402-425.

60. Cruickshanks KJ, Klein R, Klein BE, Wiley TL, Nondahl DM, Tweed TS. Cigarette Smoking And Hearing Loss: The Epidemiology Of Hearing Loss Study. *JAMA* 1998;279:1715-1719.

61. Doty Richard L. Handbook of Olfaction And Gustation. Second Edition, 2003. Informa Healthcare.

62. Shils Maurice E (author), Shike Moshe (editor), Ross Catherine A (editor), Caballero Benjamin (editor), Cousins Robert (editor). Modern Nutrition In Health And Disease, Tenth edition, 2005. Lippincott Williams And Wilkins.

63. Bernard Rudy A, Halpern Bruce P. Taste Changes In Vitamin A Deficiency. *The Journal of General Physiology*, 1968.

64. Wolf G, Johnson BC. Vitamin A And Mucopolysaccharide Biosynthesis. *Vitamin Hormones*, 1960;18:439.

65. Leopold Donald L, Holbrook Eric H, Noell Courtney A. Disorders Of Taste And Smell. emedicine/WebMD, 2009.

66. Henkin R, Kelser HR, Joffe IR, et el. *Lancet* 1967;2:1268.

67.   Mattes RD, Heller AD, Rivlin RS. Abnormalties In Suprathreshold Taste Function In Early Hypothyroidism In Humans. In: Melselman HI, Rivlin RS, eds. Clinical Measurement Of Taste And Smell, New York: Macmillan, 1986.

68.   Osaki T, Oshim AM, Tomita Y, et el. *Journal Oral Pathol Med* 1996;25:38-43

69.   Hadjivassiliou M, Grunewald RA, Chattopadhyay AK, Davies-Jones GA, Gibson A, Jarrat JA, et el. Clinical, Radiological, Neurophysiological, And Nuropathological Characteristics Of Gluten Ataxia. *Lancet* 1998;352:1582-5.

70.   Pruessner Harold T, MD. Detecting Celiac Disease In Your Patients. *American Family Physician.* March 1st, 1998.

71.   Feldman Mark, MD, Friedman Lawrence S, MD, Sleisenger, Marvin H, MD, Gastrointestinal and Liver Disease Pathophysiology/Diagnosis/Management 7th Edition, Volume11, 2002,Saunders

72.   Canadian Celiac Association Health Survey (2007) http://tinyurl.com/n3fbj7 Also in Digestive Diseases And Sciences April 2007:52(4):1087-1095.

73.   Barrett KE. Gastrointestinal Physiology. Lange Medical Books/McGraw-Hill 2006.

74.   Nelson David A, JR.,MD., MS. University of Arkansas for Medical Sciences, Little Rock, Arkansas. Gluten-Sensitive Enteropathy (Celiac Disease): More Common Than You Think. *American Family Physician,* December 15, 2002

75.   Lee Eric S, Pulido Jose S. Nonischemic Central Retinal Vein Occlusion Associated With Celiac Disease. Mayo Clinic Proceedings. February 1st, 2005. HighBeam Research, Inc. http://www.highbeam.com

76.   Age-Related Eye Disease Study—Results. National Eye Institute. http://www.nei.nih.gov/amd/

77.   Stye. http://en.wikipedia.org/wiki/Stye

78.   Henri-Bhargava Alexandre, Melmed Calvin, Glikstein Rafael, and Schipper Hyman M. Neurologic Impairment Due to Vitamin E and Copper Deficiencies in Celiac Disease. *Neurology,* Vol. 71, Issue 11, 860-861, September 9, 2008

79.   Types Of Neuropathy-Inflammatory: Celiac Disease. www.millercenter.uchicago.edu Jack Miller Center For Peripheral Neuropathy.

80.   Mayo Clinic Staff. Peripheral Neuropathy. www.mayoclinic.com

81.   Dunlop, William M., M.D.; James G. Watson, III, M.D., F.A.C.P.; and Hume David M., M.D., F.A.C.S. Anemia and Neutropenia Caused by Copper Deficiency. Annals of Internal medicine. 1 April 1974 | Volume 80 Issue 4 | Pages 470-476

82. Hadjivassilou M and Grünwald RA, Davies-Jones GAB. Gluten Sensitivity As a Neurological Illness. *Journal of Neurology,* Neurosurgery, and Psychiatry 2002;72:560-563

83. Kagnoff MF. AGA Institute Medical Position Statement on the Diagnosis and Management of CD. Gastroenterology, *Official Journal of the American Gastroenterological Association* (AGA). December 2006.

84. Alessio Fasano, M.D. Physiological, Pathological, and Therapeutic Implications of Zonulin-Mediated Intestinal Barrier Modulation. *American Journal of Pathology,* 2008;173:1243-1252.

85. Sandyk R., MD, Brennan M.J.W., MB, BCh, PhD. Isolated Ocular Myopathy And Celiac Disease In Childhood. Neurology 1983;33:792. *American Academy Of Neurology.*

86. Bigar Francis, Wiffen Steven J., Bourne William M. Corneal Manifestations of Systemic Diseases. Ophthalmologica. *International Journal of Ophthalmology.* Vol. 215, No. 1, 2001.

87. Hadjivassiliou M, Chattopadhyay AK, Davies-Jones GA, Gibson A, Grunewald RA, Lobo AJ. Neuromuscular Disorder As a Presenting Feature of Coeliac Disease. *J Neurol Neurosurg Psychiatry* 1997;63:770-5.

88. Hadjivassiliou M, Maki M, Saunders DS, Williamson CA, Grunewald RA, Woodroof NM, Korponay-Szabo IR. Autoantibody Targeting of Brain and Intestinal Transglutaminase in Gluten Ataxia. *Neurology* 2006 Feb.14;66(3):373-7.

Chapter 7

1. Pruessner Harold T, MD. Detecting Celiac Disease In Your Patients. *American Family Physician.* March 1st, 1998.

2. Feldman Mark, MD, Friedman Lawrence S, MD, Sleisenger, Marvin H, MD, Gastrointestinal and Liver Disease Pathophysiology/Diagnosis/Management 7th Edition, Volume11, 2002,Saunders

3. Abenavoli L, Proietti I, Leggio L, Ferrulli A, Vonghia L, Capizzi R, Rotoli M, Amerio PL, Gasbarrini g, Addolorato G. Cutaneous Manifestations In Celiac disease. *World Journal Of Gastroenterology.* 2006 February 14;12(6):843-852.

4. Jones FA. The skin: a mirror of the gut. *Geriatrics* 1973; 28: 75-81

5. Holdstock DJ, Oleesky S. Vasculitis in coeliac diseases. *Br Med J* 1970; 4: 369

6. Meyers S, Dikman S, Spiera H, Schultz N, Janowitz HD. Cutaneous vasculitis complicating coeliac disease. *Gut* 1981; 22: 61-64

7. Similä S, Kokkonen J, Kallioinen M. Cutaneous Vasculitis As A Manifestation Of Celiac Disease. *Acta Paediatrica* Volume 71 Issue 6, Pages 1051-1054.

8. Brickman CM, Tsokos GC, Chused TM, Balow JE, Lawley TJ, Santaella M, Hammer CH, Linton GF, Frank MM. Immunoregulatory disorders associated with hereditary angioedema. II. Serologic and cellular abnormalities. *J Allergy Clin Immunol* 1986; 77: 758-767

9. Farkas H, Gyeney L, Nemesanszky E, Kaldi G, Kukan F, Masszi I, Soos J, Bely M, Farkas E, Fust G, Varga L. Coincidence of hereditary angioedema (HAE) with Crohn's disease. *Immunol Invest* 1999; 28: 43-53

10. Farkas H, Visy B, Fekete B, Karadi I, Kovacs JB, Kovacs IB, Kalmar L, Tordai A, Varga L. Association of celiac disease and hereditary angioneurotic edema. *Am J Gastroenterol* 2002; 97: 2682-2683

11. Hautekeete ML, DeClerck LS, Stevens WJ. Chronic urticaria associated with coeliac disease. *Lancet* 1987; 1: 157

12. Gabrielli M, Candelli M, Cremonini F, Ojetti V, Santarelli L, Nista EC, Nucera E, Schiavino D, Patriarca G, Gasbarrini G, Pola P, Gasbarrini A. Idiopathic chronic urticaria and celiac disease. *Dig Dis Sci* 2005; 50: 1702-1704

13. Hodgson HJ, Davies RJ, Gent AE, Hodson ME. Atopic disorders and adult coeliac disease presenting with symptoms of worsening astma. *Lancet* 1986; 2: 1157-1158

14. Cooper BT, Holmes GK, Cooke WT. Coeliac disease and immunological disorders. *Br Med J* 1978; 1: 537-539

15. Scala E, Giani M, Pirrotta L, Guerra EC, De Pita O, Puddu P. Urticaria and adult celiac disease. *Allergy* 1999; 54: 1008-1009

16. Pedrosa Delgado M, Martín Muñoz F, Polanco Allué I, Martín Esteban M. Cold urticaria and celiac disease. *J Investig Allergol Clin Immunol.* 2008;18(2):123-5.

17. Wojnarowska F, Marsden RA, Bhogal B, Black MM. Chronic bullous disease of childhood, childhood cicatricial pemphigoid, and linear IgA disease of adults. A comparative study demonstrating clinical and immunopathologic overlap. *J Am Acad Dermatol* 1988; 19: 792-805

18. Lawley TJ, Strober W, Yaoita H, Katz SI. Small intestinal biopsies and HLA types in dermatitis herpetiformis patients with granular and linear IgA skin deposits. *J Invest Dermatol* 1980; 74: 9-12

19. Chorzelski TP, Jablonska S. Diagnostic significance of the immunofluorescent pattern in dermatitis herpetiformis. *Int J Dermatol* 1975; 14: 429-436

20. Leonard JN, Griffiths CE, Powles AV, Haffenden GP, Fry L. Experience with a gluten free diet in the treatment of linear IgA disease. *Acta Derm Venereol* 1987; 67: 145-148

21. Egan CA, Smith EP, Taylor TB, Meyer LJ, Samowitz WS, Zone JJ. Linear IgA bullous dermatosis responsive to a gluten-free diet. *Am J Gastroenterol* 2001; 96: 1927-1929

22. Durand JM, Lefevre P, Weiller C. Erythema nodosum and coeliac disease. *Br J Dermatol* 1991; 125: 291-292

23. Bartyik K, Varkonyi A, Kirschner A, Endreffy E, Turi S, Karg E. Erythema nodosum in association with celiac disease. *Pediatr Dermatol* 2004; 21: 227-230

24. Douglas JG, Gillon J, Logan RF, Grant IW, Crompton GK. Sarcoidosis and coeliac disease: an association? *Lancet* 1984; 2: 13-15

25. Blackford S, Wright S, Roberts DL. Necrolytic migratory erythema without glucagonoma: the role of dietary essential fatty acids. *Br J Dermatol* 1991; 125: 460-462

26. Goodenberger DM, Lawley TJ, Strober W, Wyatt L, Sangree MH Jr, Sherwin R, Rosenbaum H, Braverman I, Katz SI. Necrolytic Migratory Erythema without glucagonoma: report of two cases. *Arch Dermatol* 1979; 115: 1429-1432

27. Kelly CP, Johnston CF, Nolan N, Keeling PW, Weir DG. Necrolytic migratory erythema with elevated plasma enteroglucagon in celiac disease. *Gastroenterology* 1989; 96: 1350-1353

28. Thorisdottir K, Camisa C, Tomecki KJ, Bergfeld WF. Necrolytic migratory erythema: a report of three cases. *J Am Acad Dermatol* 1994; 30: 324-329

29. Tasanen K, Raudasoja R, Kallioinen M, Ranki A. Erythema elevatum diutinum in association with coeliac disease. *Br J Dermatol* 1997; 136: 624-627

30. Collin P, Korpela M, Hallstrom O, Viander M, Keyrilainen O, Maki M. Rheumatic complaints as a presenting symptom in patients with coeliac disease. *Scand J Rheumatol* 1992; 21: 20-23

31. Rodriguez-Serna M, Fortea JM, Perez A, Febrer I, Ribes C, Aliaga A. Erythema elevatum diutinum associated with celiac disease: response to a gluten-free diet. *Pediatr Dermatol* 1993; 10: 125-128

32. Michaelsson G, Gerden B, Hagforsen E, Nilsson B, Pihl-Lundin I, Kraaz W, Hjelmquist G, Loof L. Psoriasis patients with antibodies to gliadin can be improved by a gluten-free diet. *Br J Dermatol* 2000; 142: 44-51

33. Cardinali C, Degl'innocenti D, Caproni M, Fabbri P. Is the search for serum antibodies to gliadin, endomysium and tissue transglutaminase meaningful in psoriatic patients? Relationship between the pathogenesis of psoriasis and coeliac disease. *Br J Dermatol* 2002; 147: 187-188

34. Woo WK, McMillan SA, Watson RG, McCluggage WG, Sloan JM, McMillan JC. Coeliac disease-associated antibodies correlate with psoriasis activity. *Br J Dermatol* 2004; 151: 891-894

35. Michaelsson G, Gerden B, Ottosson M, Parra A, Sjoberg O, Hjelmquist G, Loof L. Patients with psoriasis often have increased serum levels of IgA antibodies to gliadin. *Br J Dermatol* 1993; 129: 667-673

36. Addolorato G, Parente A, de Lorenzi G, D'angelo Di Paola ME, Abenavoli L, Leggio L, Capristo E, De Simone C, Rotoli M, Rapaccini GL, Gasbarrini G. Rapid regression of psoriasis in a coeliac patient after gluten-free diet. A case report and review of the literature. *Digestion* 2003; 68: 9-12

37. Abenavoli L, Leggio L, Ferrulli A, Vonghia L, Gasbarrini G, Addolorato G. Association between psoriasis and coeliac disease. *Br J Dermatol* 2005; 152: 1393-1394

38. Ojetti V, Aguilar Sanchez J, Guerriero C, Fossati B, Capizzi R, De Simone C, Migneco A, Amerio P, Gasbarrini G, Gasbarrini A. High prevalence of celiac disease in psoriasis. *Am J Gastroenterol* 2003; 98: 2574-2575

39. Damasiewicz-Bodzek A, Wielkoszynski T. Serologic Markers Of Celiac Disease In Psoriatic Patients. *J Eur Acad Dermatol Venereol*. 2008 Sep;22(9):1055-61.

40. Gorgos Diana. Patients With Psoriasis At Higher Risk For Celiac Disease. *Dermatology Nursing* June 1st, 2004.

41. Volta U, Bardazzi F, Zauli D, Defranceschi L, Tosti A, Molinaro N, Ghetti S, Tetta C, Grassi A, Bianchi FB. Serological Screening For Coeliac Disease In Vitiligo And Alopecia Areata. *Br J Dermatol* 1997 May;136(5):801-2.

42. Vitiligo: Autoimmune Silent and Non-Silent Celiac Sign. *stanford.wellsphere.com/.../vitiligo-autoimmune-silent-and-non-silent...sign/736565 -*

43. Collin P, Reunala T. Recognition and management of the cutaneous manifestations of celiac disease: a guide for dermatologist. *Am J Clin Dermatol* 2003; 4: 13-20

44. Reunala T, Collin P. Diseases associated with dermatitis herpetiformis. *Br J Dermatol* 1997; 136: 315-318

45. Triolo G, Triolo G, Accardo-Palumbo A, Carbone MC, Giardina E, La Rocca G. Behcet's disease and coeliac disease. *Lancet* 1995; 346: 1495

46. Buderus S, Wagner N, Lentze MJ. Concurrence of celiac disease and juvenile dermatomyositis: result of a specific immunogenetic susceptibility? *J Pediatr Gastroenterol Nutr* 1997; 25: 101-103

47. Falcini F, Porfirio B, Lionetti P. Juvenile dermatomyositis and celiac disease. *J Rheumatol* 1999; 26: 1419-1420

48. Marie I, Lecomte F, Hachulla E, Antonietti M, Francois A, Levesque H, Courtois H. An uncommon association: celiac disease and dermatomyositis in adults. *Clin Exp Rheumatol* 2001; 19: 201-203

49. Iannone F, Lapadula G. Dermatomyositis and celiac disease association: a further case. *Clin Exp Rheumatol* 2001; 19: 757-758

50. Evron E, Abarbanel JM, Branski D, Sthoeger ZM. Polymyositis, arthritis, and proteinuria in a patient with adult celiac disease. *J Rheumatol* 1996; 23: 782-783

51. Mustajoki P, Vuoristo M, Reunala T. Celiac disease or dermatitis herpetiformis in three patients with porphyria. *Dig Dis Sci* 1981; 26: 618-621

52. Twaddle S, Wassif WS, Deacon AC, Peters TJ. Celiac disease in patients with variegate porphyria. *Dig Dis Sci* 2001; 46: 1506-1508

53. Moore MR, Disler PB. Drug sensitive diseases-I-acute porphyrias. *Adverse Drug React Bull* 1988; 129: 484-487

54. Menni S, Boccardi D, Brusasco A. Ichthyosis revealing coeliac disease. *Eur J Dermatol* 2000; 10: 398-399

55. Schattner A. A 70-year-old man with isolated weight loss and a pellagra-like syndrome due to celiac disease. *Yale J Biol Med* 1999; 72: 15-18

56. Lewis FM, Lewis-Jones S, Gipson M. Acquired cutis laxa with dermatitis herpetiformis and sarcoidosis. *J Am Acad Dermatol* 1993; 29: 846-848

57. Bodvarsson S, Jonsdottir I, Freysdottir J, Leonard JN, Fry L, Valdimarsson H. Dermatitis herpetiformis–an autoimmune disease due to cross-reaction between dietary glutenin and dermal elastin? *Scand J Immunol* 1993; 38: 546-550

58. Montalto M, Diociaiuti A, Alvaro G, Manna R, Amerio PL, Gasbarrini G. Atypical mole syndrome and congenital giant naevus in a patient with celiac disease. *Panminerva Med* 2003; 45: 219-221

59. Wright DH. The major complications of coeliac disease. *Baillieres Clin Gastroenterol* 1995; 9: 351-369

60. Marghoob AA, Schoenbach SP, Kopf AW, Orlow SJ, Nossa R, Bart RS. Large congenital melanocytic nevi and the risk for the development of malignant melanoma. A prospective study. *Arch Dermatol* 1996; 132: 170-175

61. Marghoob AA, Kopf AW, Rigel DS, Bart RS, Friedman RJ, Yadav S, Abadir M, Sanfilippo L, Silverman MK, Vossaert KA. Risk of cutaneous malignant melanoma in patients with 'classic' atypical-mole syndrome. A case-control study. *Arch Dermatol* 1994; 130: 993-998

62. Ackerman AB, Sood R, Koenig M. Primary acquired melanosis of the conjunctiva is melanoma in situ. *Mod Pathol* 1991; 4: 253-263

63. Corazza GR, Masina M, Passarini B, Neri I, Varotti C. Ipetricosi lanuginosa acquisita associata a sindrome celiaca. *G Ital Dermatol Venereol* 1988; 123: 611-612

64. Jones HJ, Mason DH. Oral manifestation of systemic disease. 2nd ed. London: Baillier Tindall, 1990.

65. Ferguson R, Basu MK, Asquith P, Cooke WT. Jejunal mucosal abnormalities in patients with recurrent aphthous ulceration. *Br Med J* 1976; 1: 11-13

66. Fortune F, Buchanan JA. Oral lichen planus and coeliac disease. *Lancet* 1993; 341: 1154-1155

67. Francesco Stefanini G, Resta F, Marsigli L, Gaddoni G, Baldassarri L, Caprio GP, Degli Azzi I, Giuseppe Foschi F, Gasbarrini G. Prurigo Nodularis (Hyde's Prurigo) Disclosing Celiac Disease. *Hepatogastroenterology* 1999 Jul-Aug;46(28):2281-4

68. Randle HW, Winkelmann RK. Pityriasis Rubra Pilaris And Celiac Sprue With Malabsorption. *Cutis* 1980 June;25(6):626-7

69. Acne, Celiac Disease and Gluten Sensitivities
http://www.acne.org/messageboard/root-acne-celiac-t138946.html

70. Menni S, Boccardi D, Brusasco A. Ichthyosis Revealing Coeliac Disease. *Eur J Dermatol* 2000 Jul-Aug;10(5):398-9

71. Green PH, Fleischauer AT, Bhagat G, Goyal R, Jabri B, Neugut AI. Risk Of Malignancy In Patients With Celiac Disease. *Am J Med* 2003 Aug 15;115(3):191-195

72. http://sclero.org/medical/symptoms/associated/a-to-z.html and
http://sclero.org/medical/symptoms/associated/celiac-disease/a-to-z.html

73. Gibney MJ, Marinos E, Olle L, Dowsett J. Clinical Nutrition. Blackwell Publishing 2005.

74. Gibney MJ, Vorster HH, Kok FJ. Introduction to Human Nutrition. Blackwell Publishing 2002.

75. Corazza GR, Andreani ML, Venturo N, Bernardi M, Tosti A, Gasbarrini G. Celiac disease And Alopecia Areata: Report Of A new Association. *Gastroenterology* 1995;109: 1333-1337.

76. Naveh Y, Rosenthal E, Ben-Arieh Y, Etzioni A. Celiac Disease-Associated Alopecia In Childhood. *J Pediatr* 1999;134: 362-364.

77. Philippe Humbert, Fabien Pelletier, Brigitte Dreno, Eve Puzenat, François Aubin. Gluten intolerance and skin diseases. *European Journal Of Dermatology.* Volume 16, Numéro 1, 4-11, January-February 2006.

78. Balch Phyllis A. Prescription For Nutritional Healing. Penguin Group Inc., 2006.

79. Fawcett Robert S, Linford Sean, Stulberg Daniel. Nail Abnormalities: Clues To Systemic Disease. March 15, 2004.

80. Kagnoff MF. AGA Institute Medical Position Statement on the Diagnosis and Management of CD. *Gastroenterology,* Official Journal of the American Gastroenterological Association (AGA). December 2006.

81. Alessio Fasano, M.D. Physiological, Pathological, and Therapeutic Implications of Zonulin-Mediated Intestinal Barrier Modulation. *American Journal of Pathology,* 2008;173:1243-1252.

Chapter 8

1. Pruessner Harold T, MD. Detecting Celiac Disease In Your Patients. *American Family Physician.* March 1st, 1998.

2. Feldman Mark, MD, Friedman Lawrence S, MD, Sleisenger, Marvin H, MD, Gastrointestinal and Liver Disease Pathophysiology/Diagnosis/Management 7th Edition, Volume11, 2002,Saunders

3. Rickets http://www.nlm.nih.gov/medlineplus/ency/article/000344.htm

4. Osteomalacia http://www.nlm.nih.gov/medlineplus/ency/article/000376.htm

5. Osteoporosis http://www.nlm.nih.gov/medlineplus/ency/article/000360.htm

6. Cimaz R, , Bazzi P, Prelle A. Myopathy associated with rickets and celiac disease. *Acta Paediatr* 2000 Apr;89(4):496-7.

7. Lejarraga H, et el. Normal Growth Velocity Before Diagnosis Of Celiac Disease. *J Pediatr Gastrenterol Nutr* 2000;30:552-556.

8. Mehmet D. Demirag, Berna Goker, Seminur Haznedaroglu, Mehmet A. Ozturk, Tarkan Karakan, Reha Kuruoglu· Osteomalacic Myopathy Associated with

Coexisting Coeliac Disease and Primary Biliary Cirrhosis. *Med Princ Pract* 2008;17:425-428

9. Costantine Albany, MD, Zhanna Servetnyk, MD, PhD. Disabling Osteomalacia And Myopathy As The Only Presenting Features Of Celiac Disease: A Case Report. Department of Medicine, St. Luke's Roosevelt Hospital Centre, Columbia University College of Physicians And Surgeons.

10. Harzy T, et el. An Unusual Case of Osteomalacia As The Presenting Feature Of Coeliac Disease. *Rheumatol Int,* 2005. 26(1):p.90-91.

11. Basu RA,et el. Coeliac Disease Can Still present With Osteomalacia! Rheumatology (Oxford), 2000. 39(3):p335-336.

12. Hurtado-Valenzuela JG, Sotelo-Cruz N, López-Cervantes G, de la Barca AM. Tetany caused by chronic diarrhea in a child with celiac disease: A case report. *Cases J.* 2008 Sep 23;1(1):176.

13. Meyer D, Stavropoulos S, Diamond B, Shane E, Green PHR. Osteoporosis In A North American Adult Population With Celiac Disease. *Am J Gastroenterol* 2001, 96:112-119.

14. Vazquez H, Mazure R, Gonzalez D, Flores D, Pedreira S, Niveloni S, Smecuol E, Maurino E, Bai JC. Risk Of Fractures In Celiac Disease Patients: A Cross-Sectional, Case Control Study. *Am J Gastroenterol* 2000;95(1):183-189.

15. Ferretti J, Mazure R, Tanoue P, Marino A, Cointry G, Vazquez H, Niveloni S, Pedreira S, Maurino E, Zanchetta J, Bai JC. Analysis Of The Structure And Strength Of Bones In Celiac Disease Patients. *Am J Gastroenterol* 2003;98(2):382-90.

16. Kemppainen T. Osteoporosis in adult patients with celiac disease. **Bone**, Volume 24, Issue 3, Pages 249-255.

17. Stazi AV, Trecca A, Trinti B. Osteoporosis in celiac disease and in endocrine and reproductive disorders. *World J Gastroenterol.* 2008 Jan 28;14(4):498-505.

18. David A Nelson, JR., MD., MS., University of Arkanas for Medical Sciences, Little Rock, Arkansas. Gluten-Sensitive Enteropathy (Celiac Disease): More Common Than You Think. *American Family Physician*, December 15, 2002.

19. Feldman Mark, MD, Friedman Lawrence S, MD, Sleisenger, Marvin H, MD, Gastrointestinal and Liver Disease Pathophysiology/Diagnosis/Management 7th Edition, Volume11, 2002,Saunders

20. Kagnoff MF. AGA Institute Medical Position Statement on the Diagnosis and Management of CD. Gastroenterology, *Official Journal of the American Gastroenterological Association* (AGA). November 2006.

21. Unsure of Author, The American Journal of Managed Care. 2003;9:825-831.

22. Hafström, et el. A Vegan diet free Of gluten Improves The signs And symptoms Of Rheumatoid Arthritis: The Effects on Arthritis correlate With A reduction In Antibodies To Food Antigens. *Rheumatology* 2001;40:1175-9

23. Lubrano et el. The Arthritis of Celiac Disease: Prevalence And Pattern In 200 Adult Patients. *British Journal of Rheumatology.* 1996;35:1314-8.

24. Bourne JT, Kumar P, Huskisson EC, Mageed R, Unsworth DJ, Wojtulewski JA. Arthritis And Celiac disease. *Ann Rheum Dis* 1985, September;44(9):592-598.

25. Collin P, Korpela M, Hallstrom O, et el. Rheumatic Complaints As A Presenting Symptom In Patients With Celiac Disease. *Scan J Rheumatol* 1992;21:20-3.

26. Usai P. Adult Celiac disease is Frequently Associated With Sarcoilitis. *Dig Dis Sci* 1995;40:1906-8.

27. Carinini C, Brostroff J. Gut and Joint Disease. Annals of Allergy 1985;55:624-625.

28. Keiffer M et al. Wheat gliadin fractions and other cereal antigens reactive with antibodies in the sera of celiac patients. *Clin Exp Immunol 1982;50:651-60.*

29. Parke AI et al. Celiac Disease and Rheumatoid arthritis. *Annals of Rheum Dis* 1984;43:378-380.

30. U. Lindqvist, Å. Rudsander, Å. Boström, B. Nilsson and G. Michaëlsson IgA antibodies to gliadin and coeliac disease in psoriatic arthritis. *Rheumatology* 2002; 41: 31-37.

31. Sandyk R., MD, Brennan M.J.W., MB, BCh, PhD. Isolated Ocular Myopathy And Celiac Disease In Childhood. *Neurology* 1983;33:792. American Academy Of Neurology.

32. Wong M, et el. Proximal Myopathy And Bone Pain As The Presenting Features Of Coeliac Disease. *Ann Rheum Dis*, 2002, 61(1):p87-8.

33. Kleopa KA, Kyriacou K, Zamba-Papanicolaou E, Kyriakides T. Reversible inflammatory and vacuolar myopathy with vitamin E deficiency in celiac disease. *Muscle Nerve*. 2005 Feb;31(2):260-5.

34. Little C, Stewart AG, Fennesy MR. Platelet serotonin release in rheumatoid arthritis: a study in food intolerant patients. *Lancet* 1983;297-9.

35. Albert Selva-O'Callaghan, MD, PhD, Francesc Casellas, MD, PhD, Ines de Torres, MD, PhD, Eduard Palou, MD, PhD, Josep M. Grau-Junyent, MD, PhD, Miquel Vilardell-Tarrés, MD, PhD Celiac disease and antibodies associated with celiac disease in patients with inflammatory myopathy. *Muscle & Nerve,* Volume 35 Issue 1, Pages 49 – 54.

36. Erkan Kozanoglu, Sibel Basaran and M. Kamil Goncu˙ Proximal myopathy as an unusual presenting feature of celiac disease. *Journal Clinical Rheumatology.* Issue Volume 24, Number 1 / February, 2005. Pages 76-78

37. Vivek Jain, Rajeshwar Reddy Angitii, Surjit Singh, Babu Ram Thapa and Lata Kumar Proximal Muscle Weakness—An Unusual Presentation of Celiac Disease. Department of Pediatrics, Postgraduate Institute of Medical Education and Research PGIMER), Chandigarh, India

38. Alawneh K, Ashley C, Carlson JA. Neutrophilic myositis as a manifestation of celiac disease: a case report. Journal of Tropical Pediatrics 2002 48(6):380-381; doi:10.1093/tropej/48.6.380. © 2002 by Oxford University Press

http://www.ncbi.nlm.nih.gov/pubmed/18180977

39. Hardoff D, Sharf B, Berger A. Myopathy as a presentation of coeliac disease. *Dev Med Child Neurol.* 1980 Dec;22(6):781-3.

40. Canadian Celiac Association Health Survey (2007) http://tinyurl.com/n3fbj7 Also in *Digestive Diseases And Sciences* April 2007:52(4):1087-1095.

41. Roubenoff R, Coleman Laura A. Nutrition And Rheumatic Disease. Humana Press, 2008.

42. Selva-O'Callaghan A, et el. Celiac disease And Antibodies Associated With Celiac Disease In Patients With Inflammatory Myopathy. *Muscle Nerve,* 2006;volume 35, issue 1,page 49-54.

43. WebMd Arthritis Basics http://www.webmd.com/osteoarthritis/guide/arthritis-basics

44. Slot D, Locht H. Arthritis As Presenting Symptom In Silent Adult Celiac Disease. *Scandinavian Journal Of Rheumatology.* 2000;29:260-3

45. Stenson W, et el. Increased Prevalence Of Celiac Disease And Need For Routine Screening Among Patients With Osteoporosis. *Archives Of Internal Medicine* February 28, 2005;165(4).

46. Panush RS. Possible role of food sensitivity in arthritis. *Ann Allergy.* 1988 Dec;61(6 Pt 2):31-5.

47.   Toğrol RE, Nalbant S, Solmazgül E, Ozyurt M, Kaplan M, Kiralp MZ, Dinçer U, Sahan B. The significance of coeliac disease antibodies in patients with ankylosing spondylitis: a case-controlled study. *J Int Med Res.* 2009 Jan-Feb;37(1):220-6.

48.   Hernandez L, Green PH. Extraintestinal manifestations of celiac disease. *Curr Gastroenterol Rep.* 2006 Oct;8(5):383-9.

49.   www.arthritis.org/

50.   Carinini C, Brostroff J. Gut And Joint Disease. *Annals Of Allergy.* 1985;55:624-625.

51.   Williams SF, Mincey BA, Calamia KT. Inclusion body myositis associated with celiac sprue and idiopathic thrombocytopenic purpura. *South Med J.* 2003 Jul;96(7):721-3.

52.   M Hadjivassiliou, A K Chattopadhyay, G A B Davies-Jones, A Gibson, R A Grünewald, A J Lobo Neuromuscular disorder as a presenting feature of coeliac disease. *J Neurol Neurosurg Psychiatry* 1997;63:770-775 (December)

53.   April Chang-Miller, M.D. Can a gluten-free diet help reduce signs and symptoms of polymyositis?

       http://www.mayoclinic.com/health/polymyositis/AN00572

54.   Evron E, Abarbanel JM, Branski D, Sthoeger ZM. Polymyositis, arthritis, and proteinuria in a patient with adult celiac disease. *J Rheumatol.* 1996 Apr;23(4):782-3.

55.   Meini A, Morandi L, Mora M, Bernasconi P, Monafo V, Pillan MN, Ugazio AG, Plebani A. An unusual association: celiac disease and Becker muscular dystrophy. *Am J Gastroenterol.* 1996 Jul;91(7):1459-60.

56.   Stenhammar L, Klintberg B, Tevebring J, Henriksson KG. Muscular dystrophy misdiagnosed as hepatic disease in a child with coeliac disease. *Acta Paediatr.* 1995 Jun;84(6):707-8.

57.   Dubowitz Victor. The Floppy Infant. Cambridge University Press. 2 Edition, 1993.

58.   Falcini F, Porfirio B, Lionetti P. Juvenile dermatomyositis and celiac disease. *J Rheumatol* 1999; 26: 1419-1420

59.   Marie I, Lecomte F, Hachulla E, Antonietti M, Francois A, Levesque H, Courtois H. An uncommon association: celiac disease and dermatomyositis in adults. *Clin Exp Rheumatol* 2001; 19: 201-203

60.   Iannone F, Lapadula G. Dermatomyositis and celiac disease association: a further case. *Clin Exp Rheumatol* 2001; 19: 757-758

61. Philippe Humbert, Fabien Pelletier, Brigitte Dreno, Eve Puzenat, François Aubin. Gluten intolerance and skin diseases. *European Journal Of Dermatology*. Volume 16, Numéro 1, 4-11, January-February 2006.

62. Chernoff Ronni. Geriatric Nutrition: The Health Professionals Handbook. Jones And Bartlett Publishers Inc. 3rd edition, 2006.

63. Kamhi Ellen, Zampierson Eugene R. Arthritis: Reverse Underlying Causes Of Arthritis With Clinically Proven Alternative Therapies. Celestial Arts. 2nd Edition, 2006.

64. Gibney MJ, Marinos E, Olle L, Dowsett J. Clinical Nutrition. Blackwell Publishing 2005.

65. Gibney MJ, Vorster HH, Kok FJ. Introduction to Human Nutrition. Blackwell Publishing 2002.

66. Carolyn S. Chen, MD, Ethan U. Cumbler, MD, and Andrzej T. Triebling, MD, PhD Coagulopathy Due to Celiac Disease Presenting as Intramuscular Hemorrhage. *J Gen Intern Med.* 2007 November; 22(11): 1608–1612.

67. Orbach H, Amitai N, Barzilai O, Boaz M, Ram M, Zandman-Goddard G, Shoenfeld Y. Autoantibody screen in inflammatory myopathies high prevalence of antibodies to gliadin. *Ann N Y Acad Sci.* 2009 Sep;1173:174-9.

68. Kagnoff MF. AGA Institute Medical Position Statement on the Diagnosis and Management of CD. Gastroenterology, *Official Journal of the American Gastroenterological Association* (AGA). December 2006.

69. Alessio Fasano, M.D. Physiological, Pathological, and Therapeutic Implications of Zonulin-Mediated Intestinal Barrier Modulation. American Journal of Pathology, 2008;173:1243-1252.

70. Smith Roger, Wordsworth Paul. Clinical And Biochemical Disorders of the Skeleton. Oxford University Press, 2005.

71. Joyce B.J. van Meurs, Ph.D., Rosalie A.M. Dhonukshe-Rutten, M.Sc., Saskia M.F. Pluijm, Ph.D., Marjolein van der Klift, M.D., Ph.D., Robert de Jonge, Ph.D., Jan Lindemans, Ph.D., Lisette C.P.G.M. de Groot, Ph.D., Albert Hofman, M.D., Ph.D., Jacqueline C.M. Witteman, Ph.D., Johannes P.T.M. van Leeuwen, Ph.D., Monique M.B. Breteler, M.D., Ph.D., Paul Lips, M.D., Ph.D., Huibert A.P. Pols, M.D., Ph.D., and André G. Uitterlinden, Ph.D. Homocysteine Levels and the Risk of Osteoporotic Fracture. *New England Journal Of Medicine.* Volume 350:2033-2041, Number 20 May 13, 2004

72. Green, PH. The many faces of celiac disease: clinical presentation of celiac disease in the adult population. *Gastroenterology.* 2005;128:S74-78.

73. Brandimarte G, Tursi A, Giorgetti GM. Changing trends in clinical form of celiac disease. Which is now the main form of celiac disease in clinical practice? *Minerva Gastroenterol Dietol.* 2002;48:121-30.

74. Bagnato GF, Quattrocchi E, Gulli S et el. Unusual Polyarthritis As A Unique Clinical Manifestation Of Celiac Disease. *Rheumatol Int* 2000;20:29-30.

75. Borg AA, Dawes PT, Swan CH, Hathersall TE. Persistant Monoarthritis And Occult Celiac Disease. *Postgrad Med j* 1994;70:51-53.

76. Buderus S, Wagner N, Lentze MJ. Concurrence of celiac disease and juvenile dermatomyositis: result of a specific immunogenetic susceptibility? *J Pediatr Gastroenterol Nutr* 1997; 25: 101-103

Chapter 9

1. Pruessner Harold T, MD. Detecting Celiac Disease In Your Patients. *American Family Physician.* March 1st, 1998.

2. Feldman Mark, MD, Friedman Lawrence S, MD, Sleisenger, Marvin H, MD, Gastrointestinal and Liver Disease Pathophysiology/Diagnosis/Management 7th Edition, Volume11, 2002,Saunders

3. Eliakim Rami ; Sherer David M.; Celiac disease : Fertility and pregnancy. Division of Gastroenterology, Rambam Medical Center, Technion School of Medicine, Haifa, ISRAEL.
http://cat.inist.fr/?aModele=afficheN&cpsidt=859066

4. Rudolph Colin D., Rudolph Abraham M., Hostetter Margaret K., and Lister George E. Rudolph's Pediatrics, McGraw-Hill Professional; 21 edition, 2002.

5. Green-Hernandez Carol, Singleton Joanne K., and Aronzon Daniel Z . Primary Care Pediatrics Lippincott Williams & Wilkins; 1 edition (Jan 1 2001)

6. Hudson Tori. Women's Encyclopedia of Natural Medicine: Alternative Therapies and Integrative Medicine for Total Health and Wellness McGraw-Hill; 2 edition (Sep 20 2007)

7. Ayhan Abaci, MD; Ihsan Esen, MD; Tolga Unuvar, MD; Nur Arslan, MD; Ece Bober, MD. Two Cases Presenting With Pubertal Delay and Diagnosed as Celiac Disease. *Clinical Pediatrics.*
http://cpj.sagepub.com/cgi/content/abstract/47/6/607

8. Gianni Bona, Daniela Marinello, Giuseppina Oderda. Mechanisms of Abnormal Puberty in Coeliac Disease. *Horm Res* 2002;57:63-65.

9. Coeliac disease and birth defects in offspring. (Letters to the editor) *Gut* 2001;49:738; doi:10.1136/gut.49.5.738

10. Aubrey J. Katz M.B., B.Ch., F.C.P., Z. Myron Falchuk M.D., and Harry Shwachman M.D. The Coexistence of Cystic Fibrosis and Celiac Disease. *Pediatrics* Vol. 57 No. 5 May 1976, pp. 715-721.

11. Malena Cohen-Cymberknoh, Michael Wilschanski Concomitant cystic fibrosis and coeliac disease: reminder of an important clinical lesson. *BMJ Case Reports* 2009 [doi:10.1136/bcr.07.2008.0578]. Copyright © 2009 by the BMJ Publishing Group Ltd.

12. Venuta A, Bertolani P, Casarini R, Ferrari F, Guaraldi N, Garetti E. Coexistence of cystic fibrosis and celiac disease. Description of a clinical case and review of the literature. *Pediatr Med Chir.* 1999 Sep-Oct;21(5 Suppl):223-6.

13. Sharma KA, Kumar A, Kumar N, Aggarwal S, Prasad S. Celiac disease in intrauterine growth restriction. *Int J Gynaecol Obstet.* 2007 Jul;98(1):57-9.

14. A.Gasbarrini, E.Torre, C.Trivellini, S.De Carolis, A.Caruso, G.Gasbarrini. Recurrent spontaneous abortion and intrauterine fetal growth retardation as symptoms of coeliac disease. The Lancet, Volume 356, Issue 9227, Pages 399-400.

15. Rami Eliakim, David M. Sherer Celiac Disease: Fertility and Pregnancy. *Gynecol Obstet Invest* 2001;51:3-7.

16. Porpora, Maria Grazia MD; Picarelli, Antonio MD; Porta, Romana Prosperi MD; Di Tola, Marco BSc; D'Elia, Claudia MD; Cosmi, Ermelando Vinicio MD, PhD. Celiac Disease as a Cause of Chronic Pelvic Pain, Dysmenorrhea, and Deep Dyspareunia. *Obstetrics & Gynecology:* May 2002 – Volume 99 – Issue 5, Part 2 – p 937-939.

17. Rujner J. Age at menarche in girls with celiac disease. *Ginekol Pol.* 1999 May;70(5):359-62.

18. Pradhan M, Manisha, Singh R, Dhingra S. Celiac disease as a rare cause of primary amenorrhea: a case report. *J Reprod Med.* 2007 May;52(5):453-5.

19. P Collin, S Vilska, P K Heinonen, O Hällström, P Pikkarainen. Infertility and coeliac disease. *Gut* 1996;39:382-384; doi:10.1136/gut.39.3.382.

20. K Rostami, EAP Steegers, WY Wong, DD ... – Coeliac disease and reproductive disorders: a neglected association. *European Journal of Obstetrics and Gynecology,* 2001 – Elsevier. Science Ireland Ltd. All rights reserved.

21. Bradley, Ryan J. and; Rosen, Mitchell P. MD Subfertility and Gastrointestinal Disease: 'Unexplained' Is Often Undiagnosed. *Obstetrical & Gynecological Survey.* 59(2):108-117, February 2004.

22. Carmen Lívia da Silva Martins; Lenora Gandolfi; Pedro Luiz Tauil; Marilúcia de Almeida Rocha Picanço; Maria Ophelia Galvão de Araujo; Riccardo Pratesi Celiac disease and female infertility: a frequently neglected association. Rev. Bras. *Ginecol. Obstet.* vol.28 no.10 Rio de Janeiro Oct. 2006

23. K. Sharma, A. Kumar, N. Kumar, S. Aggarwal, S. Prasad. Celiac disease in intrauterine growth restriction. International Journal of Gynecology & Obstetrics, Volume 98, Issue 1, Pages 57-59.

24. Gian Mario Tiboni, Maria Grazia de Vita, Raffaella Faricelli, Franca Giampietro and Marco Liberati Serological testing for celiac disease in women undergoing assisted reproduction techniques. *Human Reproduction* Vol 21, No. 2 pp376-379,2206. http://humrep.oxfordjournals.org/cgi/reprint/21/2/376.pdf

25. Kotze, L M S PHD. Gynecologic and Obstetric Findings Related to Nutritional Status and Adherence to a Gluten-Free Diet in Brazilian Patients with Celiac Disease. *Journal of Clinical Gastroenterology*: August 2004 – Volume 38 – Issue 7 – pp 567-574.

26. G.F. Meloni, S. Dessole, N. Vargiu, P.A. Tomasi and S. Musumeci The prevalence of coeliac disease in infertility. *Human Reproduction,* Vol. 14, No. 11, 2759-2761, November 1999.

27. Staci AV, Mantovani A, A risk factor for female fertility and pregnancy: celiac disease. *Gynecol Endocrinol 14*:454-463, 2000.

28. JF Ludvigssona, J Ludvigssona.Coeliac disease in the father affects the newborn.. *Gut* 2001;49:169-175.

29. Gasbarrini A, Torre ES, Trivellini C, De Caroliss, Caruso A, Gasbarrini G. Recurrent Spontaneous Abortion And intrauterine Fetal growth Retardation As Symptoms of celiac Disease. *Lancet* 356: 399-400, 2000.

30. SE Ferguson, GN Smith, MC Walker Maternal plasma homocysteine levels in women with preterm premature rupture of membranes. Medical Hypotheses, Volume 56, Issue 1, Pages 85-90.

31. James L. Mills, John M. Scott, Peadar N. Kirke, Joseph M. McPartlins, Mary R. Conley, Donald G. Weir, Anne M. Molloy and Young Jack Lee, Homocysteine and Neural Tube Defects. *The Journal of Nutrition*.

32. Nelson David A. Gluten-Sensitive Enteropathy (Celiac Disease): More Common Than You Think. *American Family Physician,* December 15th, 2002.

33. Ciacca C, Cirillo M, Auriemma G, Di Dato G, Sabbatini F, Mazzaca G. Celiac Disease And Pregnancy Outcome. *Am J Gastroenterol* 91(4): 718-722, 1996.

34. Norgard B, Fonager K, Sorensen HT, Olsen J. Birth Outcomes Of Women With Celiac Disease: A Nationwide Historical Cohort Study. *Am J Gastroenterol* 94:2435-2440, 1999.

35. Ludvigsson JF, Montgomery SM, Ekbom A. Celiac Disease And Risk Of Adverse Fetal Outcome: A Population Based Cohort Study. *Gastroenterology* 129:454-463, 2005.

36. Kotze LMS PhD. Gynecologic and Obstetric Findings Related to Nutritional Status and Adherence to a Gluten-Free Diet in Brazilian Patients with Celiac Disease. *Journal of Clinical Gastroenterology:* August 2004 - Volume 38 - Issue 7 - pp 567-574.

37. Sher, K S : Jayanthi, V : Probert, C S : Stewart, C R : Mayberry, J F. Infertility, obstetric and gynaecological problems in coeliac sprue. *Dig-Dis.* 1994 May-Jun; 12(3): 186-90.

38. Molteni N, Bardella MT, Bianchi PA. Obstetric and gynecological problems in women with untreated celiac sprue. *J Clin Gastroenterol 1*990; 12: 37-9.

39. Gibney MJ, Marinos E, Olle L, Dowsett J. Clinical Nutrition. Blackwell Publishing 2005.

40. Gibney MJ, Vorster HH, Kok FJ. Introduction to Human Nutrition. Blackwell Publishing 2002.

41. S. E. Ferguson, G. N. Smith and M. C. Walker. Maternal plasma homocysteine levels in women with preterm premature rupture of membranes. Medical Hypotheses Volume 56, Issue 1, January 2001, Pages 85-90.

42. Edward J. Massaro and John M. Rogers. Folate And Human Development. Humana Press; 1 edition (Mar 10 2002)

43. Robert A. DiSilvestro. Handbook Of Minerals As Nutritional Supplements. CRC Press LLC, 2005.

44. Shils, Maurice E Shils, Moshe Shike, and A. Catharine Ross. Modern Nutrition In Health And Disease. Lippincott Williams & Wilkins; 10 edition (Aug 1 2005)

45. Namanjeet Ahluwalia and Hélène Grandje. Nutrition, an Under-Recognized Factor in Bacterial Vaginosis. American Society for Nutrition *J. Nutr.* 137:1997-1998, September 2007.

46. Corenthian J Booker, MD, Coauthor(s): Serdar H Ural, MD. Prenatal Nutrition. http://emedicine.medscape.com/article/259059-overview

47. Devlin Shane MD, Andrews Christopher MD, beck Paul MD, Celiac Disease. *CME Update* May 2004.

48. Kagnoff MF. AGA Institute Medical Position Statement on the Diagnosis and Management of CD. Gastroenterology, *Official Journal of the American Gastroenterological Association* (AGA). December 2006.

49. Sher KS, Jayanthi V, Probert CS, Stewart CR, Mayberry JF. Infertility, obstetric and gynaecological problems in celiac sprue. *Dig Dis* 1994; 12:186-90.

50. Hadjivassiliou M, Gibson A, Davies-Jones GA, Lobo AJ, Stephenson TJ, Milford-Ward A. Does Cryptic Gluten Sensitivity Play A Part In Neurological Illness? *Lancet.* 1996 Feb. 10;347(8998):369-71.

51. M Hadjivassiliou, A K Chattopadhyay, G A B Davies-Jones, A Gibson, R A Grünewald, A J Lobo. Neuromuscular disorder as a presenting feature of coeliac disease. *J Neurol Neurosurg Psychiatry* 1997;63:770-775 (December)

52. Alessio Fasano, M.D. Physiological, Pathological, and Therapeutic Implications of Zonulin-Mediated Intestinal Barrier Modulation. *American Journal of Pathology,* 2008;173:1243-1252.

53. Ferguson R, Holmes GKT, Cooke WT. Celiac disease, fertility and pregnancy. *Scand J Gastroenterol* 1982; 17: 65-8.

54. Susan M. Lark. Menstrual Cramps. Celestial Arts; REV edition (Sep 1 2004). http://tinyurl.com/yde8gpj

55. Jonathan Brostoff and Stephen J. Challacombe. Food Allergy And Intolerance. A Saunders Ltd. Title; 2 edition (Aug 5 2002).

56. Perkin. Food Allergies And Adverse Reactions. Aspen Publishers, Inc.; 1 edition (Sep 21 1990)

57. Wong M, et el. Proximal Myopathy And Bone Pain As The Presenting Features Of Coeliac Disease. *Ann Rheum Dis,* 2002, 61(1):p87-8.

58. Carroccio A, Iacono G, Montalto G, Cavataio F, Marco C Di, Balsamo V, Notar-bartolo A. Exocrine Pancreatic Function in Children With Coeliac Disease Before and After a Gluten-free Diet. *Gut.* Vol 32(7): 796-799, Jul 1991.

59. M Hadjivassiliou,a A K Chattopadhyay,b G A B Davies-Jones,a A Gibson,a R A Grünewald,a A J Loboc Neuromuscular disorder as a presenting feature of coeliac disease. *J Neurol Neurosurg Psychiatry* 1997;63:770-775 (December)

60. Rashtak, M. Ettore, H. Homburger, J. Murray. Comparative Usefulness of Deamidated Gliadin Antibodies in the Diagnosis of Celiac Disease. *Clinical Gastroenterology and Hepatology,* Volume 6, Issue 4, Pages 426-432

61. Green, PH. The many faces of celiac disease: clinical presentation of celiac disease in the adult population. *Gastroenterology.* 2005;128:S74-78.

62. Brandimarte G, Tursi A, Giorgetti GM. Changing trends in clinical form of celiac disease. Which is now the main form of celiac disease in clinical practice? *Minerva Gastroenterol Dietol.* 2002;48:121-30.

63. Alessio Fasano and Carlo Catassi. Current approaches to diagnosis and treatment of celiac disease: an evolving spectrum. *Gastroenterology* 2001:120636-651.

Chapter 10

1. Pruessner Harold T, MD. Detecting Celiac Disease In Your Patients. *American Family Physician*. March 1st, 1998.

2. Feldman Mark, MD, Friedman Lawrence S, MD, Sleisenger, Marvin H, MD, Gastrointestinal and Liver Disease Pathophysiology/Diagnosis/Management 7th Edition, Volume11, 2002,Saunders

3. M Hadjivassiliou, A K Chattopadhyay, G A B Davies-Jones, A Gibson, R A Grünewald, A J Lobo. Neuromuscular disorder as a presenting feature of coeliac disease. *J Neurol Neurosurg Psychiatry* 1997;63:770-775 (December)

4. Alessio Fasano, M.D. Physiological, Pathological, and Therapeutic Implications of Zonulin-Mediated Intestinal Barrier Modulation. *American Journal of Pathology,* 2008;173:1243-1252.

5. Ostojska J, Okniska-Hoffmann E, Gutkowska J, Radzikowski A. Chronic urinary tract infection and celiac disease in children. *Pediatr Pol. 1979* Nov;54(11):1263-71.

6. C. Ciacci, G. Spagnuolo, R. Tortora, C. Bucci, D. Franzese, F. Zingone, M. Cirillo. Urinary Stone Disease in Adults With Celiac Disease: Prevalence, Incidence and Urinary Determinants. The Journal of Urology, Volume 180, Issue 3, Pages 974-979

7. Gama R, Schweitzer FA. Renal calculus: a unique presentation of coeliac disease. *BJU Int.* 1999 Sep;84(4):528-9.

8. Codaccioni JL, Pierron H, Perrimond H, Boyer J, Unal D. Unusual development during a 1-year period of multiple complications (steatorrhea, nephropathy, statural retardation, cerebral accidents) in a 15-year-old child diabetic since the age of 4. abete. 1968 Apr-Jun;16(2):146-52.

9. Woodrow G, Innes A, Boyd SM, Burden RP. A Case Of IgA Nephropathy With Coeliac Disease Responding To A Gluten-free Diet. *Nephrol Dial Transplant* (1993) 8: 1382-1383.

10. Kenar D. Jhaveri, Vivette D. D'Agati, Robert Pursell and David Serur. Coeliac sprue-associated membranoproliferative glomerulonephritis (MPGN). NDT Advance Access published online on July 22, 2009. *Nephrology Dialysis Transplantation*, doi:10.1093/ndt/gfp353

11. R Coppo, A Amore and D Roccatello. Dietary antigens and primary immuno-globulin A nephropathy. *Journal of the American Society of Nephrology*, Vol 2, S173-S180, Copyright © 1992 by American Society of Nephrology

12. Gaboardi F, Perletti L, Cambié M, Mihatsch MJ. Dermatitis herpetiformis and nephrotic syndrome. *Clin Nephrol.* 1983 Jul;20(1):49-51.

13. Mai Ots, Oivi Uibo, Kaja Metsküla, Raivo Uibo, Vello Salupere. IgA-Antigliadin Antibodies in Patients with IgA Nephropathy: The Secondary Phenomenon? *Am J Nephrol* 1999;19:453-458 (DOI: 10.1159/000013497)

14. Jérôme Laurent, Anne Branellec, Jean-Marie Heslan, Guy Rostoker, Charles Bruneau, Chantal André, Liliane Intrator, Gilbert Lagrue. An Increase in Circulating IgA Antibodies to Gliadin in IgA Mesangial Glomerulonephritis. *Am J Nephrol* 1987;7:178-183 (DOI: 10.1159/000167460)

15. S Meyers, S Dikman, H Spiera, N Schultz, and H D Janowitz. Cutaneous vasculitis complicating coeliac disease. *Gut.* 1981 January; 22(1): 61–64.

16. DeCoteau WE, Gerrard JW, Cunningham TA. Glomerulitis in dermatitis herpetiformis. *Lancet.* 1973 Sep 22;2(7830):679–680.

17. Moorthy AV, Zimmerman SW, Maxim PE. Dermatitis herpetiformis and celiac disease: association with glomerulonephritis, hypocomplementia, and circulating immune complexes. *JAMA.* 1978 May 12;239(19):2019–2020.

18. Hilde Kloster Smerud, Bengt Fellström, Roger Hällgren, Sonia Osagie, Per Venge and Gudjón Kristjánsson· Gluten sensitivity in patients with IgA nephropathy. *Nephrology Dialysis Transplantation* 2009 24(8):2476-2481; doi:10.1093/ndt/gfp133.

19.	Pekka Collin, M.D., Jaana Syrjänen, M.D., Jukka Partanen, Ph.D, Amos Pasternack, M.D., Katri Kaukinen, M.D., Jukka Mustonen, M.D. Celiac disease and HLA DQ in patients with IgA nephropathy. *The American Journal of Gastroenterology* Volume 97 Issue 10, Pages 2572 – 2576 Published Online: 11 Aug 2004.

20.	Peeker R, Atanasiu L, Logadottir Y. Intercurrent autoimmune conditions in classic and non-ulcer interstitial cystitis. *Scand J Urol Nephrol.* 2003;37(1):60-3.

21.	E. Stadlmaier , A. Spary, M. Tillich and E. Pilger Midaortic syndrome and celiac disease: a case of local vasculitis. *Journal Clinical Rheumatology* Publisher Springer London Volume 24, Number 3 / June, 2005

22.	S Meyers, S Dikman, H Spiera, N Schultz, and H D Janowitz. Cutaneous vasculitis complicating coeliac disease. *Gut.* 1981 January; 22(1): 61–64.

23.	A Fornasieri, R A Sinico, P Maldifassi, P Bernasconi, M Vegni, G D'Amico. IgA-antigliadin antibodies in IgA mesangial nephropathy (Berger's disease). *Br Med J (Clin Res Ed)* 1987;295:78-80 (11 July), doi:10.1136/bmj.295.6590.78

24.	Laurent J, Branellec A, Heslan JM, Rostoker G, Bruneau C, André C, Intrator L, Lagrue G. An increase in circulating IgA antibodies to gliadin in IgA mesangial glomerulonephritis. *Am J Nephrol.* 1987;7(3):178-83.

25.	Nagy J, Scott H, Brandtzaeg P. Antibodies to dietary antigens in IgA nephropathy. *Clin Nephrol.* 1988 Jun;29(6):275-9.

26.	Kovács T, Mette H, Per B, Kun L, Schmelczer M, Barta J, Jean-Claude D, Nagy J. Relationship between intestinal permeability and antibodies against food antigens in IgA nephropathy. *Orv Hetil.* 1996 Jan 14;137(2):65-9.

27.	Kovács T, Kun L, Schmelczer M, Wagner L, Davin JC, Nagy J. Do intestinal hyperpermeability and the related food antigens play a role in the progression of IgA nephropathy? I. Study of intestinal permeability. *Am J Nephrol.* 1996;16(6):500-5.

28.	Davin JC, Forget P, Mahieu PR. Increased intestinal permeability to (51 Cr) EDTA is correlated with IgA immune complex-plasma levels in children with IgA-associated nephropathies. *Acta Paediatr Scand.* 1988 Jan;77(1):118-24.

29.	Coppo R. The pathogenetic potential of environmental antigens in IgA nephropathy. *Am J Kidney Dis.* 1988 Nov;12(5):420-4.

30.	Jonas F. Ludvigsson, Scott M. Montgomery, Ola Olén, Anders Ekbom, Johnny Ludvigsson and Michael Fored. Coeliac disease and risk of renal disease - a general population cohort study. *Nephrology Dialysis Transplantation* 2006 21(7):1809-1815.

31. Coppo R, Amore A, Roccatello D. Dietary antigens and primary immunoglobulin A nephropathy. *J Am Soc Nephrol.* 1992 Apr;2(10 Suppl):S173-80.

32. Russell MW, Mestecky J, Julian BA, Galla JH. IgA-associated renal diseases: antibodies to environmental antigens in sera and deposition of immunoglobulins and antigens in glomeruli. *J Clin Immunol.* 1986 Jan;6(1):74-86.

33. Sato M, Kojima H, Takayama K, Koshikawa S. Glomerular deposition of food antigens in IgA nephropathy. *Clin Exp Immunol.* 1988 Aug;73(2):295-9.

34. Govind K Makharia, Chalamalasetty Sreenivasa Baba, Rajesh Khadgawat, Suman Lal, MS Tevatia, Kaushal Madan, Siddhartha Dattagupta. Celiac Disease: Variations Of Presentations In Adults. Original Article.

    http://medind.nic.in/ica/t07/i4/icat07i4p162.pdf

35. J. S. Cameron. The Nephrotic Syndrome. Informa HealthCare; 1 edition (Dec 29 1987)

36. Nelson David A. Gluten-Sensitive Enteropathy (Celiac Disease): More Common Than You Think. *American Family Physician,* December 15th, 2002.

37. Kagnoff MF. AGA Institute Medical Position Statement on the Diagnosis and Management of CD. Gastroenterology, *Official Journal of the American Gastroenterological Association* (AGA). December 2006.

38. Hadjivassiliou M, Gibson A, Davies-Jones GA, Lobo AJ, Stephenson TJ, Milford-Ward A. Does Cryptic Gluten Sensitivity Play A Part In Neurological Illness? *Lancet.* 1996 Feb. 10;347(8998):369-71.

39. M Hadjivassiliou, A K Chattopadhyay, G A B Davies-Jones, A Gibson, R A Grünewald, A J Lobo. Neuromuscular disorder as a presenting feature of coeliac disease. *J Neurol Neurosurg Psychiatry* 1997;63:770-775 (December)

40. Abenavoli L, Proietti I, Leggio L, Ferrulli A, Vonghia L, Capizzi R, Rotoli M, Amerio PL, Gasbarrini g, Addolorato G. Cutaneous Manifestations In Celiac disease. *World Journal Of Gastroenterology.* 2006 February 14;12(6):843-852.

41. Devlin Shane MD, Andrews Christopher MD, beck Paul MD, Celiac Disease. *CME Update* May 2004.

42. Enerbäck L, Fall M, Aldenborg F. Histamine and mucosal mast cells in interstitial cystitis. *Agents Actions.* 1989 Apr;27(1-2):113-6.

43. T. Lundeberg, H. Liedberg, L. Nordling, E. Theodorsson, A. Owzarski, P. Ekman, Interstitial Cystitis: Correlation with Nerve Fibres, Mast Cells and Histamine.

British Journal of Urology Volume 71 Issue 4, Pages 427 – 429, 1998 *British Journal of Urology.* Published Online: 26 Nov 2008

44. Chernoff Ronni. Geriatric Nutrition: The Health Professionals Handbook. Jones And Bartlett Publishers Inc. 3rd edition, 2006.

45. Gibney MJ, Marinos E, Olle L, Dowsett J. Clinical Nutrition. Blackwell Publishing 2005.

46. Gibney MJ, Vorster HH, Kok FJ. Introduction to Human Nutrition. Blackwell Publishing 2002.

47. Henri-Bhargava Alexandre, Melmed Calvin, Glikstein Rafael, and Schipper Hyman M. Neurologic Impairment Due to Vitamin E and Copper Deficiencies in Celiac Disease. *Neurology,* Vol. 71, Issue 11, 860-861, September 9, 2008

48. Mayo Clinic Staff. Peripheral Neuropathy. www.mayoclinic.com

49. Dunlop William M., M.D.; James G. Watson , III, M.D., F.A.C.P.; and Hume David M. , M.D., F.A.C.S. Anemia and Neutropenia Caused by Copper Deficiency. *Annals of Internal medicine.* 1 April 1974 | Volume 80 Issue 4 | Pages 470-476

50. S. Rashtak, M. Ettore, H. Homburger, J. Murray. Comparative Usefulness of Deamidated Gliadin Antibodies in the Diagnosis of Celiac Disease. *Clinical Gastroenterology and Hepatology,* Volume 6, Issue 4, Pages 426-432.

51. IgA Antigliadin Antibodies in Children with IgA Mesangial Glomerulonephritis. *The Lancet,* Volume 331, Issue 8594, Pages 1109-1110

52. Brandimarte G, Tursi A, Giorgetti GM. Changing trends in clinical form of celiac disease. Which is now the main form of celiac disease in clinical practice? *Minerva Gastroenterol Dietol.* 2002;48:121-30.

53. Alessio Fasano and Carlo Catassi. Current approaches to diagnosis and treatment of celiac disease: an evolving spectrum. *Gastroenterology* 2001:120636-651.

54. Scholey J, Freeman HJ. Celiac sprue-associated immune complex glomerulonephritis. *J Clin Gastroenterol.* 1986 Apr;8(2):181-3.

55. Coppo R, Basolo B, Rollino C, Roccatello D, Martina G, Amore A, Bongiorno G, Piccoli G. Mediterranean diet and primary IgA nephropathy. *Clin Nephrol.* 1986 Aug;26(2):72-82.

Chapter 11

1. Clinical guideline: Guidelines For The Diagnosis And Treatment Of Children: Recommendations of The North American Society For Gastroenterology, Hepatology, And Nutrition. *Journal of Pediatric Gastroenterology And Nutrition* 40: 1-9. January 2005 Lippincott Williams and Wilkins, Phildelphia.

2. Pruessner Harold T, MD. Detecting Celiac Disease In Your Patients. *American Family Physician.* March 1st, 1998.

3. Feldman Mark, MD, Friedman Lawrence S, MD, Sleisenger, Marvin H, MD, Gastrointestinal and Liver Disease Pathophysiology/Diagnosis/Management 7th Edition, Volume11, 2002,Saunders

4. Ackerman Z, Eliashiv S, Reches A, Zimmerman J. Neurological manifestations in celiac disease and vitamin E deficiency. *J Clin Gastroenterol.* 1989 Oct;11(5):603–605

5. Hoffman RM, Jaffe PE. Plummer-Vinson syndrome. A case report and literature review. *Arch Intern Med.* 1995;155:2008-2011.

6. Dickey W, McConnell B. Celiac disease presenting as the Paterson-Brown Kelly (Plummer-Vinson) syndrome. *Am J Gastroenterol.* 1999;94:527-529.

7. Hadjivassiliou M, Grunewald RA, Chattopadhyay AK, Davies-Jones GA, Gibson A, Jarrat JA, et el. Clinical, Radiological, Neurophysiological, And Neuropathological Characteristics Of Gluten Ataxia. *Lancet* 1998;352:1582-5.

8. Henri-Bhargava Alexandre, Melmed Calvin, Glikstein Rafael, and Schipper Hyman M. Neurologic Impairment Due to Vitamin E and Copper Deficiencies in Celiac Disease. *Neurology,* Vol. 71, Issue 11, 860-861, September 9, 2008

9. Gibney MJ, Vorster HH, Kok FJ. Introduction to Human Nutrition. Blackwell Publishing 2002.

10. Gibney MJ, Marinos E, Olle L, Dowsett J. Clinical Nutrition. Blackwell Publishing 2005.

11. Dickey W. Epilepsy, Cerebral Calcifications, and Coeliac Disease. Lancet 1994;344:1585-6

12. Hadjivassiliou M, Chattopadhyay AK, Davies-Jones GA, Gibson A, Grunewald RA, Lobo AJ. Neuromuscular Disorder As a Presenting Feature of Coeliac Disease. *J Neurol Neurosurg Psychiatry* 1997;63:770-5.

13. Pratesi R, Gandolfi L, Friedman H, Farage L, de Castro CA, Catassi C. Serum IgA Antibodies From Patients With Coeliac Disease React Strongly With Human Brain Blood Vessel Structures. *Scand J Gastroenterol* 1998;33:817-21.

14. Gobbi G, Bouquet F, Greco L, et al. Coeliac Disease, Epilepsy, and Cerebral Calcifications. The Italian Working Group On Coeliac Disease and Epilepsy. *Lancet* 340:439, 1992.

15. Pallis CA, Lewis LP,. Neurological Complications of Coeliac Disease and Tropical Sprue. *The Neurology of Gastroentestinal Disease*. Vol.138. London, W.B. Saunders, 1974.

16. Hadjivassiliou M, Maki M, Saunders DS, Williamson CA, Grunewald RA, Woodroof NM, Korponay-Szabo IR. Autoantibody Targeting of Brain and Intestinal Transglutaminase in Gluten Ataxia. *Neurology* 2006 Feb.14;66(3):373-7.

17. Wilkinson ID, Hadjivassiliou M, Dickson JM, Wallis L, Grunwald RA, Coley SC, Widjaja E, Griffiths PD. Cerebellar Abnormalities On Proton MR Spectroscopy in Gluten Ataxia. *J Neurol Neurosurg Psychiatry.* 2005 Jul;76(7):1011-3.

18. Hadjivassiliou M, Davies-Jones GA, Saunders DS, Grunwald RA. Dietary treatment of Gluten Ataxia. *J Neuro Neurosurg Psychiatry.* 2003 Sep;74(9):1221-4.

19. Hadjivassiliou M, Grünwald R, Sharrack B, Sanders D, Lobo A, Williamson C, Woodroofe N, Wood N, Davies-Jones A. Gluten Ataxia in Perspective: Epidemiology, Genetic susceptibility, And Clinical Characteristics. *Brain* 2003 Mar;126(pt 3): 685-91.

20. Hadjivassilou M, Boscolo S, Davies-Jones GA, Grunwald RA, Not T, Sanders DS, Simpson JE, Tongiorgi E, Williamson CA, Woodroofe NM. The Humoral Response in the Pathogenesis of Gluten Ataxia. *Neurology* 2002 Apr 23;58(8):1221-6.

21. Hadjivassilou M, Grünwald RA, Lawden M, Davies-Jones GA, Powell T, Smith CM. Headache and CNS White Matter Abnormalties Associated with Gluten Sensitivity. *Neurology* 2001 Feb 13;56(3):385-8.

22. Hadjivassilou M and Grünwald R. The Neurology of Gluten Sensitivity: Science vs. Conviction. *Practical Neurology* 2004 4, 124-126.

23. Cooke WT, Thomas-Smith W. Neurological Disorders Associated with Adult Coeliac Disease. *Brain* 1966;89:683-722.

24. Lu CS, Thompson PD, Quin NP, et al. Ramsay Hunt syndrome and Coeliac disease: A New Association. *Mov Disord* 1986;209-19

25. Hadjivassilou M and Grünwald RA, Davies-Jones GAB. Gluten Sensitivity As a Neurological Illness. *Journal of Neurology, Neurosurgery, and Psychiatry* 2002;72:560-563

26. Hadjivassilou M, Grünwald RA, Davies-Jones GAB. Causes of Cerebellar Degeneration: Gluten Ataxia in Perspective. *J Neurol Sci* 2001;187(suppl1):S520.

27. Hahn JS, Sum JM, Crowley RS, et al. Coeliac Disease Presenting as Gait Disturbance and Ataxia in Infancy. *J Child Neurol* 1998;13:351-3.

28. Gabrielli M, Cremonini F, Fiore G, Addolorato G, Padalino C, Candelli M, De Leo ME, Santarelli L, Giacovazzo M, Gasbarrini A, Pola P, Gasbarrini A. Association between migraine and Celiac disease: results from a preliminary case-control and therapeutic study. *Am J Gastroenterol.* 2003 Mar;98(3):625-9.

29. F. Morello, G. Ronzani and F. Cappellari Migraine, cortical blindness, multiple cerebral infarctions and hypocoagulopathy in celiac disease. *Journal Neuological Sciences*. Volume 24, Number 2 / June, 2003

30. Bushara K. Neurological Presentation Of Celiac Disease. *Gastroenterology* Vol 128, Issue 4, pages 592-597.

31. Spina M, Incorpora G, Trigilia T, Branciforte F, Franco G, Di Gregorio F. Headache as atypical presentation of celiac disease: report of a clinical case. *Pediatr Med Chir.* 2001 Mar-Apr;23(2):133-5.

32. Lucio Giordano, MD Monica Valotti, BSc Adonella Bosetti, BSc Patrizia Accorsi, MD Luigi Caimi, MD Luisa Imberti, MD. Celiac Disease-Related Antibodies in Italian Children With Epilepsy. *Pediatric Neurology* – Volume 41, Issue 1 (July 2009)

33. Hugo A. Arroyo, MD, Susana De Rosa, MD, Victor Ruggieri, MD, María T. G. de Dávila, MD, Natalio Fejerman, MD. Epilepsy, Occipital Calcifications, and Oligosymptomatic Celiac Disease in Childhood. *Journal of Child Neurology,* Vol. 17, No. 11, 800-806 (2002).

34. M. Antigoni, I. Xinias, P. Theodouli, E. Karatza, F. Maria, C. Panteliadis, K. Spiroglou. Increased Prevalence of Silent Celiac Disease Among Greek Epileptic Children. Pediatric Neurology, Volume 36, Issue 3, Pages 165-169.

35. Antigoni Mavroudi, MD, Eliza Karatza, MD, Theodouli Papastavrou, MD, Christos Panteliadis, MD, Kleomenis Spiroglou, MD. Successful Treatment of Epilepsy and Celiac Disease With a Gluten-Free Diet. *Pediatric Neaurology* Volume 33, Issue 4, Pages 292-295 (October 2005).

36. Elizabeth Harper, Harold Moses, and Andre Lagrange. Occult celiac disease presenting as epilepsy and MRI changes that responded to gluten-free diet. *Neurology,* Vol. 68, Issue 7, 533-534, February 13, 2007

37. Alberto Fois, Marina Vascotto[1], Rosanna Maria Di Bartolo[1] and Virginia Di Marco[1] Celiac disease and epilepsy in pediatric patients. *Journal Child's Nervous System.* Volume 10, Number 7 / September, 1994

38. Canales P, Mery VP, Larrondo FJ, Bravo FL, Godoy J. Epilepsy and celiac disease: favorable outcome with a gluten-free diet in a patient refractory to antie-pileptic drugs. *Neurologist.* 2006 Nov;12(6):318-21.

39. A.Mavroudi, E.Karatza, T.Papastavrou, C.Panteliadis, K.Spiroglou. Successful Treatment of Epilepsy and Celiac Disease With a Gluten-Free Diet. Pediatric Neurology, Volume 33, Issue 4, Pages 292-295

40. Khalafalla O. Bushara, MD, Martha Nance, MD and Christopher M. Gomez, MD PhD. Antigliadin antibodies in Huntington's disease. *Neurology* 2004;62:132-133

41. Kitiyakara T, Jackson M, Gorard DA. Refractory coeliac disease, small-bowel lymphoma and chorea. *J R Soc Med.* 2002 Mar;95(3):133-4.

42. Victor S. C. Fung, MB, BS, Andrew Duggins, MB, BS, John G. L. Morris, DM (Oxon), Ivan T. Lorentz, MB, BS. Progressive myoclonic ataxia associated with celiac disease presenting as unilateral cortical tremor and dystonia. *Movement Disorders* Volume 15 Issue 4, Pages 732 – 734, 2001.

43. Hahn et al. Celiac Disease Presenting as Gait Disturbance and Ataxia in Infancy. J Child Neurol.1998; 13: 351-353.

44. Tunc T, Okuyucu E, Ucleri S, Sonmez T, Coskun O, Selvi E, Inan LE. bclinical celiac disease with cerebellar ataxia. 2004, N° 2 (Vol. 104/2). *Ministry of Health, Ankara Research and Training Hospital Department of Neurology, Ankara, Turkey*

45. M. T. Pellecchia, R. Scala, A. Filla, G. De Michele, C. Ciacci, and P. Barone. Idiopathic cerebellar ataxia associated with celiac disease: lack of distinctive neurological features. *J Neurol Neurosurg Psychiatry.* 1999 January; 66(1): 32–35.

46. Finelli PF, McEntee WJ, Ambler M, Kestenbaum D. Adult celiac disease presenting as cerebellar syndrome. *Neurology.* 1980 Mar;30(3):245–249.

47. Kaplan JG, Pack D, Horoupian D, DeSouza T, Brin M, Schaumburg H. Distal axonopathy associated with chronic gluten enteropathy: a treatable disorder. *Neurology.* 1988 Apr;38(4):642–645.

48. Kelkar P, Ross MA, Murray J. Mononeuropathy multiplex associated with celiac sprue. *Muscle Nerve.* 1996 Feb;19(2):234–236.

49. Ward ME, Murphy JT, Greenberg GR. Celiac disease and spinocerebellar degeneration with normal vitamin E status. *Neurology.* 1985 Aug;35(8):1199–1201.

50. Collin P, Pirttilä T, Nurmikko T, Somer H, Erilä T, Keyriläinen O. Celiac disease, brain atrophy, and dementia. *Neurology.* 1991 Mar;41(3):372–375.

51. Mauro A, Orsi L, Mortara P, Costa P, Schiffer D. Cerebellar syndrome in adult celiac disease with vitamin E deficiency. *Acta Neurol Scand.* 1991 Aug;84(2):167–170.

52. T Matsuzaka, H Tanaka, M Fukuda, M Aoki, Y Tsuji, and H Kondoh. Relationship between vitamin K dependent coagulation factors and anticoagulants (protein C and protein S) in neonatal vitamin K deficiency. *Arch Dis Child.* 1993 March; 68(3 Spec No): 297–302.

53. Jorge O, Jorge A, Camus G. Celiac disease associated with antiphospholipid syndrome. *Rev Esp Enferm Dig.* 2008 Feb;100(2):102-3.

54. Hall WH. Proximal muscle atrophy in adult celiac disease. *Am J Dig Dis.* 1968 Aug;13(8):697–704.

55. Bhatia KP, Brown P, Gregory R, Lennox GG, Manji H, Thompson PD, Ellison DW, Marsden CD. Progressive myoclonic ataxia associated with coeliac disease. The myoclonus is of cortical origin, but the pathology is in the cerebellum. *Brain.* 1995 Oct;118 (:1087–1093.

56. Cooke WT, Smith WT. Neurological disorders associated with adult coeliac disease. *Brain.* 1966 Dec;89(4):683–722.

57. Tietge UJ, Schmidt HH, Manns MP. Neurological complications in celiac disease. *Am J Gastroenterol.* 1997 Mar;92(3):540.

58. Gobbi G, Bouquet F, Greco L, Lambertini A, Tassinari CA, Ventura A, Zaniboni MG. Coeliac disease, epilepsy, and cerebral calcifications. The Italian Working Group on Coeliac Disease and Epilepsy. *Lancet.* 1992 Aug 22;340(8817):439–443.

59. Ghezzi A, Filippi M, Falini A, Zaffaroni M. Cerebral involvement in celiac disease: a serial MRI study in a patient with brainstem and cerebellar symptoms. *Neurology.* 1997 Nov;49(5):1447–1450.

60. Hermaszewski RA, Rigby S, Dalgleish AG. Coeliac disease presenting with cerebellar degeneration. *Postgrad Med J.* 1991 Nov;67(793):1023–1024.

61. Chinnery PF, Reading PJ, Milne D, Gardner-Medwin D, Turnbull DM. CSF antigliadin antibodies and the Ramsay Hunt syndrome. *Neurology.* 1997 Oct;49(4):1131–1133.

62. Kristoferitsch W, Pointner H. Progressive cerebellar syndrome in adult coeliac disease. *J Neurol.* 1987 Feb;234(2):116–118.

63. Hadjivassiliou M, Chattopadhyay AK, Davies-Jones GA, Gibson A, Grünewald RA, Lobo AJ. Neuromuscular disorder as a presenting feature of coeliac disease. *J Neurol Neurosurg Psychiatry.* 1997 Dec;63(6):770–775.

64. Muller AF, Donnelly MT, Smith CM, Grundman MJ, Holmes GK, Toghill PJ. Neurological complications of celiac disease: a rare but continuing problem. *Am J Gastroenterol.* 1996 Jul;91(7):1430–1435.

65. Matthias Kieslich, MD, Germán Errázuriz, MD, Hans Georg Posselt, MD, Walter Moeller-Hartmann, MD, Friedhelm Zanella, MD, and Hansjosef Boehles, MD. *Brain* White-Matter Lesions in Celiac Disease: A Prospective Study of 75 Diet-Treated Patients. *PEDIATRICS Vol.* 108 No. 2 August 2001, p. e21.

66. Addolorato G et al (2004) Regional cerebral hypoperfusion in patients with celiac disease *Am J Med* 116 (312-317)

67. B. Emanuel, A. Lieberman. Electroencephalogram changes in celiac disease. The Journal of Pediatrics, Volume 62, Issue 3, Pages 435-437.

68. Gefel Dov; Doncheva Maria; Ben-Valid Eli; el Wahab-Daraushe Abed; Lugassy Gilles; Sela Ben-Ami. Recurrent stroke in a young patient with celiac disease and hyperhomocysteinemia. *The Israel Medical Association Journal* : IMAJ 2002;4(3):222-3.

69. Audia, S (S); Duchêne, C (C); Samson, M (M); Muller, G (G); Bielefeld, P (P); Ricolfi, F (F); Giroud, M (M); Besancenot, J-F (JF). Stroke in young adults with celiac disease. Case Reports; English Abstract; Journal Article. La Revue de médecine interne / fondée … par la Société nationale francaise de médecine interne (Rev Med Interne), published in France.

70. Fiona C. Goodwin, MB, R.Mark Beattie, BSc, MB, BS, John Millar, BM, BS, Fenella J. Kirkham, BA, MB, BChir Celiac disease and childhood stroke. *Pediatric Neurology* Volume 31, Issue 2, Pages 139-142 (August 2004).

71. El Moutawakil B, Chourkani N, Sibai M, Moutaouakil F, Rafai M, Bourezgui M, Slassi I. Celiac disease and ischemic stroke. *Rev Neurol* (Paris). 2009 Jan 12.

72. Dubey Saroj, Agarwal Naresh and A.S. Puri. Atypical celiac disease with IgA deficiency presenting as Plummer–Vinson syndrome: a case report. *Journal Esophagus* Volume 3, Number 1 / April, 2006 Pages 23-25.

73. W Dickey MD and B McConnell MD Celiac disease presenting as the Paterson-Brown Kelly (Plummer-Vinson) syndrome. *American Journal of Gastroenterology* (1999) 94, 527–529; doi:10.1111/j.1572-0241.1999.889_r.x

74.   Marios Hadjivassiliou MD, Pascale Aeschlimann Bsc, Alexander Strigun Msc, David S. Sanders MD, Nicola Woodroofe PhD, Daniel Aeschlimann PhD. Autoantibodies in gluten ataxia recognize a novel neuronal transglutaminase. *Annals of Neurology* Volume 64, Issue 3, pages 332–343, 28 September 2008.

75.   F Alehan, F Ozçay, I Erol, O Canan, T Cemil. Increased Risk For coeliac Disease in paediatric Patients With Migraine. *Cephalalgia* Volume 28, Issue 9, pages 945–949, September 2008

76.   M. Hadjivassiliou, MD;, R.A. Grünewald, DPhil;, M. Lawden, MD;, G.A.B. Davies–Jones, MD;, T. Powell, FRCP; and C.M.L. Smith, FRCPath. Headache and CNS white matter abnormalities associated with gluten sensitivity. Neurology 2001;56:385-388

77.   Nathanel Zelnik MD, Avi Pacht MD, Raid Obeid MD, Aaron Lerner MD. Range of Neurological Disorders In Patients With Celiac Disease. *Pediatrics* Vol. 113 No. 6 June 2004, pp.1672-1676.

78.   Armando D'Angelo, Silvana Viganò D'Angelo. Protein S deficiency. *Haematologica,* Vol 93, Issue 4, 498-501.

79.   Wheat allergy and ataxia. Ataxia Center, University of Minnesota. http://www.ataxiacenter.umn.edu/aboutataxia/sporadic/wheat/home.html

80.   Lea ME, Harbord M, Sage MR. Bilateral Occipital Calcification Associated With Celiac Disease, Folate Deficiency, And Epilepsy. *AJNR 16*:1498-1500, Aug 1995.

81.   Tunc T, Okuyucu E, Ucleri S, Sonmez T, Coskun O, Selvi E, Inan LE. Subclinical celiac disease with cerebellar ataxia. *Acta Neurol Belg.,* 2004 Jun;104(2):84-6.

82.   Hernández MA, Colina G, Ortigosa L. Epilepsy, cerebral calcifications and clinical or subclinical coeliac disease. Course and follow up with gluten-free diet. *Seizure.* 1998 Feb;7(1):49-54.

83.   Díaz RM, González-Rabelino G, Delfino A. Epilepsy, cerebral calcifications and coeliac disease. The importance of an early diagnosis. *Rev Neurol.* 2005 Apr 1-15;40(7):417-20.

84.   Bilic E, Bilic E, Sepec BI, Vranjes D, Zagar M, Butorac V, Cerimagic D. Stiff-person syndrome in a female patient with type 1 diabetes, dermatitis herpeti-formis, celiac disease, microcytic anemia and copper deficiency Just a coincidence or an additional shared pathophysiological mechanism? *Clin Neurol Neurosurg.* 2009 May 25.

85.   I D Wilkinson, M Hadjivassiliou, J M Dickson, L Wallis, R A Grünewald, S C Coley, E Widjaja, P D Griffiths. Cerebellar abnormalities on proton MR spectro-

scopy in gluten ataxia. *Journal of Neurology Neurosurgery and Psychiatry* 2005;76:1011-1013.

86. Hadjivassiliou M, Grünewald R. Reply to : Gluten Ataxia "In Perspective".*Brain* Vol 126, No. 9, E5, September 2003.

87. Helge Topka. Chapter 2: Normal functions of the cerebellum. Klockgether Thomas. Handbook of Ataxia disorders. Informa Healthcare; 1 edition (Aug 18 2000)

88. Jay H. Stein, Merle A. Sande, Nathan J. Zvaifler, and John H. Klippel. *Internal Medicine* A Mosby Title; 5 edition (Feb 1 1998)

89. School of Medicine News: University of Maryland School of Medicine Scientists Pinpoint Critical Molecule to Celiac, Possibly Other Autoimmune Disorders. Tuesday, September 29, 2009.

    http://somvweb.som.umaryland.edu/absolutenm/templates/?a=915

90. Giuseppe Gobbi, Gianna Bertani and the Italian Working Group (IWG) Chapter 10: on Celiac Disease and Epilepsy. Gobbi G Epilepsy & Other Neurological Disorders in Coeliac Disease *John Libbey & Co;* 1 edition (1997).

91. *Paul V, Henkerr J, Todt H, Eysold R. Z.Klin.Med., 1985; 40: 707-709.*

92. B. Emanuel, A. Lieberman. Electroencephalogram changes in celiac disease. The Journal of Pediatrics, Volume 62, Issue 3, Pages 435-437

93. Regional cerebral hypoperfusion in patients with celiac disease. The American Journal of Medicine, Volume 116, Issue 5, Pages 312-317

94. R. L. Chin, MD, H. W. Sander, MD, T. H. Brannagan, MD, P. H.R. Green, MD, A. P. Hays, MD, A. Alaedini, PhD and N. Latov, MD PhD. Celiac Neuropathy. Neurology 2003;60:1581-1585.

95. Wilkinson ID, Hadjivassiliou M, Dickson JM, Wallis L, Grünwald RA, Coley SC, Widjaja E, Griffiths PD. Cerebellar Abnormalities On Proton MR Spectroscopy in Gluten Ataxia. *J Neurol Neurosurg Psychiatry.* 2005 Jul;76(7):1011-3.

96. Cervio E, Volta U, Verri M, Boschi F, Pastoris O, Granito A, Barbara G, Parisi C, Felicani C, Tonini M, DeGiorgio R. Sera Of Patients With Celiac Disease And Neurologic Disorders Evoke A Mitrochondrial-Depend. *Gastroenterology* (2007) 133: 195-206.

97. Vojdani Aristo, PhD., MT.; O'Bryan Thomas, D.C., C.C.N., D.A.C.B.N.. The Immunology Of Gut Sensitivity Beyond The Intestinal Tract. 1

98.   Marios Hadjivassiliou, David S. Sanders, Nicola Woodroofe, Claire Williamson and Richard A. Grünewald. Gluten Ataxia. Springer new York, volume 7, number 3/September 2008.

99.   Katrin Bürk, MD, Marie-Louise Farecki, Georg Lamprecht, MD, Guenter Roth, PhD, Patrice Decker, PhD, Michael Weller, MD, Hans-Georg Rammensee, PhD, Wolfang Oertel, MD. Neurological Symptoms In Patients With Biopsy Proven Celiac Disease. *Movement Disorders,* Volume 24, Issue 16, pages 2358-2362, 2009.

100. Cervio E, Volta U, Verri M, et el. Sera of Patients With Celiac Disease And neurological Disorders Evoke A Mitochondrial-dependent apoptosis in vitro. *Gastroenterology,* 2007;133:195-206.

101. A.Alaedini. Ganglioside reactive antibodies in the neuropathy associated with celiac disease. Journal of Neuroimmunology, Volume 127, Issue 1, Page 145.

102. Volta U, De Giorgio R, Granito A, Stanghellini V, Barbara G, Avoni P, Liguori R, Petrolini N, Fiorini E, Montagna P, Corinaldesi R, Bianchi FB. Anti-ganglioside antibodies in coeliac disease with neurological disorders. *Dig Liver Dis*. 2006 Mar;38(3):183-7. Epub 2006 Feb 7.

103. E Myrsky, K Kaukinen, M Syrjänen, I R Korponay-Szabó, M Mäki, and K Lindfors Coeliac disease-specific autoantibodies targeted against transglutaminase 2 disturb angiogenesis. *Clin Exp Immunol*. 2008 April; 152(1): 111–119.

104. Snell Richards S. Clinical Neuroanatomy. Lippincott Williams & Wilkins; 7 edition (Jan 1 2009)

105. Fujimoto S, Yokochi K, Togari H, Nishimura Y, Inukai K, Futamura M, Sobajima H, Suzuki S, Wada Y. Neonatal cerebral infarction: symptoms, CT findings and prognosis. *Brain* Dev. 1992 Jan;14(1):48-52.

106. Zsolt Barta, Gabriella Mekkel, Margit Zeher, and K. O. Bushara. Antigliadin antibodies in Huntington's disease. Neurology, Vol. 63, Issue 4, -a August 24, 2004.

107. Deepak Gupta and Naureen Mirza Systemic lupus erythematosus, celiac disease and antiphospholipid antibody syndrome: a rare association. *Journal Rheumatology International,* Volume 28, Number 11 / September, 2008.

108. R Shamir, Y Shoenfeld, M Blank, R Eliakim, N Lahat, E Sobel, E Shinar, A Lerner.The prevalence of coeliac disease antibodies in patients with the antiphospholipid syndrome.

109. Pengiran Tengah CD, Lock RJ, Unsworth DJ, Wills AJ. Multiple sclerosis and occult gluten sensitivity. *Neurology.* 2004 Jun 22;62(12):2326-7.

110. Reichelt KL, Jensen D. IgA antibodies against gliadin and gluten in multiple sclerosis. *Acta Neurol Scand.* 2004 Oct;110(4):239-41.

111. Shor DB, Barzilai O, Ram M, Izhaky D, Porat-Katz BS, Chapman J, Blank M, Anaya JM, Shoenfeld Y. Gluten sensitivity in multiple sclerosis: experimental myth or clinical truth? *Ann N Y Acad Sci.* 2009 Sep;1173:343-9.

112. Leong EM, Semple SJ, Angley M, Siebert W, Petkov J, McKinnon RA. Complementary and alternative medicines and dietary interventions in multiple sclerosis: what is being used in South Australia and why? Quality Use of Medicines and Pharmacy Research Centre, Sansom Institute, University of South Australia, North Terrace, Adelaide, SA 5000, Australia. *Complement Ther Med.* 2009 Aug;17(4):216-23. Epub 2009 Apr 21.

   http://www.ncbi.nlm.nih.gov/pubmed/19632549

113. Ferrò MT, Franciotta D, Riccardi T, D'Adda E, Mainardi E, Montanelli A. A case of multiple sclerosis with atypical onset associated with autoimmune hepatitis and silent coeliac disease. *Neurol Sci.* 2008 Feb;29(1):29-31.

114. Hernández-Lahoz C, Rodríguez S, Tuñón A, Saiz A, Santamarta E, Rodrigo L. Neurologia. Sustained clinical remission in a patient with remittent-recurrent multiple sclerosis and celiac disease gluten-free diet for 6 years. *Neurologia.* 2009 Apr;24(3):213-5.

115. Ghezzi A, Zaffaroni M. Neurological manifestations of gastrointestinal disorders, with particular reference to the differential diagnosis of multiple sclerosis. *Neurol Sci.* 2001 Nov;22 Suppl 2:S117-22.

116. Shor DB, Barzilai O, Ram M, Izhaky D, Porat-Katz BS, Chapman J, Blank M, Anaya JM, Shoenfeld Y. Gluten sensitivity in multiple sclerosis: experimental myth or clinical truth? Center for Autoimmune Diseases, Department of Medicine B, Sheba Medical Center, Ramat-Gan, Israel. *Ann N Y Acad Sci.* 2009 Sep;1173:343-9.author reply 933-4.

117. http://wildhorse.insinc.com/directms03oct2007/ Video by Potential Therapeutic Characteristics of Pre-agricultural Diets in the Prevention and Treatment of Multiple Sclerosis . This presentation is narrated by Dr Loren Cordain of the Colorado State University, USA.

118. Hadjivassiliou M, Aeschlimann P, Strigun A, Sanders DS, Woodroofe N, Aeschlimann D. Autoantibodies in gluten ataxia recognize a novel neuronal trans-glutaminase. *Ann Neurol* 2008 Sep;64(3):332-43.

119. Bansal AK, Lindemann MJ, Ramsperger V, Kumar V. Celiac G+ antibody assay for the detection of autoantibodies in celiac disease. *Ann N Y Acad Sci.* 2009 Sep;1173:36-40. http://www.ncbi.nlm.nih.gov/pubmed/19758129

120. Turner MR, Chohan G, Quaghebeur G, Greenhall RC, Hadjivassiliou M, Talbot K. A case of celiac disease mimicking amyotrophic lateral sclerosis. Nat Clin Pract Neurol. 2007 Oct;3(10):581-4.

121. Michiaki Koga, Nobuhiro Yuki, Koichi Hirata. Antiganglioside antibody in patients with Guillain-Barré syndrome who show bulbar palsy as an initial symptom. *J Neurol Neurosurg Psychiatry* 1999;66:513-516 (April).

122. William F. Brown, Charles F. Bolton, and Michael J. Aminoff. Neuromuscular Function and Disease: Basic, Clinical, and Electrodiagnostic Aspects, 2-Volume Set. A Saunders Title; 1 edition (April 16 2002)

123. Maurizio Gabrielli, M.D., Filippo Cremonini, M.D., Giuseppe Fiore, M.D., Giovanni Addolorato M.D, Cristiano Padalino M.D, Marcello Candelli M.D, Maria Elena De Leo M.D, Luca Santarelli M.D, Mario Giacovazzo M.D, Antonio Gasbarrini M.D, Paolo Pola M.D, Antonio Gasbarrini M.D. Association Between Migraine and Celiac Disease: Results From a Preliminary Case-Control and Therapeutic Study. *The American Journal of Gastroenterology* Volume 98 Issue 3, 2004, Pages 625 – 629.

124. Hadjivassiliou M, Aeschlimann P, Strigun A, Sanders DS, Woodroofe N, Aeschlimann D. Autoantibodies in gluten ataxia recognize a novel neuronal trans-glutaminase. *Ann Neurol.* 2008 Sep;64(3):332-43.

125. Volta U, De Giorgio R, Petrolini N, Stangbellini V, Barbara G, Granito A, De Ponti F, Corinaldesi R, Bianchi FB. Clinical findings and anti-neuronal antibodies in coeliac disease with neurological disorders. *Scand J Gastroenterol.* 2002 Nov;37(11):1276-81.

126. Klockgether T. Handbook of Ataxia Disorders Informa Healthcare; 1 edition (Aug 18 2000)

127. P.Rush, R.Inman, M.Bernstein, P.Carlen, L.Resch. Isolated vasculitis of the central nervous system in a patient with celiac disease. The American Journal of Medicine, Volume 81, Issue 6, Pages 1092-1094

128. S Meyers, S Dikman, H Spiera, N Schultz, H D Janowitz. Cutaneous vasculitis complicating coeliac disease. *Gut* 1981;22:61-64; doi:10.1136/gut.22.1.61

129. V. Alegre, R. Winkelmann, J. Diez-Martin, P. Banks. Adult celiac disease, small and medium vessel cutaneous necrotizing vasculitis, and T cell lymphoma† Journal of the American Academy of Dermatology, Volume 19, Issue 5, Pages 973-978

130. Gene V. Ball and S. Louis Bridges Jr. Vasculitis. Oxford University Press; Second Edition edition (Jan 15 2008)

131. Prause, Christian; Ritter, Maria; Probst, Christian; Daehnrich, Cornelia; Schlumberger, Wolfgang; Komorowski, Lars; Lieske, Ruediger; Richter, Thomas; Hauer, Almuthe C; Stern, Martin; Uhlig, Holm H; Laass, Martin W; Zimmer, Klaus-Peter; Mothes, Thomas. Antibodies Against Deamidated Gliadin as New and Accurate Biomarkers of Childhood Coeliac Disease. *Journal Of Pediatric Gastroenterology And Nutrition.* July 2009-Volume 49-Issue 1-p 52-58.

132. S. Rashtak, M. Ettore, H. Homburger, J. Murray. Comparative Usefulness of Deamidated Gliadin Antibodies in the Diagnosis of Celiac Disease. *Clinical Gastroenterology and Hepatology*, Volume 6, Issue 4, Pages 426-432.

133. Dogan M, Peker E, Cagan E, Akbayram S, Acikgoz M, Caksen H, Uner A, Cesur Y. Stroke And Dilated Cardiomyopathy Associated With Celiac Disease. *World Journal Gastroenterol*, 2010 May 14;16 (18): 2302-4.

134. Brandimarte G, Tursi A, Giorgetti GM. Changing trends in clinical form of celiac disease. Which is now the main form of celiac disease in clinical practice? *Minerva Gastroenterol Dietol.* 2002;48:121-30.

135. Hadjivassiliou M, Sanders DS, Grünewald RA, Woodroofe N, Boscolo S, Aeschlimann D. Gluten sensitivity: from gut to brain. *Lancet Neurol.* 2010 Mar;9(3):318-30.

136. De George JJ and Carbonetto S. Wheat germ agglutinin inhibits nerve fiber growth and concanavalin A stimulates nerve fiber initiation in culture of dorsal root ganaglia neurons. *Developmental Brain Research* 28, 169-75, 1986.

137. Borges LF, Sidman RL.Axonal transport of lectins in the peripheral nervous system. *Journal Of Neuroscience,* 2, pg. 647-53, 1982.

138. Tchernychev B, Wilchek M.. Natural human antibodies to dietary lectins. *FEBS* Lett.1996 Nov 18;397(2-3):139-42.

139. Dolapchieva S. Distribution of concanavalin A and wheat germ agglutinin binding sites in the rat peripheral nerve fibres revealed by lectin/glycoprotein-gold histochemistry. *TheHistochem Journal.*1996 Jan;28(1):7-12.

140. Brunngraber EC. Possible role of glycoproteins in neurol function. *Perspectives in Biology And Medicine,* 12, pg. 467-70, 1969.

141. De George JJ and Carbonetto S. Wheat germ agglutinin inhibits nerve fiber growth and concanavalin A stimulates nerve fiber initiation in culture of dorsal root ganaglia neurons. *Developmental Brain Research* 28, 169-75, 1986.

142. Brunngraber EC. Possible role of glycoproteins in neurol function. *Perspectives in Biology And Medicine,* 12, pg. 467-70, 1969.

143. De George JJ and Carbonetto S. Wheat germ agglutinin inhibits nerve fiber growth and concanavalin A stimulates nerve fiber initiation in culture of dorsal root ganaglia neurons. *Developmental Brain Research* 28, 169-75, 1986.

144. http://dogtorj.com

145. Carolyn S. Chen, MD, Ethan U. Cumbler, MD, and Andrzej T. Triebling, MD, PhD Coagulopathy Due to Celiac Disease Presenting as Intramuscular Hemorrhage. *J Gen Intern Med.* 2007 November; 22(11): 1608–1612.

146. Borges LF, Sidman RL.Axonal transport of lectins in the peripheral nervous system. *Journal Of Neuroscience*, 2, pg. 647-53, 1982.

147. Broadwell RD, Balin BJ, Salcman M.. Transcytotic pathway for blood-borne protein through the blood-brain barrier. *Proceedings from the National Academy of Sciences* U S A. 1988 Jan;85(2):632-6.

148. Begbic R, King TP. The interaction of dietary lectin with porcine small intestine and production of lectin-specific antibodies. In Lectins Biology, Biochemistry, *Clinical Biochemistry* (Bog-Hansen TC, Breborovicz J eds). Vol 4, pages 15-27. Walter de Gruyter, Berlin and New York, 1985.

149. Dolapchieva S. Distribution of concanavalin A and wheat germ agglutinin binding sites in the rat peripheral nerve fibres revealed by lectin/glycoprotein-gold histochemistry. *The Histo Chem Journal.*1996 Jan;28(1):7-12.

150. Kepes JJ, Chou SM, Price LW., Jr Progressive multifocal leukoencephalopathy with 10-year survival in a patient with nontropical sprue. Report of a case with unusual light and electron microscopic features. *Neurology.* 1975 Nov;25(11):1006–1012.

151. De George JJ and Carbonetto S. Wheat germ agglutinin inhibits nerve fiber growth and concanavalin A stimulates nerve fiber initiation in culture of dorsal root ganaglia neurons. *Developmental Brain Research* 28, 169-75, 1986.

152. Dolapchieva S. Distribution of concanavalin A and wheat germ agglutinin binding sites in the rat peripheral nerve fibres revealed by lectin/glycoprotein-gold histochemistry. *The Histo Chem Journal.*1996 Jan;28(1):7-12.

153. Fabian RH, Coulter JD. Transneuronal transport of lectins. *Brain Research* 344, 41-48, 1985.

Chapter 12

1. Pruessner Harold T, MD. Detecting Celiac Disease In Your Patients. *American Family Physician*. March 1st, 1998.

2. Feldman Mark, MD, Friedman Lawrence S, MD, Sleisenger, Marvin H, MD, Gastrointestinal and Liver Disease Pathophysiology/Diagnosis/Management 7th Edition, Volume11, 2002,Saunders

3. Green, PH. The many faces of celiac disease: clinical presentation of celiac disease in the adult population. *Gastroenterology.* 2005;128:S74-78.

4. Medicinenet.com. How Are Malabsorption And Malnutrition Evaluated In Celiac Disease. http://www.medicinenet.com/celiac_disease/page7.htm

5. Gibney MJ, Marinos E, Olle L, Dowsett J. Clinical Nutrition. Blackwell Publishing 2005.

6. Gibney MJ, Vorster HH, Kok FJ. Introduction to Human Nutrition. Blackwell Publishing 2002.

7. Ludvigsson JF, Reutfors J, Osby U, Ekbom A, Montgomery SM. Coeliac disease and risk of mood disorders–a general population-based cohort study. *J Affect Disord*. 2007 Apr;99(1-3):117-26. Epub 2006 Oct 6.

8. Pynnönen PA, Isometsä ET, Aronen ET, Verkasalo MA, Savilahti E, Aalberg VA. Mental disorders in adolescents with celiac disease. *Psychosomatics.* 2004 Jul-Aug;45(4):325-35.

9. Päivi A Pynnönen, Erkki T Isometsä, Matti A Verkasalo, Seppo A Kähkönen, Ilkka Sipilä, Erkki Savilahti, and Veikko A Aalberg. Gluten-free diet may alleviate depressive and behavioural symptoms in adolescents with coeliac disease: a prospective follow-up case-series study. *BMC Psychiatry.* 2005; 5: 14.

10. William Eaton, professor, Preben Bo Mortensen, professor, Esben Agerbo, assistant professor, Majella Byrne, assistant professor, Ole Mors, associate

professor, and Henrik Ewald, professor. Coeliac disease and schizophrenia: population based case control study with linkage of Danish national registers. BMJ. 2004 February 21; 328(7437): 438–439.

11. Bryan D Kraft and Eric C Westman. Schizophrenia, gluten, and low-carbohydrate, ketogenic diets: a case report and review of the literature. *Nutr Metab* (Lond). 2009; 6: 10.

12. O. Dhodanand Kowlessar, Lorraine J. Haeffner, and Gordon D. Benson· Abnormal Tryptophan Metabolism in Patients with Adult Celiac Disease, with Evidence for Deficiency of Vitamin B$_6$. J Clin Invest. 1964 May; 43(5): 894–903.

13. M I Torres, M A López-Casado, P Lorite, and A Ríos. Tryptophan metabolism and indoleamine 2,3-dioxygenase expression in coeliac disease. Clin Exp Immunol. 2007 June; 148(3): 419–424.

14. Ciacci C, Iovino P, Amoruso D, Siniscalchi M, Tortora R, Di Gilio A, Fusco M, Mazzacca G. Grown-up coeliac children: the effects of only a few years on a gluten-free diet in childhood. *Aliment Pharmacol Ther.* 2005 Feb 15;21(4):421-9.

15. Dr. David Perlmutter, MD, FACN, ABIHM. Gluten sensitivity (Celiac Disease), ADHD, and other neurological problems in children. http://tinyurl.com/c2pzoo

16. Niederhofer H, Pittschieler K. A preliminary investigation of ADHD Symptoms In persons With celiac Disease. *Journal of Attention Disorders*, 2006 Nov;10(2):200-4. http://jad.sagepub.com/cgi/content/abstract/10/2/200

17. G Addolorato, DD Giuda, GD Rossi, V Valenza, et el. Regional cerebral hypoperfusion in patients with celiac disease. The American Journal of Medicine, Volume 116, Issue 5, Pages 312-317

18. Nathanel Zelnik MD, Avi Pacht MD, Raid Obeid MD, Aaron Lerner MD. Range of Neurological Disorders In Patients With Celiac Disease. *Pediatrics* Vol. 113 No. 6 June 2004, pp.1672-1676.

19. Rosa A: Depressive symptoms in adult coeliac disease. *Scand J Gastroenterology* 1998; 33:247–250

20. Hallert C, Martensson J, Allgen LG: Brain availability of monoamine precursors in adult coeliac disease. *Scand J Gastroenterol* 1982; 17:87–89

21. Hallert C, Derefeldt T: Psychic disturbances in adult coeliac disease, I: clinical observations. *Scand J Gastroenterol* 1982; 17:17–19

22. Hallert C, Åström J, Walan A: Reversal of psychopatology in adult coeliac disease with the aid of pyroxidine (vitamin B6). *Scand J Gastroenterol* 1983; 18:229–304

23. Addolorato G, Stefanini GF, Capristo E, Caputo F, Gasbarrini A, Gasbarrini G: Anxiety and depression in adult untreated celiac subjects and in patients affected by inflammatory bowel disease: a personality "trait" or a reactive illness? *Hepato-gastroenterology* 1996; 43:1513–1517.

24. Hjiej H, Doyen C, Couprie C, Kaye K, Contejean Y. Substitutive and dietetic approaches in childhood autistic disorder: interests and limits. *Encephale*. 2008 Oct;34(5):496-503. Epub 2008 Mar 4.

25. Päivi A. Pynnönen, M.D., Erkki T. Isometsä, M.D., Ph.D., Matti A. Verkasalo, M.D., Erkki Savilahti, M.D., Ph.D., and Veikko A. Aalberg, M.D., Ph.D. Untreated Celiac Disease and Development of Mental Disorders in Children and Adolescents. *Psychosomatics* 43:331-334, August 2002.

26. A J Wakefield FRCS, A Anthony PhD, MBBS, MSc, S H Murch PhD, FRCP, FRCPCH, M Thomson MBChB, MRCP, FRCPCH, S M Montgomery PhD, S Davies MRCPath, J J O'Leary MD, DPhil, MRCPath, M Berelowitz FRCPsych and J A Walker-Smith MD, FRCP, FRACP, FRCPCH Enterocolitis in children with developmental disorders. *The American Journal of Gastroenterology* (2000) 95, 2285-2295; doi:10.1111/j.1572-0241.2000.03248.x

27. http://www.nature.com/ajg/journal/v95/n9/abs/ajg2000579a.html

28. William W. Eaton, Ph.D., Majella Byrne, Ph.D., Henrik Ewald, Dr.Med.Sc., Ole Mors, Ph.D., Chuan-Yu Chen, Ph.D., Esben Agerbo, M.S., and Preben Bo Mortensen, M.D., Dr.Med.Sc. Association of Schizophrenia and Autoimmune Diseases: Linkage of Danish National Registers. *Am J Psychiatry* 163:521-528, March 2006. http://ajp.psychiatryonline.org/cgi/content/abstract/163/3/521

29. O. Dhodanand Kowlessar, Lorraine J. Haeffner, and Gordon D. Benson. Abnormal Tryptophan Metabolism in Patients with Adult Celiac Disease, with Evidence for Deficiency of Vitamin B_6 *J Clin Invest*. 1964 May; 43(5): 894–903.

30. PA Pynnonen, ET Isometsa, MA Verkasalo, E Savilahti, VA Aalberg. Untreated Celiac Disease And Development Of Mental Disorders In Children And Adolescents. *Psychosomatics* 43:331-334, August 2002.

http://psy.psychiatryonline.org/cgi/reprint/43/4/331.pdf

31. Hallert C, Derefeldt T. Psychic disturbances in adult coeliac disease. I. Clinical observations. *Scand J Gastroenterol*. 1982 Jan;17(1):17-9.

32. Hallert C, Aström J. Psychic disturbances in adult coeliac disease. II. Psychological findings. *Scand J Gastroenterol*. 1982 Jan;17(1):21-4.

http://www.ncbi.nlm.nih.gov/pubmed/7134834

33. Hallert C, Aström J, Sedvall G. Psychic disturbances in adult coeliac disease. III. Reduced central monoamine metabolism and signs of depression. *Scand J Gastroenterol.* 1982 Jan;17(1):25-8.

34. C. Ciacci, A. Iavarone, G. Mazzacca, A. De Rosa. Depressive Symptoms in Adult Coeliac Disease. *Scandinavian Journal of Gastroenterology* 1998, Vol. 33, No. 3, Pages 247-250

35. Hallert C, Sedvall G. Improvement in central monoamine metabolism in adult coeliac patients starting a gluten-free diet. *Psychol Med.* 1983 May;13(2):267-71.

36. A Hernanz and I Polanco. Plasma precursor amino acids of central nervous system monoamines in children with coeliac disease. *Gut. 1*991 December; 32(12): 1478–1481. http://www.ncbi.nlm.nih.gov/pmc/articles/PMC1379246/

37. Smith KA, Fairburn CG, Cowen PJ. Relapse of depression after rapid depletion of tryptophan. *Lancet.* 1997 Mar 29;349(9056):915-9.

38. Lahat, Shapiro, Karban, Gerstein, Kinarty & Lerner. Cytokine Profile in Coeliac Disease. *Scandinavian Journal Of Immunology,* Volume49 Issue 4, Pages 441-447.

39. Olga J.G. Schiepers, Marieke C. Wichersand Michael Maes. Cytokines and major depression. *Progress in Neuro-Psychopharmacology and Biological Psychiatry.* Volume 29, Issue 2, February 2005, Pages 201-217.

40. Maes M, Smith R. Immune Activation And Major Depression: A hypothesis. *Perspectives In Depression* 1999;7:6-8.

41. Ziad Kronfol, M.D., and Daniel G. Remick, M.D. Cytokines and the Brain: Implications for Clinical Psychiatry. *Am J Psychiatry* 157:683-694, May 2000

42. Maes M, Kubera M, Leunis JC. The gut-brain barrier in major depression: intestinal mucosal dysfunction with an increased translocation of LPS from gram negative enterobacteria (leaky gut) plays a role in the inflammatory pathophysiology of depression. *Neuro Endocrinol* Lett. 2008 Feb;29(1):117-24.

    http://www.ncbi.nlm.nih.gov/sites/entrez?
    Db=pubmed&Cmd=DetailsSearch&Term=18283240[uid]

43. Repo-Tiihonen E, Halonen P, Tiihonen J, Virkkunen M. Total serum cholesterol level, violent criminal offences, suicidal behavior, mortality and the appearance of conduct disorder in Finnish male criminal offenders with antisocial personality disorder. *Eur Arch Psychiatry Clin Neurosci.* 2002 Feb;252(1):8-11.

44. Jian Zhang, Matthew F. Muldoon, Robert E. McKeown and Steven P. Cuffe. Association of Serum Cholesterol and History of School Suspension among

School-age Children and Adolescents in the United States. *American Journal of Epidemiology* 2005 161(7):691-699.

45. Ludovico Abenavoli, MD, Lorenzo Leggio, MD, Daniela Di Giuda, MD, Giovanni Gasbarrini, MD, Giovanni Addolorato, MD. Neurologic Disorders in Patients With Celiac Disease: Are They Mediated by Brain Perfusion Changes? *PEDIATRICS* Vol. 114 No. 6 December 2004, pp. 1734.

46. Hadjivassiliou M, Grunewald RA, Chattopadhyay AK, Davies-Jones GA, Gibson A, Jarrat JA, et el. Clinical, Radiological, Neurophysiological, And Neuropathological Characteristics Of Gluten Ataxia. *Lancet 1*998;352:1582-5.

47. Dickey W. Epilepsy, Cerebral Calcifications, and Coeliac Disease. *Lancet* 1994;344:1585-6

48. Gobbi G, Bouquet F, Greco L, et al. Coeliac Disease, Epilepsy, and Cerebral Calcifications. The Italian Working Group On Coeliac Disease and Epilepsy. *Lancet* 340:439, 1992.

49. Hadjivassilou M and Grünwald R. The Neurology of Gluten Sensitivity: Science vs. Conviction. *Practical Neurology* 2004 4, 124-126.

50. Hugo A. Arroyo, MD, Susana De Rosa, MD, Victor Ruggieri, MD, María T. G. de Dávila, MD, Natalio Fejerman, MD. Epilepsy, Occipital Calcifications, and Oligosymptomatic Celiac Disease in Childhood. *Journal of Child Neurology,* Vol. 17, No. 11, 800-806 (2002).

51. Kepes JJ, Chou SM, Price LW., Jr Progressive multifocal leukoencephalopathy with 10-year survival in a patient with nontropical sprue. Report of a case with unusual light and electron microscopic features. *Neurology.* 1975 Nov;25(11):1006–1012.

52. Collin P, Pirttilä T, Nurmikko T, Somer H, Erilä T, Keyriläinen O. Celiac disease, brain atrophy, and dementia. *Neurology.* 1991 Mar;41(3):372–375.

53. Ghezzi A, Filippi M, Falini A, Zaffaroni M. Cerebral involvement in celiac disease: a serial MRI study in a patient with brainstem and cerebellar symptoms. *Neurology.* 1997 Nov;49(5):1447–1450.

54. Matthias Kieslich, MD, Germán Errázuriz, MD, Hans Georg Posselt, MD, Walter Moeller-Hartmann, MD, Friedhelm Zanella, MD, and Hansjosef Boehles, MD. Brain White-Matter Lesions in Celiac Disease: A Prospective Study of 75 Diet-Treated Patients. *PEDIATRICS* Vol. 108 No. 2 August 2001, p. e21.

55. Addolorato G et al (2004) Regional cerebral hypoperfusion in patients with celiac disease *Am J Med* 116 (312-317)

56. B. Emanuel, A. Lieberman. Electroencephalogram changes in celiac disease. The Journal of Pediatrics, Volume 62, Issue 3, Pages 435-437.

57. Lea ME, Harbord M, Sage MR. Bilateral Occipital Calcification Associated With Celiac Disease, Folate Deficiency, And Epilepsy. *AJNR* 16:1498-1500, Aug 1995.

58. Tunc T, Okuyucu E, Ucleri S, Sonmez T, Coskun O, Selvi E, Inan LE. Subclinical celiac disease with cerebellar ataxia. *Acta Neurol Belg.*, 2004 Jun;104(2):84-6.

59. I D Wilkinson, M Hadjivassiliou, J M Dickson, L Wallis, R A Grünewald, S C Coley, E Widjaja, P D Griffiths. Cerebellar abnormalities on proton MR spectro-scopy in gluten ataxia. *Journal of Neurology Neurosurgery and Psychiatry* 2005;76:1011-1013.

60. Helge Topka. Chapter 2: Normal functions of the cerebellum. Klockgether Thomas. Handbook of Ataxia disorders. *Informa Healthcare;* 1 edition (Aug 18 2000)

61. Paul V, Henkerr J, Todt H, Eysold R. Z.Klin.Med., 1985; 40: 707-709.

62. B. Emanuel, A. Lieberman. Electroencephalogram changes in celiac disease. The Journal of Pediatrics, Volume 62, Issue 3, Pages 435-437

63. Regional cerebral hypoperfusion in patients with celiac disease. The American Journal of Medicine, Volume 116, Issue 5, Pages 312-317

64. R. L. Chin, MD, H. W. Sander, MD, T. H. Brannagan, MD, P. H.R. Green, MD, A. P. Hays, MD, A. Alaedini, PhD and N. Latov, MD PhD. Celiac Neuropathy. Neurology 2003;60:1581-1585.

65. Wilkinson ID, Hadjivassiliou M, Dickson JM, Wallis L, Grunwald RA, Coley SC, Widjaja E, Griffiths PD. Cerebellar Abnormalities On Proton MR Spectroscopy in Gluten Ataxia. *J Neurol Neurosurg Psychiatry.* 2005 Jul;76(7):1011-3.

66. Vojdani Aristo, PhD., MT. O'Bryan Thomas, D.C., C.C.N., D.A.C.B.N. The Immunology Of Gut Sensitivity Beyond The Intestinal Tract.

67. E Myrsky, K Kaukinen, M Syrjänen, I R Korponay-Szabó, M Mäki, and K Lindfors. Coeliac disease-specific autoantibodies targeted against transglutaminase 2 disturb angiogenesis. *Clin Exp Immunol.* 2008 April; 152(1): 111–119.

68. Hadjivassiliou M, Aeschlimann P, Strigun A, Sanders DS, Woodroofe N, Aeschlimann D. Autoantibodies in gluten ataxia recognize a novel neuronal trans-glutaminase. Ann Neurol. 2008 Sep;64(3):332-43.

69. Bansal AK, Lindemann MJ, Ramsperger V, Kumar V. Celiac G+ antibody assay for the detection of autoantibodies in celiac disease. *Ann N Y Acad Sci.* 2009 Sep;1173:36-40. http://www.ncbi.nlm.nih.gov/pubmed/19758129

70. Marios Hadjivassiliou, David S. Sanders, Nicola Woodroofe, Claire Williamson and Richard A. Grünewald. Gluten Ataxia. Springer new York, volume 7, number 3/September 2008.

71. Hadjivassiliou M, Aeschlimann P, Strigun A, Sanders DS, Woodroofe N, Aeschlimann D. Autoantibodies in gluten ataxia recognize a novel neuronal transglutaminase. *Ann Neurol* 2008 Sep;64(3):332-43.

72. Hadjivassilou M and Grünwald RA, Davies-Jones GAB. Gluten Sensitivity As a Neurological Illness. Journal of Neurology, Neurosurgery, and Psychiatry 2002;72:560-563

73. Hadjivassilou M, Grünwald RA, Davies-Jones GAB. Causes of Cerebellar Degeneration: Gluten Ataxia in Perspective. *J Neurol Sci* 2001;187(suppl1):S520.

74. Hadjivassiliou M, Chattopadhyay AK, Davies-Jones GA, Gibson A, Grünewald RA, Lobo AJ. Neuromuscular disorder as a presenting feature of coeliac disease. *J Neurol Neurosurg Psychiatry.* 1997 Dec;63(6):770–775.

75. School of Medicine News: University of Maryland School of Medicine Scientists Pinpoint Critical Molecule to Celiac, Possibly Other Autoimmune Disorders. Tuesday, September 29, 2009.

   http://somvweb.som.umaryland.edu/absolutenm/templates/?a=915

76. L. Corvaglia, M.D., R. Catamo, M.D., G. Pepe, M.D., R. Lazzari, M.D., E. Corvaglia, M.D. Depression in adult untreated celiac subjects: diagnosis by the pediatrician. *The American Journal of Gastroenterology* Volume 94 Issue 3, Pages 839 – 843.

77. A. De Santis , G. Addolorato , A. Romito , S. Caputo , A. Giordano , G. Gambassi , C. Taranto , R. Manna & G. Gasbarrini. Schizophrenic symptoms and SPECT abnormalities in a coeliac patient: regression after a gluten-free diet. *Journal of Internal Medicine* Volume 242 Issue 5, Pages 421 – 423.

78. A. E. Kalaydjian, W. Eaton, N. Cascella, A. Fasano The gluten connection: the association between schizophrenia and celiac disease. *Acta Psychiatrica Scandinavica* Volume 113 Issue 2, Pages 82 – 90.

   http://www3.interscience.wiley.com/journal/118626206/abstract

79. Dohan FC, Grasberger JC, Lowell FM, Johnston HT Jr, Arbegast AW. Relapsed schizophrenics: more rapid improvement on a milk- and cereal-free diet. *Br J Psychiatry.* 1969 May;115(522):595-6.

80. Ludvigsson JF, Osby U, Ekbom A, Montgomery SM. Psychiatric illness, gluten, and celiac disease.1: *Biol Psychiatry.* 1982 Sep;17(9):959-61.

81. Individuals with Celiac Disease may be at increased risk of non-affective psychosis. 1: *Scand J Gastroenterol.* 2007 Feb;42(2):179-85.Coeliac disease and risk of schizophrenia and other psychosis: a general population cohort study.

82. Graff H, Handford A. Celiac syndrome in the case histories of five schizophreics. *Psychiatr Q.* 1961 Apr;35:306-13.

83. S. Rashtak, M. Ettore, H. Homburger, J. Murray. Comparative Usefulness of Deamidated Gliadin Antibodies in the Diagnosis of Celiac Disease. *Clinical Gastroenterology and Hepatology*, Volume 6, Issue 4, Pages 426-432.

84. Green, PH. The many faces of celiac disease: clinical presentation of celiac disease in the adult population. *Gastroenterology.* 2005;128:S74-78.

85. Brandimarte G, Tursi A, Giorgetti GM. Changing trends in clinical form of celiac disease. Which is now the main form of celiac disease in clinical practice? *Minerva Gastroenterol Dietol.* 2002;48:121-30.

86. Alessio Fasano and Carlo Catassi. Current approaches to diagnosis and treatment of celiac disease: an evolving spectrum. *Gastroenterology* 2001:120636-651.

87. Hadjivassiliou M, Sanders DS, Grünewald RA, Woodroofe N, Boscolo S, Aeschlimann D. Gluten sensitivity: from gut to brain. *Lancet* Neurol. 2010 Mar;9(3):318-30.

88. Signs and symptoms of Depression
http://www.nimh.nih.gov/health/publications/depression/complete-index.shtml#pub3

89. Luca Mascitelli, M.D., Medical Service Comando Brigata Alpina "Julia" Udine, Italy, Francesca Pezzetta, M.D., Cardiology Service Ospedale di Tolmezzo Tolmezzo, Italy, and Mark R. Goldstein, M.D., Fountain Medical Court Bonita Springs, FL United States. Low Cholesterol and Mental Disorders in Children and Adolescents With Celiac Disease. *Psychosomatics* 50:300-301, May-June 2009

Chapter 13

1. Pruessner Harold T, MD. Detecting Celiac Disease In Your Patients. *American Family Physician*. March 1st, 1998.

2. Feldman Mark, MD, Friedman Lawrence S, MD, Sleisenger, Marvin H, MD, Gastrointestinal and Liver Disease Pathophysiology/Diagnosis/Management 7th Edition, Volume11, 2002,Saunders

3. F.M. Stevens, C.E. Connolly, J.P. Murray, C.F. McCarthy. Lung Cavities in Patients with Coeliac Disease. *Digestion* 1990;46:72-80

4. Williams AJ, Asquith P, Stableforth DE. Susceptibility to tuberculosis in patients with coeliac disease. *Tubercle.* 1988 Dec;69(4):267-74.

5. J F Ludvigsson, J Wahlstrom, J Grunewald, A Ekbom, S M Montgomery. Coeliac disease and risk of tuberculosis: a population based cohort study. Published Online First: 17 October 2006. doi:10.1136/thx.2006.059451
    Thorax 2007;62:23-28

6. Goel NK, McBane RD, Kamath PS. Cardiomyopathy associated with celiac disease. *Mayo Clin Proc.* 2005 May;80(5):674-6.
    http://www.ncbi.nlm.nih.gov/pubmed/15887437

7. Nidhi Narula, Pawan Rawal, Rohit Manoj Kumar and Babu Ram Thapa. Association of Celiac Disease with Cardiomyopathy and Pulmonary Hemosiderosis. Oxford Journals. Journal of Tropical Pediatrics Advance Access published online on November 6, 2009. *Journal of Tropical Pediatrics,* doi:10.1093/tropej/fmp088.
    http://tropej.oxfordjournals.org/cgi/content/abstract/fmp088v1

8. Mario Curione, Maria Barbato, Pietro Cugini, Silvia Amato, Silvia Da Ros, Simonetta Di Bona. Association of cardiomyopathy and celiac disease: an almost diffuse but still less know entity. *Arch Med Sci* 2008; 4, 2: 103–107.
    http://www.termedia.pl/magazine.php?
    magazine_id=19&article_id=10658&magazine_subpage=ABSTRACT

9. Lodha, Ankur MD; Haran, Mehandi MD; Hollander, Gerald MD; Frankel, Robert MD; Shani, Jacob MD. Celiac Disease Associated with Dilated Cardiomyopathy. *Southern Medical Journal:* October 2009 – Volume 102 – Issue 10 – pp 1052-1054.

10. Tarcisio Not, Elena Faleschini, Alberto Tommasini, Alessandra Repetto, Michele Pasotti, Valentina Baldas, Andrea Spano, Daniele Sblattero, Roberto Marzari, Carlo Campana, Antonello Gavazzi, Luigi Tavazzi, Federico Biagi, Gino Roberto Corazza, Alessandro Ventura and Eloisa Arbustini. Celiac disease in patients with sporadic and inherited cardiomyopathies and in their relatives. *European Heart Journal* 2003 24(15):1455-1461.

11. M. Curione, M. Barbato, F. Viola, P. Francia, L. De Biase and S. Cucchiara Idiopathic dilated cardiomyopathy associated with coeliac disease: the effect of a gluten-free diet on cardiac performance. *Digestive and Liver Disease* Volume 34, Issue 12, December 2002, Pages 866-869. http://tinyurl.com/y9hhwjt

12. Ricardo Schmit T De Bem, Shirley Ramos Da Ro Sa Utiyama, Renato Mitsunori Nisihara, Jerônimo Antônio fortunato, josuÉ Augusto Tondo, Eliane Ribeiro Carmes, Raquel Almada E. Souza, Julio CÉsar Pisani and Heda Maria Barska Dos

Santos Amarante. Celiac Disease Prevalence in Brazilian Dilated Cardiomyopathy Patients. *Journal Digestive Diseases and Sciences* Issue Volume 51, Number 5 / May, 2006

http://www.springerlink.com/content/t13467701v3648nu/

13.   Ravi Mahadeva, Christopher Flower, John Shneerson Bronchiectasis in association with coeliac disease. *Thorax* 1998;53:527-529; doi:10.1136/thx.53.6.527

14.   Tugcin B. Polat, Nafiye Urganci, Yalim Yalcin, Cenap Zeybek, Celal Akdeniz, Abdullah Erdem, Elnur Imanov and Ahmet Celebi Cardiac functions in children with coeliac disease during follow-up: Insights from tissue Doppler imaging. *Digestive and Liver Disease* Volume 40, Issue 3, March 2008, Pages 182-187.

15.   Wei, L., Spiers, E., Reynolds, N., Walsh, S. Fahey, T. MacDonald, T. M., The association between coeliac disease and cardiovascular disease. Alimentary Pharmacology & Therapeutics. 27(6):514-519, March 15, 2008.

http://tinyurl.com/yeyw2aw

16.   Siry M, Burges C, Stiens R, Schneider H, Steiff J. [First diagnosis of celiac disease in a 67-year old female patient]. *Dtsch Med Wochenschr.* 2000 Aug 4;125(31-32):932-6.

17.   Loren A. Laine, MD; Kenneth M. Holt, MD. Recurrent Pericarditis and Celiac Disease. JAMA. 1984;252(22):3168.

18.   R. Faizallah, F. C. Costello, Frank I. Lee and Robin Walker. Adult celiac disease and recurrent pericarditis. *Journal Digestive Diseases and Sciences* Volume 27, Number 8 / August, 1982

19.   Dawes PT, Atherton ST. Coeliac disease presenting as recurrent pericarditis. *Lancet.* 1981 May 9;1(8228):1021-2.

20.   D. Pratil, M. T. Bardella, M. Peracchi, L. Porretti, M. Cardillo, C. Pagliari, C. Tarantin, E. Della Torre, M. Scalamogna, P. A. Sianchi, G. Sirchia, D. Conte and North Italy Transplant Programme Working Group (NITp) High frequency of anti-endomysial reactivity in candidates to heart transplant. *Digestive and Liver Disease* Volume 34, Issue 1, January 2002, Pages 39-43. http://tinyurl.com/ye75v9p

21.   Andrea Frustaci, MD; Lucio Cuoco, MD; Cristina Chimenti, MD; Maurizio Pieroni, MD; Giuseppina Fioravanti, CTER; Nicola Gentiloni, MD; Attilio Maseri, MD; Giovanni Gasbarrini, MD. Celiac Disease Associated With Autoimmune Myocarditis. (Circulation. 2002;105:2611.)

22. Malena Cohen-Cymberknoh[1], Michael Wilschanski[2] Concomitant cystic fibrosis and coeliac disease: reminder of an important clinical lesson. *BMJ Case Reports* 2009 [doi:10.1136/bcr.07.2008.0578].

23. Davidson DC, Shannon RS. Letter: Cystic fibrosis and coeliac disease. *Arch Dis Child.* 1974 Jun;49(6):501.

24. Franklin JL, Asquith P, Rosenberg IH. The occurrence of cystic fibrosis and celiac sprue within a single sibship. *Am J Dig Dis.* 1974 Feb;19(2):149-55.

25. Hide DW, Burman D. An infant with both cystic fibrosis and coeliac disease. *Arch Dis Child.* 1969 Aug;44(236):533-5.

26. Goodchild MC, Nelson R, Anderson CM. Cystic fibrosis and coeliac disease: coexistence in two children. *Arch Dis Child* 1973 Sep;48(9):684-91.

27. Katz AJ, Falchuk ZM, Schwachman H. The coexistence of cystic fibrosis and celiac disease. *Pediatrics.* 1976 May;57(5):715-21.

28. Santer R, Harms HK. [Cystic fibrosis and celiac disease. Report of two cases]. *Monatsschr Kinderheilkd.* 1990 Sep;138(9):623-6.

29. Chiaravalloti G, Baracchini A, Rossomando V, Ughi C, Ceccarelli M. [Celiac disease and cystic fibrosis: casual association?]. Minerva Pediatr. 1995 Jan-Feb;47(1-2):23-6.

30. Venuta A, Bertolani P, Casarini R, Ferrari F, Guaraldi N, Garetti E. [Coexistence of cystic fibrosis and celiac disease. Description of a clinical case and review of the literature]. *Pediatr Med Chir.* 1999 Sep-Oct;21(5 Suppl):223-6.

31. G. Fluge, H. Olesen, M. Gilljam, P. Meyer, T. Pressler, O. Storrösten, F. Karpati, L. Hjelte. Co-morbidity of cystic fibrosis and celiac disease in Scandinavian cystic fibrosis patients. Journal of Cystic Fibrosis, Volume 8, Issue 3, Pages 198-202.

32. Conn DL, McDuffie FC, Holley KE, Schroeter AL. Immunologic mechanisms in systemic vasculitis. *Mayo Clin Proc.* 1976 Aug;51(8):511-8.

33. Vázquez Gomis RM, Izquierdo Fos I, Zapata A, Parra G, Chicano Marin FJ. [Dilated myocardiopathy as a form of presentation of coeliac disease in childhood.]. *An Pediatr (Barc).* 2009 Oct 9.

34. Prati D, Bardella MT, Peracchi M, Porretti L, Scalamogna M, Conte D. Antiendomysial antibodies in patients with end-stage heart failure. *Am J Gastroenterol.* 2002 Jan;97(1):218-9.

35. Nisheeth K. Goel, MD; Robert D. McBane, MD; and Patrick S. Kamath, MD. Cardiomyopathy Associated With Celiac Disease. *Mayo Clinic Proc.* 2005;80(5):674-676.

36. Ph. Camus, T.V. Colby. The Lung In Inflammatory Bowel Disease. *Eur Respir* J 2000; 15:5-10.

37. O.C. Ioachimescu, S. Sieber, A. Kotch. Idiopathic Pulmonary Haemosiderosis Revisited. *Eur Respir* J 2004;24;162-169.

38. Mario Curione, maria Barbato, Pietro Cugini, Silvia Amato, Silvia Da Ros, Simonetta Di Bona. Association of Cardiomyopathy And Celiac Disease: An Almost Diffuse But Still Less Known Entity. *Arch Med Sci* 2008; 4, 2:103-107.

39. Ackerman Z, Eliashiv S, Reches A, Zimmerman J. Neurological manifestations in celiac disease and vitamin E deficiency. *J Clin Gastroenterol.* 1989 Oct;11(5):603–605

40. Henri-Bhargava Alexandre, Melmed Calvin, Glikstein Rafael, and Schipper Hyman M. Neurologic Impairment Due to Vitamin E and Copper Deficiencies in Celiac Disease. *Neurology*, Vol. 71, Issue 11, 860-861, September 9, 2008

41. Gibney MJ, Vorster HH, Kok FJ. Introduction to Human Nutrition. Blackwell Publishing 2002.

42. Gibney MJ, Marinos E, Olle L, Dowsett J. Clinical Nutrition. Blackwell Publishing 2005.

43. Vincent Cottin, Gael Clérici, Nicole Fabien, Hugues Rousset and Jean-François Cordier. Celiac disease revealed by diffuse alveolar hemorrhage and heart block. *Respiratory Medicine* Extra Volume 2, Issue 3, 2006, Pages 89-91.

44. Maddalena Peracchi MD, Cristina Trovato MD, Massimo Longhi MD, Maurizio Gasparin DSc, Dario Conte MD, Cristina Tarantino BSc, Daniele Prati MD and Maria Teresa Bardella MD Tissue transglutaminase antibodies in patients with end-stage heart failure. *The American Journal of Gastroenterology* (2002) 97, 2850–2854; doi:10.1111/j.1572-0241.2002.07033.x.

45. Alessandro Luciani, Valeria Rachela Villella, Angela Vasaturo, Ida Giardino, Valeria Raia, Massimo Pettoello-Mantovani, Maria D'Apolito, Stefano Guido, Teresinha Leal[l], Sonia Quaratino and Luigi Maiuri. SUMOylation of Tissue Trans-glutaminase as Link between Oxidative Stress and Inflammation[1.] Published online July 22, 2009, The Journal of Immunology, 2009, 183, 2775 –2784.

46. Wong M, et el. Proximal Myopathy And Bone Pain As The Presenting Features Of Coeliac Disease. *Ann Rheum Dis,* 2002, 61(1):p87-8.

47. Kleopa KA, Kyriacou K, Zamba-Papanicolaou E, Kyriakides T. Reversible inflammatory and vacuolar myopathy with vitamin E deficiency in celiac disease. *Muscle Nerve.* 2005 Feb;31(2):260-5.

48. Albert Selva-O'Callaghan, MD, PhD, Francesc Casellas, MD, PhD, Ines de Torres, MD, PhD, Eduard Palou, MD, PhD, Josep M. Grau-Junyent, MD, PhD, Miquel Vilardell-Tarrés, MD, PhD. Celiac disease and antibodies associated with celiac disease in patients with inflammatory myopathy. *Muscle & Nerve*, Volume 35 Issue 1, Pages 49 – 54. Published

49. Hadjivassiliou M, Maki M, Saunders DS, Williamson CA, Grunewald RA, Woodroof NM, Korponay-Szabo IR. Autoantibody Targeting of Brain and Intestinal Transglutaminase in Gluten Ataxia. *Neurology* 2006 Feb.14;66(3):373-7.

50. T Matsuzaka, H Tanaka, M Fukuda, M Aoki, Y Tsuji, and H Kondoh. Relationship between vitamin K dependent coagulation factors and anticoagulants (protein C and protein S) in neonatal vitamin K deficiency. *Arch Dis Child.* 1993 March; 68(3 Spec No): 297–302.

51. Jorge O, Jorge A, Camus G. Celiac disease associated with antiphospholipid syndrome. *Rev Esp Enferm Dig.* 2008 Feb;100(2):102-3.

52. Armando D'Angelo, Silvana Viganò D'Angelo. Protein S deficiency. *Haematologica, V*ol 93, Issue 4, 498-501 doi:10.3324/haematol.12691

53. E Myrsky, K Kaukinen, M Syrjänen, I R Korponay-Szabó, M Mäki, and K Lindfors. Coeliac disease-specific Autoantibodies Targeted Against Transglutaminase 2 Disturb Angiogenesis.. *Clin Exp Immunol.* 2008 April; 152(1): 111–119.

54. Deepak Guptaand Naureen MirzaSystemic lupus erythematosus, celiac disease and antiphospholipid antibody syndrome: a rare association. *Journal Rheumatology International*, Volume 28, Number 11 / September, 2008.

55. R Shamir, Y Shoenfeld, M Blank, R Eliakim, N Lahat, E Sobel, E Shinar, A Lerner. The prevalence of coeliac disease antibodies in patients with the antiphospholipid syndrome.

56. P.Rush, R.Inman, M.Bernstein, P.Carlen, L.Resch. Isolated vasculitis of the central nervous system in a patient with celiac disease. The American Journal of Medicine, Volume 81, Issue 6, Pages 1092-1094

57. S Meyers, S Dikman, H Spiera, N Schultz, H D Janowitz. Cutaneous vasculitis complicating coeliac disease. *Gut* 1981;22:61-64; doi:10.1136/gut.22.1.61

58. V. Alegre, R. Winkelmann, J. Diez-Martin, P. Banks. Adult celiac disease, small and medium vessel cutaneous necrotizing vasculitis, and T cell lymphoma† Journal of the American Academy of Dermatology, Volume 19, Issue 5, Pages 973-978.

59. Siiri E. Iismaa, Bryony M. Mearns, Laszlo Lorand and Robert M. Graham. Transglutaminases and Disease: Lessons From Genetically Engineered Mouse Models and Inherited Disorders. *Physiol. Rev.* 89: 991-1023, 2009.

60. Luigi Maiuri, Alessandro Luciani, Ida Giardino, Valeria Raia, Valeria R. Villella, Maria D'Apolito, Massimo Pettoello-Mantovani, Stefano Guido, Carolina Ciacci, Mariano Cimmino, Olivier N. Cexus, Marco Londei and Sonia Quaratino. Tissue Transglutaminase Activation Modulates Inflammation in Cystic Fibrosis via PPAR Down-Regulation The Journal of Immunology, 2008, 180, 7697–7705.

61. Vincent Cottin, Gael Clérici, Nicole Fabien, Hugues Rousset and Jean-François Cordier. Celiac disease revealed by diffuse alveolar hemorrhage and heart block. *Respiratory Medicine* Extra Volume 2, Issue 3, 2006, Pages 89-91.

62. Hadjivassilou M and Grünwald RA, Davies-Jones GAB. Gluten Sensitivity As a Neurological Illness. *Journal of Neurology, Neurosurgery, and Psychiatry* 2002;72:560-563

63. School of Medicine News: University of Maryland School of Medicine Scientists Pinpoint Critical Molecule to Celiac, Possibly Other Autoimmune Disorders. Tuesday, September 29, 2009.

    http://somvweb.som.umaryland.edu/absolutenm/templates/?a=915

64. Diet and Human Immune Function by David A. Hughes, L. Gail Darlington, and Adrianne Bendich. Humana Press; 1 edition (Dec 4 2003)

65. Rashtak, M. Ettore, H. Homburger, J. Murray. Comparative Usefulness of Deamidated Gliadin Antibodies in the Diagnosis of Celiac Disease. *Clinical Gastroenterology and Hepatology,* Volume 6, Issue 4, Pages 426-432

66. Dogan M, Peker E, Cagan E, Akbayram S, Acikgoz M, Caksen H, Uner A, Cesur Y. Stroke And Dilated Cardiomyopathy Associated With Celiac Disease. *World Journal Gastroenterol*, 2010 May 14;16 (18): 2302-4.

67. Neil GA, Lukie BE, Cockcroft DW, Murphy F. Lymphocytic interstitial pneumonia and abdominal lymphoma complicating celiac sprue. *J Clin Gastroenterol.* 1986 Jun; 8 (3 Pt 1): 282-5.

68. Elisa Romagnoli, Elena Boldrini and Antonello Pietrangelo. Association between celiac disease and idiopathic dilated cardiomyopathy: a case report. *Intern Emerg Med.* 2010 Aug 25.

69. Najada AS, Dahabreh MM.. Pulmonary haemosiderosis in a 13-year-old girl with coeliac disease after 3 months on a gluten-free diet: case report and review of the literature. Ann *Trop Paediatr.* 2010;30(3):249-53.

70. Peter Thomas. Fibrosing Alveolitis. *Can Med Assoc J.* 1978 November 18; 119(10): 1211–1216.

Chapter 14

1. Clinical guideline: Guidelines For The Diagnosis And Treatment Of Children: Recommendations of The North American Society For Gastroenterology, Hepatology, And Nutrition. *Journal of Pediatric Gastroenterology And Nutrition* 40: 1-9. January 2005 Lippincott Williams and Wilkins, Phildelphia.

2. Pruessner Harold T, MD. Detecting Celiac Disease In Your Patients. *American Family Physician.* March 1st, 1998.

3. Feldman Mark, MD, Friedman Lawrence S, MD, Sleisenger, Marvin H, MD, Gastrointestinal and Liver Disease Pathophysiology/Diagnosis/Management 7th Edition, Volume11, 2002, Saunders

4. Alessio Fasano. Systemic Autoimmune Disorders in Celiac Disease: Autoimmune Diseases Associated with Celiac Disease.

   http://www.medscape.com/viewarticle/547107_4

5. C. O'leary, C.H. Walsh, P. Wieneke, P. O'regan, B. Buckley, D.J. O'halloran, J.B. Ferriss, E.M.M. Quigley, P. Annis, F. Shanahan and C.C. Cronin. Coeliac disease and autoimmune Addison's disease: a clinical pitfall. *Q J Med* 2002; 95: 79-82.

6. Elfström et al. Risk of primary adrenal insufficiency in patients with celiac disease. J Clin Endocrinol Metab .2007

7. Corrado Betterle, Francesca Lazzarotto, Aglaura Cinzia Spadaccino, Daniela Basso[1], Mario Plebani[1], Beniamino Pedini, Silvia Chiarelli[2] and Mariapaola Albergoni[3] Celiac disease in North Italian patients with autoimmune Addison's disease. *European Journal of Endocrinology,* Vol 154, Issue 2, 275-279

8. Logan RF, Ferguson A, Finlayson ND, Weir DG. Primary biliary cirrhosis and coeliac disease: an association? *Lancet.* 1978 Feb 4;1(8058):230-3.

9. Primary biliary cirrhosis and coeliac disease. *Lancet.* 1978 Apr 1;1(8066):713–714.11.

10. Shanahan F, O'Regan PF, Crowe JP. Primary Biliary Cirrhosis associated with Coeliac Disease. *Ir Med J.* 1983 Jun;76(6):282–282.

11. Schrijver G, Van Berge Henegouwen GP, Bronkhorst FB. Gluten-sensitive coeliac disease and primary biliary cirrhosis syndrome. *Neth J Med.* 1984;27(6):218–221

12. P. Ginn and R. D. Workman. Primary biliary cirrhosis and adult celiac disease. *West J Med.* 1992 May; 156(5): 547–549.

13. Mirza, E. Bonilla and P. E. Phillips. Celiac disease in a patient with systemic lupus erythematosus: a case report and review of literature. *Journal Clinical Rheumatology* Issue Volume 26, Number 5 / May, 2007

14. Mondher Zitouni, Wafa Daoud, Maryam Kallel and Sondés Makni. Systemic lupus erythematosus with celiac disease: a report of five cases. *Joint Bone Spine* Volume 71, Issue 4, July 2004, Pages 344-346.

15. Freeman HJ. Adult celiac disease followed by onset of systemic lupus erythematosus. *J Clin Gastroenterol.* 2008 Mar;42(3):252-5.

16. Deepak Gupta and Naureen Mirza· Systemic lupus erythematosus, celiac disease and antiphospholipid antibody syndrome: a rare association. *Journal Rheumatology International* Issue Volume 28, Number 11 / September, 2008

17. Abenavoli L, Proietti I, Leggio L, Ferrulli A, Vonghia L, Capizzi R, Rotoli M, Amerio PL, Gasbarrini g, Addolorato G. Cutaneous Manifestations In Celiac disease. *World Journal Of Gastroenterology.* 2006 February 14;12(6):843-852

18. Edoardo Rosato, Daniela De Nitto, Carmelina Rossi, Valerio Libanori, Giuseppe Donato, Marco Di Tola, Simonetta Pisarri, Felice Salsano and Antonio Picarelli. High Incidence of Celiac Disease in Patients with Systemic Sclerosis. *The Journal of Rheumatology.* http://www.jrheum.org/content/36/5/965.abstract

19. Jorge O, Jorge A, Camus G. Celiac disease associated with antiphospholipid syndrome. Rev Esp Enferm Dig. 2008 Feb;100(2):102-3.

20. Szodoray P, Barta Z, Lakos, Szakall S, Zeher M. Coeliac Disease In Sjogren's Syndrome-A Study of 111 Hungarian Patients. *Rheumatol Int* 2004 Sep;24(5):278-82. Epub 2003 Sep 17.

21. Matz Jenilee. The Link Between Type 1 Diabetes and Celiac Disease. http:www.myoptumhealth.com

22. Hilde Kloster Smerud, Bengt Fellström, Roger Hällgren, Sonia Osagie, Per Venge and Gudjón Kristjánsson Gluten sensitivity in patients with IgA nephropathy. *Nephrology Dialysis Transplantation* 2009 24(8):2476-2481; doi:10.1093/ndt/gfp133.

23. Pekka Collin, M.D., Jaana Syrjänen, M.D. , Jukka Partanen, Ph.D , Amos Pasternack, M.D. , Katri Kaukinen, M.D. , Jukka Mustonen, M.D. Celiac disease and HLA DQ in patients with IgA nephropathy. *The American Journal of Gastroenterology* Volume 97 Issue 10, Pages 2572 – 2576

24. Goel NK, McBane RD, Kamath PS. Cardiomyopathy associated with celiac disease. *Mayo Clin Proc.* 2005 May;80(5):674-6.
http://www.ncbi.nlm.nih.gov/pubmed/15887437

25. Nidhi Narula, Pawan Rawal, Rohit Manoj Kumar and Babu Ram Thapa. Association of Celiac Disease with Cardiomyopathy and Pulmonary Hemosiderosis. Oxford Journals. Journal of Tropical Pediatrics Advance Access published online on November 6, 2009. *Journal of Tropical Pediatrics,* doi:10.1093/tropej/fmp088.
http://tropej.oxfordjournals.org/cgi/content/abstract/fmp088v1

26. Mario Curione, Maria Barbato, Pietro Cugini, Silvia Amato, Silvia Da Ros, Simonetta Di Bona. Association of cardiomyopathy and celiac disease: an almost diffuse but still less know entity. *Arch Med Sci* 2008; 4, 2: 103–107.
http://www.termedia.pl/magazine.php?
magazine_id=19&article_id=10658&magazine_subpage=ABSTRACT

27. Jorge O, Jorge A, Camus G. Celiac disease associated with antiphospholipid syndrome. *Rev Esp Enferm Dig.* 2008 Feb;100(2):102-3.

28. R Shamir, Y Shoenfeld, M Blank, R Eliakim, N Lahat, E Sobel, E Shinar, A Lerner. The prevalence of coeliac disease antibodies in patients with the antiphospholipid syndrome.

29. P.Rush, R.Inman, M.Bernstein, P.Carlen, L.Resch. Isolated vasculitis of the central nervous system in a patient with celiac disease. The American Journal of Medicine, Volume 81, Issue 6, Pages 1092-1094

30. S Meyers, S Dikman, H Spiera, N Schultz, H D Janowitz. Cutaneous vasculitis complicating coeliac disease. *Gut* 1981;22:61-64; doi:10.1136/gut.22.1.61

31. V. Alegre, R. Winkelmann, J. Diez-Martin, P. Banks. Adult celiac disease, small and medium vessel cutaneous necrotizing vasculitis, and T cell lymphoma† Journal of the American Academy of Dermatology, Volume 19, Issue 5, Pages 973-978.

32. Ola Olén, Scott M. Montgomery, Göran Elinder, Anders Ekbom and Jonas F. Ludvigsson Increased risk of immune thrombocytopenic purpura among inpatients with coeliac disease. *Scandinavian Journal of Gastroenterology* 2008, Vol. 43, No. 4, Pages 416-422.

33. L. Stenhammar, C. G. Ljunggren. Thrombocytopenic Purpura and Coeliac Disease. *Acta Pædiatrica* Volume 77 Issue 5, Pages 764 – 766

34. Alessio Fasano, M.D. Physiological, Pathological, and Therapeutic Implications of Zonulin-Mediated Intestinal Barrier Modulation. *American Journal of Pathology,* 2008;173:1243-1252.

35. Matsueda K, Rosenberg IH. Malabsorption with idiopathic hypoparathyroidism responding to treatment for coincident celiac sprue. Dig Dis Sci 27:269–273, 1982.

36. Rensch M.J. et el. The Prevalence Of Celiac Disease Autoantibodies In Patients With Systemic Lupus Erythematosus. *American Journal Of Gastroenterology* 96 (2001):1113-5.

37. Hadjivassilou et el. Gluten Sensitivity Masquerading As Systemic Lupus Erythematosus. Annals Of Rheumatic Diseases 63 (2004): 1501-3.

38. Kumar V, Valeski JE, Wortsman J. Celiac disease and hypoparathyroidism: cross-reaction of endomysial antibodies with parathyroid tissue. Clin Diagn Lab Immunol 3:143–146, 1996.

39. Peter Elfström, Scott M. Montgomery, Olle Kämpe, Anders Ekbom, and Jonas F. Ludvigsson. Risk of primary adrenal insufficiency in patients with celiac disease. *Journal of Clinical Endocrinology & Metabolism* doi:10.1210/jc.2007-0960.

40. *Inflamm bowel Dis*. 2005 Jul;11(7):662-666.

41. Tursi A, Giorgetti GM, Brandimarte G, Elisei W. High prevalence of celiac disease among patients affected by Crohn's disease. *Inflamm Bowel Dis*. 2005 Jul;11(7):662-6.

42. Alessio Fasano and Carlo Catassi. Current approaches to diagnosis and treatment of celiac disease: an evolving spectrum. *Gastroenterology* 2001:120636-651.

43. Dr. Rob for MSN Health and Fitness. Raynard's Syndrome. http://health.msn.com/health-topics/articlepage.aspx?cp-documentid=100234985

44. William Dickey. A Case of Sequential Development of Celiac Disease and Ulcerative Colitis: Discussion of Diagnosis. www.medscape.com/viewarticle/560764_3

45. Raymakers JA. Autonomous hyperparathyroidism in a patient with adult coeliac disease. *Neth J Med* 31:308–311, 1987.

46. Valdez R, Appelman HD, Bronner MP, Greenson JK. Diffuse duodenitis associated with ulcerative colitis. *Am J Surg Pathol*. 2000 Oct;24(10):1407-13.

47. Collin P, Hakanen M, Salmi J, Mäki M, Kaukinen K. Autoimmune hypopituitarism in patients with coeliac disease—symptoms confusingly similar. *Scand J Gastroenterol* 36:558–560, 2001.

48. GR Corazza, M. Frisoni, D. Vaira, G. Gasbarrini. Effect Of Gluten-Free Diet On Splenic Hypofunction Of Adult Celiac Disease. *Gut* 24, 228-230, 1983.

49. Peter Elfström, Scott M. Montgomery, Olle Kämpe, Anders Ekbom, and Jonas F. Ludvigsson. Risk of primary adrenal insufficiency in patients with celiac disease . *Journal of Clinical Endocrinology & Metabolism*, June 26th, 2007. doi:10.1210/jc.2007-0960

50. Rabszlyn A, Green PH, Berti I, Fasano A, Perman JA, Horvath K. Macroamylasmia In Patients With Celiac Disease. Am J Gastroenterol, 2001 Apr;96(4):1096-100.

51. Elizabeth Hwang, Russell McBride, Alfred I Neugut, and Peter HR Green. Sarcoidosis in Patients with Celiac Disease. *Digestive Diseases and Sciences*, Volume 53, Number 4, 977-981.

52. Zeglaoui, H, Landolsi, H, Mankai, A, Ghedira, I, Bouajina, E. Type 1 Diabetes Mellitis, Celiac Disease, Lupus Erythematosus, And Scleroderma in a 15 Year Old Girl. *Rheumatol Int.* 2010, Apr 30(6) 793-5.

Chapter 15

Refer to references for chapters 4-14 for symptoms and associated diseases in checklist.

1. Lejarraga H, et el. Normal Growth Velocity Before Diagnosis Of Celiac Disease. *J Pediatr Gastrenterol Nutr* 2000;30:552-556.

Chapter 16

1. Shane M. Devlin, MD, FRCPC, Christopher N. Andrews, MD, FRCPC, Paul L. Beck, MD, PHD, FRCPC. Celiac Disease. *Canadian Family Physician,* CME update for family physicians. May, 2004

2. Kamaeva OI, Reznikov IP, Pimenova NS, Dobritsyna LV. Antigliadin antibodies in the absense of celiac disease. *Klinicheskaia Meditsina,* 1998; 76 (2):33-5.

3. Hill ID, Dirks MH, Liptak GS, Colletti RB, Fasano A, Guandalini S, Hoffenberg EJ, Horvath K, Murray JA, Pivor M, Seidman EG. Guideline for the diagnosis and treatment of celiac disease in children: recommendations of the North American Society for Pediatric Gastroenterology, Hepatology and Nutrition. *J Pediatr Gastroenterol Nutr* 2005 Jan;40(1):1-19.

4. M Hadjivassiliou, RA Grünwald, GAB Davies-Jones. Gluten Sensitivity As A Neurological Illness. *J Neurol Neurosurg Psychiatry* 2002:72: 560-563.

5.   Marios Hadjivassiliou, Richard Grünwald. The Neurology Of Gluten Sensitivity: Science vs Conviction. *Pract Neurol* 2004,4:124-127.

6.   A. Balas, F Garcia-Sanchez, JL Vicario. A New DQA1 allele (DQA1*0510) In A Spanish Celiac Patient. Tissue Antigens Immune Response Genetics. Online Dec. 2009

7.   Rubio-Tapia, Alberto; Murray, Joseph A. Celiac Disease. Current Opinion in *Gastroenterology*: March 2010-Volume 26-Issue 2-pg 116-122.

8.   Carina Lagerqvist, Ingrid Dahlbom, Tony Hansson, Erik Jidell, Per Juto, Per Olcen, Hans Stenlund, Olle Hernell, Anneli Ivarsson. Antigliadin Immunoglobulin A Best In Finding Celiac Disease In Children Younger Than 18 Months. *J Pediatr Gastroenterol Nutr.* 2008 Oct;47 (5):428-435.

9.   Alessio Fasano, MD.. Celiac Disease. University Of Maryland School Of Medicine, Baltimore, MD. A*GA Instiute Focussed Clinical Updates*, May 20th and 21st, 2007.

10.   Prause, Christian; Ritter, Maria; Probst, Christian; Daehnrich, Cornelia; Schlumberger, Wolfgang; Komorowski, Lars; Lieske, Ruediger; Richter, Thomas; Hauer, Almuthe C; Stern, Martin; Uhlig, Holm H; Laass, Martin W; Zimmer, Klaus-Peter; Mothes, Thomas. Antibodies Against Deamidated Gliadin as New and Accurate Biomarkers of Childhood Coeliac Disease. *Journal Of Pediatric Gastroenterology And Nutrition*. July 2009-Volume 49-Issue 1-p 52-58.

11.   GR Corazza And V Villanacci. Coeliac Disease. *J Clin Pathol*. 2005 June; 58(6): 573-574.

12.   Mohsin Rashid and Andrea MacDonald. Importance Of Duodenal Bulb Biopsies In Children For Diagnosis Of Celiac Disease In Clinical Practice. *BMC Gastroenterology* 2009, 9:78

13.   Martin Goetz, Ralf Kiesslich. Advances Of Endomicroscopy For Gastrointestinal Physiology And Diseases. *Am J Physiol Gastrointest Liver Psysiol* 298: G797-G806, Feb. 25th, 2010.

14.   Hadjivassiliou M, Aeschlimann P, Strigun A, Sanders DS, Woodroofe N, Aeschlimann D. Autoantibodies in gluten ataxia recognize a novel neuronal transglutaminase. *Ann Neurol* 2008 Sep;64(3):332-43.

15.   Denery-Papini S, Lauriére M, Branlard G, *et al.* (2007). "Influence of the allelic variants encoded at the Gli-B1 locus, responsible for a major allergen of wheat, on IgE reactivity for patients suffering from food allergy to wheat". *J. Agric. Food Chem.* 55 (3): 799–805.

16. Volta U, Cassani F, De Franchis R, *et al.* (1984). "Antibodies to gliadin in adult coeliac disease and dermatitis herpetiformis". *Digestion* 30 (4): 263–70.

17. Volta U, Lenzi M, Lazzari R, *et al.* (1985). Antibodies to gliadin detected by immunofluorescence and a micro-ELISA method: markers of active childhood and adult coeliac disease". *Gut* 26 (7): 667–71.

18. Bateman EA, Ferry BL, Hall A, Misbah SA, Anderson R, and Kelleher P. (2004). "IgA antibodies of coeliac disease patients recognise a dominant T cell epitope of A-gliadin.". *Gut.* 53 (9): 1274–1278

19. Hadjivassiliou M, Gibson A, Davies-Jones GA, Lobo AJ, Stephenson TJ, Milford-Ward A (1996). "Does cryptic gluten sensitivity play a part in neurological illness?". *Lancet* 347 (8998): 369–71

20. Collin P, Mäki M, Keyriläinen O, Hällström O, Reunala T, Pasternack A (1992). "Selective IgA deficiency and coeliac disease". *Scand J Gastroenterol* 27 (5): 367–71.

21. Matsuo H, Morita E, Tatham AS, Morimoto K, Horikawa T, Osuna H, Ikezawa Z, Kaneko S, Kohno K, and Dekio S. (2004). "Identification of the IgE-binding epitope in omega-5 gliadin, a major allergen in wheat-dependent exercise-induced anaphylaxis.". *J Biol Chem.* 279 (13): 12135–12140

22. Agardh D (November 2007). "Antibodies against synthetic deamidated gliadin peptides and tissue transglutaminase for the identification of childhood celiac disease". *Clin. Gastroenterol. Hepatol.* 5 (11): 1276–81.

23. Mabel Aleanzila, Ana María Demonte1, Cecilia Esper1, Silvia Garcilazo1 and Marta Waggener2 Antibody Recognition against Native and Selectively Deamidated Gliadin Peptides. *Clinical Chemistry* 47: 2023-2028, 2001.

24. Antony K Akobeng. Understanding Diagnostic Tests 1: Sensitivity, Specificity And Predictive Values. *Acta Paediatrica,* December 8 2006.

25. Carolina Arguelles-Grande, Gary L Norman, Govind Bhagat, Peter HR Green. Hemolysis Interferes With The Detection Of Anti-Tissue Transglutaminase Antibodies In Celiac Disease. *Clinical Chemistry* 56:1034-1036, 2010.

26. Kaukinen K, Collin P, Huhtala H, Ruuskanen A, Mäki M, Luostarinen L. Positive serum antigliadin antibodies without celiac disease in the elderly population: does it matter? Scand J *Gastroenterol.* 2010 Jun 14.

27. Eisenmann A, Murr C, Fuchs D, Ledochowski M. Gliadin IgG antibodies and circulating immune complexes. *Scand J Gastroenterol.* 2009;44(2):168-71.

28. Kaistha A, Castells S. Celiac disease in African American children with type 1

diabetes mellitus in inner city Brooklyn. *Pediatr Endocrinol Rev.* 2008 Aug;5 Suppl 4:994-8.

29. Bonamico M, Rasore-Quartino A, Mariani P, Scartezzini P, Cerruti P, Tozzi MC, Cingolani M, Gemme G. *Acta Paediatr.* Down syndrome and coeliac disease: usefulness of antigliadin and antiendomysium antibodies. 1996 Dec;85(12):1503-5.

30. Floreani A, Chiaramonte M, Venturini R, Plebani M, Martin A, Giacomini A, Naccarato R. Antigliadin antibody classes in chronic liver disease. Ital J Gastroenterol. 1992 Oct;24(8):457-60.

31. Reichelt KL, Jensen D. IgA antibodies against gliadin and gluten in multiple sclerosis. *Acta Neurol Scand.* 2004 Oct;110(4):239-41.

32. Akçay MN, Akçay G. The presence of the antigliadin antibodies in autoimmune thyroid diseases. *Hepatogastroenterology.* 2003 Dec;50 Suppl 2:cclxxix-cclxxx.

33. Paimela L, Kurki P, Leirisalo-Repo M, Piirainen H. Gliadin immune reactivity in patients with rheumatoid arthritis. *Clin Exp Rheumatol.* 1995 Sep-Oct;13(5):603-7.

34. Kalaydjian AE, Eaton W, Cascella N, Fasano A. The gluten connection: the association between schizophrenia and celiac disease. *Acta Psychiatr Scand.* 2006 Feb;113(2):82-90.

35. Reichelt KL, Landmark J. Specific IgA antibody increases in schizophrenia. *Biol Psychiatry.* 1995 Mar 15;37(6):410-3.

36. Kamaeva OI, Reznikov IuP, Pimenova NS, Dobritsyna LV. Klin Med (Mosk). Antigliadin antibodies in the absence of celiac disease *Klin Med (Mosk).* 1998;76(2):33-5.

37. Woo WK, McMillan SA, Watson RG, McCluggage WG, Sloan JM, McMillan JC. Coeliac disease-associated antibodies correlate with psoriasis activity. *Br J Dermatol.* 2004 Oct;151(4):891-4.

38. Kull K, Uibo O, Salupere R, Metsküla K, Uibo R. High frequency of antigliadin antibodies and absence of antireticulin and antiendomysium antibodies in patients with ulcerative colitis. *J Gastroenterol.* 1999 Feb;34(1):61-5.

39. D S Sanders, M Hadjivassiliou, R A Grünewald, M Akil Gluten sensitivity masquerading as systemic lupus erythematosus. *Ann Rheum Dis* 2004;63:1501-1503.

40. Jami L Miller, MD Dermatis Herpetiformis

    http://emedicine.medscape.com/article/1062640-diagnosis

41.   Jami L Miller, MD http://emedicine.medscape.com/article/1062640-overview

42.   James Braly, Patrick Holford. Hidden Food Allergies: The Essential Guide To Uncovering Hidden Food Allergies—And Achieving Permanent Relief. Fitzhenry & Whiteside Ltd.; 1 edition (2006)

43.   HLA-DQ and Susceptibility to Celiac Disease: Evidence for Gender Differences and Parent-of-Origin Effects. Megiorni F et al. *Am Journal Gastroenterol.* 2008;103:997-1003.

44.   Dr. Scot Lewey. Ten Facts About Celiac Disease Genetic Testing. http://www.celiac.com/articles/21567/1/Ten-Facts-About-Celiac-Disease-Genetic-Testing/Page1.html

45.   Dr. Scot Lewey. Celiac Disease Genetics.

http://www.celiac.com/articles/21628/1/Celiac-Disease-Genetics/Page1.html

46.   Clinical guideline: Guidelines For The Diagnosis And Treatment Of Children: Recommendations of The North American Society For Gastroenterology, Hepatology, And Nutrition. *Journal of Pediatric Gastroenterology And Nutrition* 40: 1-9. January 2005 Lippincott Williams and Wilkins, Phildelphia.

47.   Alessio Fasano and Carlo Catassi. Current approaches to diagnosis and treatment of celiac disease: an evolving spectrum. *Gastroenterology* 2001:120636-651.

48.   Fukudome S, Yoshikawa M. Opiod Peptides Derived from Wheat Gluten: Their Isolation And Characterization. *Febs Letts.* 1992. January 13 ;296(1) : 107-11.

49.   C Zioudrou, R A Streaty and W A Klee . Opioid peptides derived from food proteins. The exorphins. *The Journal Of Biological Chemistry,* April 10, 1979. 254: 2446-2449

50.   Shattock P, Whiteley P. (2002) "Biochemical aspects in autism spectrum disorders: updating the opioid-excess theory and presenting new opportunities for biomedical intervention" "Autism Research Unit, University of Sunderland, UK.

51.   Bret A. Lashner, MD. Should Intestinal Healing Be Assessed in Treated Celiac Patients? Medscape Nurses www.medscape.com

52.   Edward J.Ciaccioa, Christina A.Tennysonb, Suzanne K. Lewisb, Suneeta Krishnareddyb, Govind Bhagatc, Peter H.R. Greenb. Distinguishing patients with celiac disease by quantitative analysis of videocapsule endoscopy images. *Computer Methos And Programs In Biomedicine.* Volume 100, Issue 1, Pages 39-48 (October 2010)

53.   Enzo Masci, MD, Barbara Parma, MD, Graziano Barera, MD, Paolo Viaggi, MD, Luca Albarello, MD, Giulia Maria Tronconi, MD, Alberto Mariani, MD, Sabrina

Testoni, MD, Tara Santoro, MD, Pier Alberto Testoni, MD. Bulb biopsies for the diagnosis of celiac disease in pediatric patients. *Gastrointestinal Endoscopy* Volume 72, Issue 3 , Pages 564-568, September 2010

54. Hadjivassiliou M, Sanders DS, Grünewald RA, Woodroofe N, Boscolo S, Aeschlimann D. Gluten sensitivity: from gut to brain. *Lancet* Neurol. 2010 Mar;9(3):318-30.

55. Brocchi E, Tomassetti P, Volta U, Piscitelli L, Bonora M, Campana D, Corinaldesi R. Adult coeliac disease diagnosed by endoscopic biopsies in the duodenal bulb. *Eur J Gastroenterol Hepatol.* 2005 Dec;17(12):1413-5.

56. Vogelsang H, Hänel S, Steiner B, Oberhuber G. Diagnostic Duodenal biopsy in celiac disease. Endoscopy. 2001 Apr;33(4):336-40. *Endoscopy.* 2001 Apr;33(4):336-40.

57. Dascha C Weir MD, Jonathan N Glickman MD, Tracey Roiff[1], Clarissa Valim MD, ScD and Alan M Leichtner MD. Variability of Histopathological Changes in Childhood Celiac Disease. *Am J Gastroenterol* 2010; 105:207–212.

58. Thijs WJ, van Baarlen J, Kleibeuker JH, Kolkman JJ. Duodenal versus jejunal biopsies in suspected celiac disease. *Endoscopy.* 2004 Nov;36(11):993-6.

59. Koskinen O, Collin P, Lindfors K, Laurila K, Maki M, Kaukinen K. Usefulness of small-bowel mucosa transglutaminase-2 specific autoantibody deposits in the diagnosis and follow-up of celiac disease. *J Clin Gastroenterol,* 2010 Aug;44(7):483-8.

60. Watson RG, 2005. Diagnosis of coeliac disease. BMJ 330:739-40.

61. Reif S, A Lerner, 2004. Tissue transglutaminase-the key players in coeliac disease: a review. *Autoimmunity reviews* 3:40-45.

62. Wong RC, RJ Wilson, RH Steele, G Radford-Smith, S Adelstein, 2002. A comparison of 13 guinea pig and human anti-tissue transglutaminase antibody ELISA kits. *J Clin Pathol* 55:488-494.

63. V Hakeem, R Fifield, H F al-Bayaty, M J Aldred, D M Walker, J Williams, and H R Jenkins. Salivary IgA antigliadin antibody as a marker for coeliac disease. *Arch Dis Child.* 1992 June; 67(6): 724–727.

64. Stenhammar L, Kilander AF, Nilsson LA, Strömberg L, Tarkowski A. Serum gliadin antibodies for detection and control of childhood coeliac disease. *Acta Paediatr Scand.* 1984 Sep;73(5):657-63.

65. Lindberg T, Nilsson LA, Borulf S, Cavell B, Fällström SP, Jansson U, Stenhammar L, Stintzing G. Serum IgA and IgG gliadin antibodies and small

intestinal mucosal damage in children. *J Pediatr Gastroenterol Nutr.* 1985 Dec;4(6):917-22.

66. M. Hadjivassiliou, MD, M. Mäki, MD, D. S. Sanders, MD, C. A. Williamson, PhD, R. A. Grünewald, DPhil, N. M. Woodroofe, MD and I. R. Korponay-Szabó, MD. Autoantibody targeting of brain and intestinal transglutaminase in gluten ataxia. *NEUROLOGY* 2006;66:373-377.

67. E K Janatuinen, T A Kemppainen, R J K Julkunen, V-M Kosma, M Mäki, M Heikkinen1, M I J Uusitupa2 . No harm from five year ingestion of oats in coeliac disease. *Gut 2002;50:332-335 doi:10.1136/gut.50.3.332*

68. V. Kumar, M. Jarzabek-Chorzelska, J. Sulej, Krystyna Karnewska, T. Farrell, and S. Jablonska. Celiac Disease and Immunoglobulin A Deficiency: How Effective Are the Serological Methods of Diagnosis? Clinical and Diagnostic Laboratory Immunology, November 2002, p. 1295-1300, Vol. 9, No. 6

69. Carolee Bateson-Koch DC ND. Allergies, Disease In Disguise. How To Heal Your Allergic Condition Permanently And Naturally. Alive Books, 1994.

70. Grodzinsky E, Hed J, Liedén G, Sjögren F, Ström M. Presence of IgA and IgG antigliadin antibodies in healthy adults as measured by micro-ELISA. Effect of various cutoff levels on specificity and sensitivity when diagnosing coeliac disease. Int Arch Allergy Appl Immunol. 1990;92(2):119-23.

71. Jos W. Meijer, Peter J. Wahab and Chris J. Mulder. Small intestinal biopsies in celiac disease: duodenal or jejunal? *Virchows Archiv* Volume 442, Number 2, 124-128.

72. Hadjivassiliou M, RA Grunwald, GAB Davies-Jones. Gluten Sensitivity: A Many Headed Hydra. Heightened Response To Gluten Is Not Confined To The Gut. BMJ 1999 June 26;318(7200):710-711.

73. Sugai E, Smecuol E, Niveloni S, Vazquez H, Label M, Mazure R, Czech A, Kogan Z, Maurino E, Bai JC. Celiac Disease. Serology In Dermatitis Herpetiformis. Which Is The Best Option For Detecting Gluten Sensitivity? Acta Gastroenterol Latinoam 2006 Dec;36(4):197-201.

Chapter 17

1. Health Canada's Position on the Introduction of Oats to the Diet of Individuals Diagnosed with Celiac Disease (CD). "Celiac disease and the safety of oats.

    http://www.hc-sc.gc.ca/fn-an/securit/allerg/cel-coe/oats_cd-avoine-eng.php

2. Canadian Celiac Association Position Statement on Oats, August 2007

http://www.celiac.ca/Articles/PABoats.html

3. Mohsin Rashid. Canadian Celiac Association Guidelines for consumption of pure and uncontaminated oats by individuals with celiac disease, June 2007.

    http://www.celiac.ca/Articles/PABoatsguidelines2007June.html

4. Päivi M. Kanerva, Tuula S. Sontag-Strohm, Päivi H. Ryöppy, Pirjo Alho-Lehto and Hannu O. Salovaara. Analysis of barley contamination in oats using R5 and ω-gliadin antibodies. *Journal of Cereal Science.* Volume 44, Issue 3, November 2006, Pages 347-352

5. A. R. Lee, D. L. Ng, E. Dave, E. J. Ciaccio, P. H. R. Green. The effect of substituting alternative grains in the diet on the nutritional profile of the gluten-free diet. Journal of Human Nutrition And Dietetics. Volume 22, issue 4, pages 359-363, August 2009.

6. Handbook of Cereal Science and Technology, 2nd Edition, Edited by Karel Kulp and Joseph G. Ponte, Jr. Marcel Dekker, Inc., New York, 2000.

7. A Consumer's Dictionary of Cosmetic Ingredients, Ruth Winter, M.S. Three Rivers Press, New York, 1999.

8. A Consumer's Dictionary of Food Additives, Ruth Winter, M.S. Three Rivers Press, New York, 1999.

9. The Gluten-Free Pantry [www.glutenfree.com]

10. E K Janatuinen, T A Kemppainen, R J K Julkunen, V-M Kosma, M Mäki, M Heikkinen1, M I J Uusitupa2 . No harm from five year ingestion of oats in coeliac disease. *Gut 2002;50:332-335 doi:10.1136/gut.50.3.332*

11. The Cooks Thesaurus [www.foodsubs.com]

12. Bob's Red Mill [www.bobsredmill.com]

13. Food Lover's Companion, 3rd Edition, Sharon Tyler Herbst Barron's, New York, 2001.

14. Celiac Disease Methods and Protocols, Edited by Michael N. Marsh, MD, DSc, FRCP Humana Press, New Jersey, 2000

15. The Bread & Circus Whole Food Bible, Christopher S. Kilham, Addison-Wesley, New York, 1991.

16. Brune M, Rossander L, Hallberg L (August 1989). "Iron absorption and phenolic compounds: importance of different phenolic structures". *Eur J Clin Nutr* 43 (8): 547–57.

17. Afsana K, Shiga K, Ishizuka S, Hara H (1 November 2003). "Ingestion of an

Indigestible saccharide, difructose anhydride III, partially prevents the tannic acid-induced suppression of iron absorption in rats". *J. Nutr.* 133 (11): 3553–60.

18. Hurrell RF, Reddy M, Cook JD (April 1999). "Inhibition of non-haem iron absorption in man by polyphenolic-containing beverages". *Br. J. Nutr.* 81 (4): 289–95.

19. Elvin-Lewis, Memory P. F.; Lewis, Walter Hepworth (1977). Medical botany: plants affecting man's health. New York: Wiley.

20. Hallert C, Grant C, Grehn S, Grännö C, Hultén S, Midhagen G, Ström M, Svensson H, Valdimarsson T. Evidence of poor vitamin status in coeliac patients on a gluten-free diet for 10 years. *Aliment Pharmacol Ther.* 2002 Jul;16(7):1333-9

21. A. Lanzini, F. Lanzarotto, V. Villanacci, A. Mora, S. Bertolazzi, D. Turini, G. Carella, A. Malagoli, G. Ferrante, B.M. Cesana, and C. Ricci. Complete recovery of intestinal mucosa occurs very rarely in adult coeliac patients despite adherence to gluten-free diet. *Aliment Pharmacol* Ther 29, 1299–1308.

22. Alessio Fasano, MD.. Celiac Disease. University Of Maryland School Of Medicine, Baltimore, MD. A*GA Instiute Focussed Clinical Updates*, May 20th and 21st, 2007.

23. Rashid, Mohsin (2007-06-08). "Guidelines for Consumption of Pure and Uncontaminated Oats by Individuals with Celiac Disease". Professional Advisory Board of Canadian Celiac Association.

    http://www.celiac.ca/Articles/PABoatsguidelines2007June.html.

24. Størsrud S, Hulthén LR, Lenner RA (July 2003). "Beneficial effects of oats in the gluten-free diet of adults with special reference to nutrient status, symptoms and subjective experiences. *Br. J. Nutr.* 90 (1): 101–7.

25. Haboubi NY, et al. (2006). Coeliac disease and oats: A systematic review. *Postgraduate Medical Journal,* 82(972): 672–678.

26. Farrell RJ, Kelly CP (2002). Celiac sprue. *New England Journal of Medicine,* 346(3): 180–188.

27. Anna-Liisa Prangli, Meeme Utt, Ija Talja, Epp Sepp, Marika Mikelsaar, Tarvo Rajasalu, Oivi Uibo, Vallo Tillmann, Raivo Uibo. Antigenic Proteins Of Lactobacillus Acidophilus That Are Recognised By Serum IgG antibodies In Children With Type 1 Diabetes And Celiac Disease. *Pediatr Allergy Immunol.* 2009 Jul 2.

28. N Y Haboubi, S Taylor, S Jones (2006). "Coeliac disease and oats: a systematic review". *The Fellowship of Postgraduate Medicine.*

http://pmj.bmj.com/cgi/content/abstract/82/972/672.

29. The Scoop on Oats"Celiac Sprue Association (CSA). February 20, 2008. http://www.csaceliacs.org/InfoonOats.php.

30. USDA Nutrient Data Base For Standard Reference.Searched Gluten-Free Grains And Flours http://www.nal.usda.gov/fnic/foodcomp/search/

31. Marye Audet. Brewer's yeast or nutritional yeast.

    http://hubpages.com/hub/BrewersYeast

32. Janis Kelly. Olive Oil Component Has A Ibuprophen-Like Activity. Medscape Nurses. http://www.medscape.com/viewarticle/538330

33. E K Janatuinen, T A Kemppainen, R J K Julkunen, V-M Kosma, M Mäki, M Heikkinen1, M I J Uusitupa2 . No harm from five year ingestion of oats in coeliac disease. *Gut 2002;50:332-335 doi:10.1136/gut.50.3.332*

34. James Braly, Patrick Holford. Hidden Food Allergies: The Essential Guide To Uncovering Hidden Food Allergies—And Achieving Permanent Relief. Fitzhenry & Whiteside Ltd.; 1 edition (2006)

35. Carolee Bateson-Koch DC ND. Allergies, Disease In Disguise. How To Heal Your Allergic Condition Permanently And Naturally. Alive Books, 1994.

36. Executive Summary. Celiac Disease And The Safety Of Oats. Health Canada's Position On The Introduction Of Oats To The Diet Of Individuals Diagnosed With Celiac Disease (CD). www.hs-sc.gc.ca/fn-an/securit/allerg/cel-coe/oats_cd-avoine-eng.php

Chapter 18

1. Park SD et al. Failure to respond to hepatitis B vaccine in children with celiac disease. J*ournal of Pediatric Gastroenterology and Nutrition* 2007;44:431-5

2. Ahishali E et al. Response to Hepatitis B Vaccination in Patients with Celiac Disease. Digestive Diseases and Sciences 2007 Dec 20. [Epub ahead of print]

3. Noh KW et al. Hepatitis B vaccine nonresponse and celiac disease. American Journal of Gastroenterology 2003;98:2289-92

4. Farrell RJ, Kelly CP (2002). Celiac sprue. New England Journal of Medicine, 346(3): 180–188.

5. Comprehensive metabolic panel

   http://www.labtestsonline.org/understanding/analytes/cmp/glance.html

6. Celiac Disease Tests

http://www.labtestsonline.org/understanding/analytes/celiac_disease/test.html

7. Devlin Shane MD, Andrews Christopher MD, beck Paul MD, Celiac Disease. *CME Update* May 2004.

8. Feldman Mark, MD, Friedman Lawrence S, MD, Sleisenger, Marvin H, MD, Gastrointestinal and Liver Disease Pathophysiology/Diagnosis/Management 7th Edition, Volume11, 2002,Saunders

9. Kagnoff MF. AGA Institute Medical Position Statement on the Diagnosis and Management of CD. Gastroenterology, Official Journal of the American Gastroenterological Association (AGA). December 2006.

10. Management After the diagnosis of CD. Accessed September 2010.

    http://www.celiacdiseasecenter.columbia.edu/C_Doctors/C07-Management.htm

11. Hallert C, Grant C, Grehn S, Grännö C, Hultén S, Midhagen G, Ström M, Svensson H, Valdimarsson T. Evidence of poor vitamin status in coeliac patients on a gluten-free diet for 10 years. *Aliment Pharmacol Ther.* 2002 Jul;16(7):1333-9.

12. A. Lanzini, F. Lanzarotto, V. Villanacci, A. Mora, S. Bertolazzi, D. Turini, G. Carella, A. Malagoli, G. Ferrante, B.M. Cesana, and C. Ricci. Complete recovery of intestinal mucosa occues very rarely in adult coeliac patients despite adherence to gluten-free diet, *Aliment Pharmacol Ther* 29, 1299–1308.

13. Alessio Fasano, MD.. Celiac Disease. University Of Maryland School Of Medicine, Baltimore, MD. A*GA Instiute Focussed Clinical Updates*, May 20th and 21st, 2007.

14. Anna-Liisa Prangli, Meeme Utt, Ija Talja, Epp Sepp, Marika Mikelsaar, Tarvo Rajasalu, Oivi Uibo, Vallo Tillmann, Raivo Uibo. Antigenic Proteins Of Lactobacillus Acidophilus That Are Recognised By Serum IgG antibodies In Children With Type 1 Diabetes And Celiac Disease. *Pediatr Allergy Immunol.* 2009 Jul 2. http://www.ncbi.nlm.nih.gov/pubmed/19573144

Chapter 19

1. Barrett KE. Gastrointestinal Physiology. Lange Medical Books/McGraw-Hill 2006.

2. Marieb Elaine. Human Anatomy And Physiology. The Benjamin/Cummings Publishing Company, Inc.,1992.

3. Fasano A, Not T, Wang W, Uzzau S, Berti I, Tommasini A, Goldblum SE. Zonulin, a newly discovered modulator of intestinal permeability, and it's expression in coeliac disease. *Lancet,* 2000 Apr 29;355(9214):1518-9

4. Marsh, Michael N.; Miller, Victor. Studies of Intestinal Lymphoid Tissue. VIII. Use of Epithelial Lymphocyte Mitotic Indices in Differentiating Untreated Celiac Sprue Mucosa from Other Childhood Enteropathies. *Journal of Pediatric Gastroenterology and Nutrition*:

5. Feldman Mark, MD, Friedman Lawrence S, MD, Sleisenger, Marvin H, MD, Gastrointestinal and Liver Disease Pathophysiology/Diagnosis/Management 7th Edition, Volume11, 2002,Saunders

6. Ghana VAST Study Team. Vitamin A Supplementaion in Northern Ghana: Effects on Clinic Attendances, hospital admissions, and child mortality. *Lancet* 1993;342:7-12.

7. Hossain S, Biswas R, Kabir I, et el. Single Dose Vitamin A Treatment In Acute Shigellosis In Bangladesh Children: Randomized Double Blind Controlled Trial. *BMJ* 1998;316:422-6.

8. Barreto M, Santos L,Assis A, et el. Effect of Vitamin A Supplementaion On Diarrhea and Acute Lower Respiratory Tract Infections In Young Children In Brazil. *Lancet* 1994;344:228-31.

9. Bhandari N, Bhan M, Sazawal S. Impact of Massive Dose of Vitamin A Given to Preschool Children With Acute Diarrhea On Subsequent Respiratory and Diarrhoeal Morbidity. *BMJ* 1994;309:1404-7.

10. Warden RA, Strazzari MJ, Dunkley PR, O'Loughlin EV. Vitamin A Deficient Rats Have Only Mild Changes In Jejunal structure and Function. *J Nutr* 1996;126:1817-26.

11. Rojanapo W, Lamb AJ, Olsen JA. The Prevalence, Metabolism And Migration of Goblet Cells in Rat Intestine Following The Induction of Rapid, Synchronous Vitamin A Deficiency. *J Nutr* 1980;110:178-88.

12. Ahmed F, Jones DB, Jackson AA. The Interaction of Vitamin A Deficiency and Rotavirus infection In the Mouse. *Br J Nutr* 1990;63:363-73.

13. Gibney MJ, Vorster HH, Kok FJ. Introduction to Human Nutrition. Blackwell Publishing 2002.

14. Gibney MJ, Marinos E, Olle L, Dowsett J. Clinical Nutrition. Blackwell Publishing 2005.

15. Drago S, El Asmar R, Di Pierro M, Grazia Clemente M, Tripathi A, Sapone A, Thakar M, Iacono G, Carroccio A, D'Agate C, Not T, Zampini L, Catassi C, Fasano A. Gliadin, zonulin and gut permeability: Effects on celiac and non-celiac

intestinal mucosa and intestinal cell lines. *Scand J Gastroenterol.* 2006 Apr;41(4):408-19.

16. Friedman SL, McQuaid KR,Grendall JH. Current Diagnosis and Treatment in Gastroenterology. Lange Medical Books/McGraw-Hill. 2nd Edition 2003.

17. Radivoj V. Krstic. Human Microscopic Anatomy: An Atlas For Students Of Mediicine And Biology. Springer; 1st ed. 1991. Corr. 3rd printing edition (Mar 18 2004).

18. Helga Fritsch and Wolfgang Kuehnel. Color Atlas of Human Anatomy: internal organs v. 2 Thieme Publishing Group; 5th Revised edition edition (Nov 21 2007).

19. Arnaldo Cantani. Pediatric Allergy, Asthma and Immunology. Springer; 1 edition (Feb 6 2008).

20. Scott H. Sicherer, M.D. Manifestations Of Food Allergies: Evaluation And management. *American Family Physician*, 1999.

21. D. D. Metcalfe, Hugh Sampson, and Ronald Simon. Food Allergy: Adverse reactions to food and food additives. Wiley-Blackwell; 3 edition (Jun 16 2003)

22. Yezid Gutierrez. Diagnostic Pathology of Parasitic Infections With Clinical Correlations. Oxford University Press; Second Edition edition (Dec 15 1999).

23. University of Maryland Medical Center. Dr. Alessio Fasano MD. Researchers Find Increased Zonulin levels Among Celiac Disease Patients, Public Release 28-Apr 2000.

24. Tursi A,Brandimarte G, Giorgetti G. High Prevalence of Small Intestinal Bacterial Overgrowth in Celiac Patients With Persistance of Gastrointestinal Symptoms After Gluten Withdrawl. *Am J Gastroenterol* 98(4):839-43

25. Alessio Fasano, M.D. Physiological, Pathological, and Therapeutic Implications of Zonulin-Mediated Intestinal Barrier Modulation. *American Journal of Pathology*, 2008;173:1243-1252.

26. Anna-Liisa Prangli, Meeme Utt, Ija Talja, Epp Sepp, Marika Mikelsaar, Tarvo Rajasalu, Oivi Uibo, Vallo Tillmann, Raivo Uibo. Antigenic Proteins Of Lactobacillus Acidophilus That Are Recognised By Serum IgG antibodies In Children With Type 1 Diabetes And Celiac Disease. *Pediatr Allergy Immunol.* 2009 Jul 2.

http://www.ncbi.nlm.nih.gov/pubmed/19573144

Chapter 20

1. Vuoristo M, MiettinenTA. The Role Of Fat And Bile Acid Malabsorption in Diarrhoea Of Coeliac Disease. *Scand J Gastroenterol* 22:289, 1987.

2. Gibney MJ, Marinos E, Olle L, Dowsett J. Clinical Nutrition. Blackwell Publishing 2005.

3. James Braly, Patrick Holford. Hidden Food Allergies: The Essential Guide To Uncovering Hidden Food Allergies—And Achieving Permanent Relief. Fitzhenry & Whiteside Ltd.; 1 edition (2006)

4. Feldman Mark, MD, Friedman Lawrence S, MD, Sleisenger, Marvin H, MD, Gastrointestinal and Liver Disease Pathophysiology/Diagnosis/Management 7th Edition, Volume11, 2002,Saunders

5. Fasano A, Not T, Wang W, Uzzau S, Berti I, Tommasini A, Goldblum SE. Zonulin, a newly discovered modulator of intestinal permeability, and it's expression in coeliac disease. *Lance*t, 2000 Apr 29;355(9214):1518-9.

6. Drago S, El Asmar R, Di Pierro M, Grazia Clemente M, Tripathi A, Sapone A, Thakar M, Iacono G, Carroccio A, D'Agate C, Not T, Zampini L, Catassi C, Fasano A. Gliadin, zonulin and gut permeability: Effects on celiac and non-celiac intestinal mucosa and intestinal cell lines. *Scand J Gastroenterol.* 2006 Apr;41(4):408-19.

7. University of Maryland Medical Center. Dr. Alessio Fasano MD. Researchers Find Increased Zonulin levels Among Celiac Disease Patients, Public Release 28-Apr 2000.

8. Rhodes RA, Tai HH, Chey WY. Impairment of Secretin Release in Celiac Sprue. *Am J Dig Dis* 23:833, 1978.

9. Maton PN, Seldon AC, Fitzpatrick ML, et al. Defective Gallbladder Emptying And Cholecystokinin Release In Celiac Disease. Reversal by Gluten-free Diet. Gastroenterology 88:391, 1985.

10. Tursi A,Brandimarte G, Giorgetti G. High Prevalence of Small Intestinal Bacterial Overgrowth in Celiac Patients With Persistance of Gastrointestinal Symptoms After Gluten Withdrawl. *Am J Gastroenterol* 98(4):839-43

11. Bateson-Koch Carolee. How to Permanently Heal Your Allergic Condition Permanently and Naturally. Alive Books 1994.

12. Alessio Fasano, M.D. Physiological, Pathological, and Therapeutic Implications of Zonulin-Mediated Intestinal Barrier Modulation. *American Journal of Pathology,* 2008;173:1243-1252.

13. Kate E Evans, John S leeds, Stephen Morley, David S Sanders. Pancreatic Insufficiency In Adult Celiac Disease: Do Patients Require Long-Term Enzyme Supplementation? *Digestive Diseases and Sciences,* Springer netherlands, May 11,

2010.

14.   Ge De Palma, J Cinova, R Stepankova, L Tuckova, Y Sanz. Pivotal Advance: Bifidobacteria And Gram-Negative Bacteria Differentially Influence Immune In The Proinflammatory Milieu Of Celiac Disease. *Journal of Leukocyte Biology*, 2009.

15.   Devlin Shane MD, Andrews Christopher MD, beck Paul MD, Celiac Disease. *CME Update* May 2004.

16.   Feldman Mark, MD, Friedman Lawrence S, MD, Sleisenger, Marvin H, MD, Gastrointestinal and Liver Disease Pathophysiology/Diagnosis/Management 7th Edition, Volume11, 2002,Saunders

17.   Kagnoff MF. AGA Institute Medical Position Statement on the Diagnosis and Management of CD. Gastroenterology, *Official Journal of the American Gastroenterological Association* (AGA). December 2006.

18.   Gary B Huffnagle with Sarah Wernick. The Probiotics Revolution. Bantam Books, 2007.

19.   Alessio Fasano, MD.. Celiac Disease. University Of Maryland School Of Medicine, Baltimore, MD. *AGA Instiute Focussed Clinical Updates,* May 20th and 21st, 2007.

20.   JH Ovelgonne, JFJG Koninkxa, A Pusztaib, S bardoczb, W Koka, SWB Ewenc, HGCJM Hendriksa, JE van Dijka. Decreased levels of heat shock proteins in gut epithelial cells after exposure to plant lectins. *Gut.* 2000 May;46(5):679-87.

21.   Wheat germ agglutinin induces NADPH-oxidase activity in human neutrophils by interaction with mobilizable receptors. *Infection and Immunity.*1999 Jul;67(7):3461-8.

22.   Gloria V. Guzyeyeva. Lectin Glycosylation As A Marker of Thin Gut inflammation. *The FASEB Journal.* 2008;22:898.3

23.   A. Pusztai, S. W. B. Ewen, G. Grant, D. S. Brown, J. C. Stewart, W. J. Peumans, E. J. M. Van Damme and S. Bardocz Antinutritive effects of wheat-germ agglutinin and other N-acetylglucosamine-specific lectins.*The British Journal of Nutrition* 1993 Jul;70(1):313-21.

24.   Tchernychev B, Wilchek M.. Natural human antibodies to dietary lectins. *FEBS Lett.*1996 Nov 18;397(2-3):139-42.

25.   Broadwell RD, Balin BJ, Salcman M.. Transcytotic pathway for blood-borne protein through the blood-brain barrier.Proceedings from the National Academy of Sciences U S A. 1988 Jan;85(2):632-6.

26. Damak S, Mosinger B, Margolskee RF. Transsynaptic transport of wheat germ agglutinin expressed in a subset of type II taste cells of transgenic mice. *BMC Neuroscience.*2008 Oct 2;9:96.

27. Dolapchieva S. Distribution of concanavalin A and wheat germ agglutinin binding sites in the rat peripheral nerve fibres revealed by lectin/glycoprotein-gold histochemistry. *TheHistochem Journal.*1996 Jan;28(1):7-12.

28. Hashimoto S, Hagino A. Wheat germ agglutinin, concanavalin A, and lens culinalis agglutinin block the inhibitory effect of nerve growth factor on cell-free phosphorylation of Nsp100 in PC12h cells. *Cell Struct and Function* 1989 Feb;14(1):87-93.

29. Liu WK, Sze SC, Ho JC, Liu BP, Yu MC. Wheat germ lectin induces G2/M arrest in mouse L929 fibroblasts. *J Cell Biochem.* 2004 Apr 15;91(6):1159-73

30. Yevdokimova NY, Yefimov AS. Effects of wheat germ agglutinin and concanavalin A on the accumulation of glycosaminoglycans in pericellular matrix of human dermal fibroblasts. A comparison with insulin.*Acta Biochim Pol.*2001;48(2):563-72.

31. Sasano H, Rojas M, Silverberg SG. Analysis of lectin binding in benign and malignant thyroid nodules. *Arch Pathol Lab Med.*1989 Feb;113(2):186-9.

32. Lebret M, Rendu F. Further characterization of wheat germ agglutinin interaction with human platelets: exposure of fibrinogen receptors. *Thromb Haemost.*1986 Dec 15;56(3):323-7.

33. Ohmori T, Yatomi Y, Wu Y, Osada M, Satoh K, Ozaki Y. Wheat germ agglutinin-induced platelet activation via platelet endothelial cell adhesion molecule-1: involvement of rapid phospholipase C gamma 2 activation by Src family kinases. *Biochemistry.* 2001 Oct 30;40(43):12992-3001

34. Prangli AL, Utt M, Talja I, Sepp E, Mikelsaar M, Rajasalu T, Uibo O, Tillmann V, Uibo R. Antigenic proteins of Lactobacillus acidophilus that are recognised by serum IgG antibodies in children with type 1 diabetes and coeliac disease. *Pediatr Allergy Immunol.* 2010 Jun;21(4 Pt 2):e772-9.

35. Anna-Liisa Prangli, Meeme Utt, Ija Talja, Epp Sepp, Marika Mikelsaar, Tarvo Rajasalu, Oivi Uibo, Vallo Tillmann, Raivo Uibo. Antigenic Proteins Of Lactobacillus Acidophilus That Are Recognised By Serum IgG antibodies In Children With Type 1 Diabetes And Celiac Disease. *Pediatr Allergy Immunol.* 2009 Jul 2. http://www.ncbi.nlm.nih.gov/pubmed/19573144

Chapter 21

1. Lindeberg, Staffan (June 2005). "Palaeolithic diet ("stone age" diet)". *Scandinavian Journal of Food & Nutrition* 49 (2): 75–7.

2. Specific Carbohydrate Diet www.breakingtheviciouscycle.info

3. Specific Carbohydrate Diet

    www.breakingtheviciouscycle.info/beginners_guide/beginners.htm.

4. Paleolithic Diet. Wikipedia http://en.wikipedia.org/wiki/Paleolithic_diet

5. Jönsson T, Ahrén B, Pacini G, Sundler F, Wierup N, Steen S, Sjöberg T, Ugander M, Frostegård J, Göransson L, Lindeberg S. A Paleolithic diet confers higher insulin sensitivity, lower C-reactive protein and lower blood pressure than a cereal-based diet in domestic pigs. Nutr Metab (Lond). 2006 Nov 2;3:39.

6. Website: http://dogtorj.com. Information about a glutamic acid or aspartic acid sensitivity.

7. Website: www.greatplainslaboratory.com/home/eng/peptide.asp.

8. A. Pusztai. Plant Lectins. Cambridge University Press, 1991.

9. James Braly, Patrick Holford. Hidden Food Allergies: The Essential Guide To Uncovering Hidden Food Allergies—And Achieving Permanent Relief. Fitzhenry & Whiteside Ltd.; 1 edition (2006)

10. Carolee Bateson-Koch DC ND. Allergies, Disease In Disguise. How To Heal Your Allergic Condition Permanently And Naturally. Alive Books, 1994.

Chapter 22

1. Hallert C, Grant C, Grehn S, Grännö C, Hultén S, Midhagen G, Ström M, Svensson H, Valdimarsson T. Evidence of poor vitamin status in coeliac patients on a gluten-free diet for 10 years. *Aliment Pharmacol Ther.* 2002 Jul;16(7):1333-9.

2. Management After the diagnosis of Celiac Disease.

    http://www.celiacdiseasecenter.columbia.edu/C_Doctors/C07-Management.htm

3. Devlin Shane MD, Andrews Christopher MD, beck Paul MD, Celiac Disease. *CME* Update May 2004.

4. Kagnoff MF. AGA Institute Medical Position Statement on the Diagnosis and Management of CD. Gastroenterology, *Official Journal of the American Gastroenterological Association* (AGA). December 2006.

Chapter 23

1. Bateson-Koch, DC, ND. *Allergies, Disease In Disguise. How To Heal Your Allergic Condition Permanently And Naturally.* Alive Books. 1994.

2. Dr. Devi S. Nambudripad, MD, DC, Lac, PhD (Acu). www.naet.com

Chapter 24

1. Bulajic M, CuperlovicM, Movsesinjan IM, Borojevil D. Interaction of dietary lectin (phytohemagglutinin) with the mucosa of rat digestive tract. *Immunofluorescence Studies. Periodicum Biologorum*, 38, 331-76, 1986.

2. Gloria V. Guzyeyeva. Lectin Glycosylation As A Marker of Thin Gut inflammation. *The FASEB Journal.* 2008;22:898.3

3. D Bernardo, J A Garrote, L Fernandez-Salazar, S Riestra, E Arranz. Is gliadin really safe for non-coeliac individuals? Production of interleukin 15 in biopsy culture from non-coeliac individuals challenged with gliadin peptides *Gut* 2007;56:889-890

4. A. Pusztai, S. W. B. Ewen, G. Grant, D. S. Brown, J. C. Stewart, W. J. Peumans, E. J. M. Van Damme and S. Bardocz. Antinutritive effects of wheat-germ agglutinin and other N-acetylglucosamine-specific lectins. *The British Journal of Nutrition* 1993 Jul;70(1):313-21.

5. Borges LF, Sidman RL.Axonal transport of lectins in the peripheral nervous system. *Journal Of Neuroscience*, 2, pg. 647-53, 1982.

6. Tchernychev B, Wilchek M.. Natural human antibodies to dietary lectins. *FEBS Lett.*1996 Nov 18;397(2-3):139-42.

7. Broadwell RD, Balin BJ, Salcman M.. Transcytotic pathway for blood-borne protein through the blood-brain barrier. *Proceedings from the National Academy of Sciences* U S A. 1988 Jan;85(2):632-6.

8. Begbic R, King TP. The interaction of dietary lectin with porcine small intestine and production of lectin-specific antibodies. In Lectins Biology, Biochemistry, *Clinical Biochemistry* (Bog-Hansen TC, Breborovicz J eds). Vol 4, pages 15-27. Walter de Gruyter, Berlin and New York, 1985.

9. Dolapchieva S. Distribution of concanavalin A and wheat germ agglutinin binding sites in the rat peripheral nerve fibres revealed by lectin/glycoprotein-gold histochemistry. *The Histo Chem Journal.*1996 Jan;28(1):7-12.

10. Boldt DH, Banwell JG. Binding of isolectins from red kidney bean (phaseolus vulgaris) to purified rat brush border membranes, *Biochimia et Biophysica Acta* 843, 230-7, 1985.

11. Hashimoto S, Hagino A. Wheat germ agglutinin, concanavalin A, and lens culinalis agglutinin block the inhibitory effect of nerve growth factor on cell-free phosphorylation of Nsp100 in PC12h cells. *Cell Struct and Function* 1989 Feb;14(1):87-93.

12. Hadjivassiliou M, Sanders DS, Grünewald RA, Woodroofe N, Boscolo S, Aeschlimann D. Gluten sensitivity: from gut to brain. *Lancet* Neurol. 2010 Mar;9(3):318-30.

13. Feldman Mark, MD, Friedman Lawrence S, MD, Sleisenger, Marvin H, MD, Gastrointestinal and Liver Disease Pathophysiology/Diagnosis/Management 7th Edition, Volume11, 2002,Saunders

14. Alessio Fasano, M.D. Physiological, Pathological, and Therapeutic Implications of Zonulin-Mediated Intestinal Barrier Modulation. *American Journal of Pathology,* 2008;173:1243-1252.

15. Alessio Fasano. Celiac Disease Insights: Clues To Solving Autoimmunity. *Scientific American,* 2009.

16. Gary B. Huffnagle, PhD with Sarah Wernick. The Probiotics Revolution. Bantam Dell, A Division Of Random House, Inc. 2007.

Chapter 25

1. Fasano A, Not T, Wang W, Uzzau S, Berti I, Tommasini A, Goldblum SE. Zonulin, a newly discovered modulator of intestinal permeability, and it's expression in coeliac disease. *Lancet,* 2000 Apr 29;355(9214):1518-9

2. Drago S, El Asmar R, Di Pierro M, Grazia Clemente M, Tripathi A, Sapone A, Thakar M, Iacono G, Carroccio A, D'Agate C, Not T, Zampini L, Catassi C, Fasano A. Gliadin, zonulin and gut permeability: Effects on celiac and non-celiac intestinal mucosa and intestinal cell lines. *Scand J Gastroenterol.* 2006 Apr;41(4):408-19.

3. Dr. Alessio Fasano MD. University of Maryland Medical Center.. Researchers Find Increased Zonulin levels Among Celiac Disease Patients, Public Release 28-Apr 2000.

4. Alessio Fasano, M.D. Physiological, Pathological, and Therapeutic Implications of Zonulin-Mediated Intestinal Barrier Modulation. American *Journal of Pathology,* 2008;173:1243-1252.

5. Alberto Rubio-Tapia, Robert A. Kyle, Edward L. Kaplan, Dwight R. Johnson, William Page, Fredrick Erdtmann, Tricia L. Brantner, W. Ray Kim, Tara K. Phelps, Brian D. Lahr, Alan R. Zinsmeister, L. Joseph Melton, Joseph A. Murray. Increased Prevalence and Mortality in Undiagnosed Celiac Disease. *Gastroenterology.* Volume 137, Issue1, Pages 88-93 (July 2009).

6. Gibney MJ, Marinos E, Olle L, Dowsett J. Clinical Nutrition. Blackwell Publishing 2005.

7. Gary B. Huffnagle, PhD with Sarah Wernick. The Probiotics Revolution. Bantam Dell, A Division Of Random House, Inc. 2007.

8. Alessio Fasano. Celiac Disease Insights: Clues To Solving Autoimmunity. *Scientific American,* 2009.

9. Fasano A, Not T, Wang W, Uzzau S, Berti I, Tommasini A, Goldblum SE. Zonulin, a newly discovered modulator of intestinal permeability, and it's expression in coeliac disease. *Lancet,* 2000 Apr 29;355(9214):1518-9.

10. Gibson PG, Henry RL, Shah S, Powell H, Wang H (September 2003). "Migration to a western country increases asthma symptoms but not eosinophilic airway inflammation". *Pediatr. Pulmonol.* 36 (3): 209–15.

11. Addo-Yobo EO, Woodcock A, Allotey A, Baffoe-Bonnie B, Strachan D, Custovic A (February 2007). "Exercise-induced bronchospasm and atopy in Ghana: two surveys ten years apart". *PLoS Med.* 4 (2): e70.

12. Marra F, Lynd L, Coombes M "et al." (2006). "Does antibiotic exposure during infancy lead to development of asthma?: a systematic review and metaanalysis". *Chest* 129 (3): 610-8.

13. Zock JP, Plana E, Jarvis D "et al." (2007). "The use of household cleaning sprays and adult asthma: an international longitudinal study". *Am J Respir Crit Care Med* 176 (8): 735–41.

14. Folkerts G, Walzl G, Openshaw PJ. Do common childhood infections 'teach' the immune system not to be allergic? *Immunol Today* 2000; 21(3):118-120.

15. Liu Z, Li N, Neu J. Tight junctions, leaky intestines, and pediatric diseases. *Acta Paediatrica,* 2005; 94:386-393.

16. Gary B. Huffnagle, PhD with Sarah Wernick. The Probiotics Revolution. Bantam Dell, A Division Of Random House, Inc. 2007.

17. Fasano A, Not T, Wang W, Uzzau S, Berti I, Tommasini A, Goldblum SE. Zonulin, a newly discovered modulator of intestinal permeability, and it's expression in coeliac disease. *Lancet,* 2000 Apr 29;355(9214):1518-9.

18. Bufford JD, Gern JE (May 2005). "The hygiene hypothesis revisited". *Immunol Allergy Clin North Am* 25 (2): 247–62, v–vi.

19. Gloria V. Guzyeyeva. Lectin Glycosylation As A Marker of Thin Gut inflammation. *The FASEB Journal.* 2008;22:898.3

20. TM McKeever, SA Lewis, C Smith, J Collins, H heatlie, M frischer, And R Hubbard. Early Exposure To Infections, Antibiotics, And The Incidence Of Allergic Disease: A Birth Cohort Study With The West Midlands General Practice Research Database. *Journal Of Allergy And Clinical Immunology.* Volume 109, Issue 1, Pages 43-50, January 2002.

21. B Björkstén, P Naaber, E Sepp, and M Mikelsaar. The Intestinal Microflora In Allergic Estonian And Swedish 2 Year Old Children. *Clinical And Experimental Allergy* 29 (3): 342-6, 1999.

22. MC Noverr, GB Huffnagle. The Microflora Hypothesis Of Allergic Diseases. *Clinical And Experimental Allergy* 35:1511, 2005.

23. MF Wang, HC Lin, YY Yang, and CH Hsu. Treatment Of Perennial Allergic Rhinitis With Lactic Acid Bacteria. *Pediatric Allergy And Immunology* 15:152, 2004.

24. H Kim, K Kwack, DY Kim, and GE Ji. Oral Probiotic Bacterial Administration Suppressed Allergic Responses In An Ovalbumin-Induced Allergy Mouse Model. *FEMS Immunology And Medical Microbiology.* Volume 45, Issue 2, pages 259-267, august 2005.

25. H Majamaa, E Isolauri. Probiotics: A Novel Approach In The Management Of Food Allergy. *Journal Of Allergy And Clinical Immunology.* Volume 99, Issue 2, pages 179-185, February 1997.

Chapter 26

1. S C Daminet. Gluten sensitive enteropathy in a family of Irish setters. *Can Vet J.* 1996 December; 37(12): 745–746.

2. Michael J Day. The Canine Model Of Dietary Hypersensitivity. *Proceeding Of The Nutrition Society.* 2004, 64, 458-464.

3. EJ Hall. Gastrointestinal Aspects Of Food Allergies. *Journal of Small Animal Practice.* Volume 35, Issue 3, pages 145-152, March 1994.

4. Chesney CJ. Systematic review of evidence for the prevalence of food sensitivity in dogs. *Vet Rec.*2001 Apr 7;148(14):445-8.

5. Ermel RW, Kock M, Griffey SM, Reinhart GA, Frick OL.. *Lab Anim Sci.* The atopic dog: a model for food allergy. 1997 Feb;47(1):40-9.

6. AJ German, EJ Hall. Immune cell populations within the intestinal mucosa of dogs with enteropathies. *Journal of Veterinary Internal Medicine.* Volume 15, Issue 1, pages 14–25, January 2001.

7. Peter Hill PhD, Diploma in Veterinary Dermatology Diagnosing cutaneous food allergies in dogs and cats - some practical considerations. *In Practice* 21: 287-294 (1999).

8. J Willis, R Harvey. Diagnosis and management of food allergy and intolerance in dogs and cats. *Aust Vet J.* 1994 Oct;71(10):322-6.

Chapter 27

1. University School Of Medicine

    http://somvweb.som.umaryland.edu/absolutenm/templates/?a=1302&z=5

2. Alberto Rubio-Tapia, Robert A. Kyle, Edward L. Kaplan, Dwight R. Johnson, William Page, Frederick Erdtmann, Tricia L. Brantner, W. Ray Kim, Tara K. Phelps, Brian D. Lahr, Alan R. Zinsmeister, Joseph Melton III, Joseph A. Murray. Increased Prevalence and Mortality in Undiagnosed Celiac Disease. *Gastroenterology*, Volume 137, Issue 1 , Pages 88-93, July 2009.

3. MR Langlois and JR Delanghe. Biological and clinical significance of haptoglobinAlberto Rubio–Tapia polymorphism in humans. *Clinical Chemistry,* Vol 42, 1589-1600.

4. LM Solid, J Kolberg, H Scott, J Ek, O Fausa, P Brandtzaeg. Antibodies to wheat germ agglutinin in coeliac disease. *Clin Exp Immunol.* 1986 January; 63(1): 95–100.

5. K. Fälth-Magnusson, K.-E. Magnusson,Elevated levels of serum antibodies to the lectin wheat germ agglutinin in celiac children lend support to the gluten-lectin theory of celiac disease. *Pediatr Allergy Immunol.* 1995 may;6(2):98-102.

6. JH Ovelgonne, JFJG Koninkxa, A Pusztaib, S bardoczb, W Koka, SWB Ewenc, HGCJM Hendriksa, JE van Dijka. Decreased levels of heat shock proteins in gut epithelial cells after exposure to plant lectins. *Gut.* 2000 May;46(5):679-87.

7. David L J Freed, Allergist. Do dietary lectins cause disease? The evidence is suggestive—and raises interesting possibilities for treatment. *BMJ.* 1999 April 17; 318(7190): 1023–1024.

8. Critical Molecule To Celiac Disease, Possibly Other Autoimmune Disorders, Pinpointed By UM Scientists.

    http://www.medicalnewstoday.com/articles/163204.php

9. Maresca M, Fantini J. Some Food Associated Mycotoxins As Potiential Risk Factors In Humans Predisposed To Chronic Intestinal Inflammatory Diseases. *Toxicon* 2010, May 11.

10. Evalotte Decker, Guido Engelmann, Annette Findeisen, Patrick Gerner, martin LaaB, Dietrich Ney. Cesarean Delivery Is Associated With Celiac Disease, But Not inflammatory Bowel Disease In Children. *Pediatrics*, May 17th, 2010.

11. Keith T Atherton. Genetically Modified Crops: Assessing Safety. CRC Press; 1 edition (Sep 12 2002)

12. Colic In Babies May Be Caused By Gut Bacteria.

    http://www.sciencedaily.com/releases/2009/07/090724144520.htm

    Their reference: From July 23, *Journal of Pediatrics*

13. Paul E Ewald. Plague Time, The New Germ Theory Of Disease. Anchor Books. 2002.

14. Alessio Fasano. Celiac Disease Insights: Clues To Solving Autoimmunity. *Scientific American,* 2009.

15. Caelie Haines, Web Editor. University Of Maryland School Of Medicine Scientists Pinpoint Critical Molecule To Celiac, Possibly Other Autoimmune Disorders. http://somvweb.som.umaryland.edu/absolutenm/templates/?a=915.   September 29th, 2009.

16. Dina Rosendorff. Worms Linked To Coeliac Relief. *ABC News.*

    http://www.abc.net.au/news/stories/2009/10/22/2721267.htm

17. AK Akobeng, AV Ramanan, I Buchan, RF Heller. Effect Of Breast Feeding On Risk Of Coeliac Disease: A Systematic Review And Meta-Analysis Of Observational Studies. *Arch Dis Child*, 2006 January 91 (1): 39-43.

18. Strachan DP (November 1989). "Hay Fever, Hygiene, And Household Size". *BMJ* 299 (6710): 1259–60.

19. Bufford JD, Gern JE (May 2005). "The hygiene hypothesis revisited". *Immunol Allergy Clin* North Am 25 (2): 247–62, v–vi.

20. Zanoni G, Navone R, Lunardi C, Tridente G, Bason C, Sivori S, Beri R, Dolcino M, Valletta E, Corrocher R, Puccetti A (2006). "In celiac disease, a subset of autoantibodies against transglutaminase binds toll-like receptor 4 and induces activation of monocytes". *PLoS Med* 3 (9): e358.

21. Salim A, Phillips A, Farthing M (1990). "Pathogenesis of gut virus infection". *Baillieres Clin Gastroenterol* 4 (3): 593–607.

22. Sompayrac Lauren. How The Immune System Works. Blackwell Publishing, 2nd edition, 2003.

23. van den Broeck HC, de Jong HC, Salentijn EM, Dekking L, Bosch D, Hamer RJ, Gilissen LJ, van der Meer IM, Smulders MJ. Presence of celiac disease epitopes in modern and old hexaploid wheat varieties: wheat breeding may have contributed to increased prevalence of celiac disease. *Theor Appl Genet.* 2010 Jul 28.

24. Farhadi A, Banan A, Fields J, Keshavarzian A. Intestinal barrier: an interface between health and disease. *Journal of gastroenterology and hepatology.* 2003; 18:479-497.

25. Liu Z, Li N, Neu J. Tight junctions, leaky intestines, and pediatric diseases. *Acta Paediatrica,* 2005; 94:386-393.

26. Gary B. Huffnagle, PhD with Sarah Wernick. The Probiotics Revolution. Bantam Dell, A Division Of Random House, Inc. 2007.

27. Fasano A, Not T, Wang W, Uzzau S, Berti I, Tommasini A, Goldblum SE. Zonulin, a newly discovered modulator of intestinal permeability, and it's expression in coeliac disease. *Lancet,* 2000 Apr 29;355(9214):1518-9.

28. G Sigthorsson, J Tibble, J Hayllar, I Menzies, A Macpherson, R Moots, D Scott, M Gumpel, and I Bjarnason. Intestinal permeability and inflammation in patients on NSAIDs. *Gut.* 1998 October; 43(4): 506–511.

29. Dr. Loren Cordain. 2007 video, "Potential Therapeutic Characteristics of Pre-agri-cultural Diets In The Prevention And Treatment Of Multiple Sclerosis" http://wildhorse.insinc.com/directms03oct2007/.

30. Folkerts G, Walzl G, Openshaw PJ. Do common childhood infections 'teach' the immune system not to be allergic? *Immunol Today* 2000; 21(3):118-120.

31. Thavagnanam S, Fleming J, Bromley A, Shields MD, Cardwell, CR (2007). "A meta-analysis of the association between Caesarean section and childhood asthma". *Clin. And Exper. Allergy* (4): 629.

32. JH Ovelgonne, JFJG Koninkxa, A Pusztaib, S bardoczb, W Koka, SWB Ewenc, HGCJM Hendriksa, JE van Dijka. Decreased levels of heat shock proteins in gut epithelial cells after exposure to plant lectins. *Gut.* 2000 May;46(5):679-87.

33. Wheat germ agglutinin induces NADPH-oxidase activity in human neutrophils by interaction with mobilizable receptors. *Infection and Immunity.*1999 Jul;67(7):3461-8.

34. Gloria V. Guzyeyeva. Lectin Glycosylation As A Marker of Thin Gut inflammation. *The FASEB Journal.* 2008;22:898.3

35. A. Pusztai, S. W. B. Ewen, G. Grant, D. S. Brown, J. C. Stewart, W. J. Peumans, E. J. M. Van Damme and S. Bardocz. Antinutritive effects of wheat-germ agglutinin and other N-acetylglucosamine-specific lectins.*The British Journal of Nutrition* 1993 Jul;70(1):313-21.

36. Tchernychev B, Wilchek M.. Natural human antibodies to dietary lectins. *FEBS Lett.*1996 Nov 18;397(2-3):139-42.

37. Broadwell RD, Balin BJ, Salcman M.. Transcytotic pathway for blood-borne protein through the blood-brain barrier.Proceedings from the National Academy of Sciences U S A. 1988 Jan;85(2):632-6.

38. Damak S, Mosinger B, Margolskee RF. Transsynaptic transport of wheat germ agglutinin expressed in a subset of type II taste cells of transgenic mice. *BMC Neuroscience.*2008 Oct 2;9:96.

39. Dolapchieva S. Distribution of concanavalin A and wheat germ agglutinin binding sites in the rat peripheral nerve fibres revealed by lectin/glycoprotein-gold histochemistry. *TheHistochem Journal.*1996 Jan;28(1):7-12.

40. Hashimoto S, Hagino A. Wheat germ agglutinin, concanavalin A, and lens culinalis agglutinin block the inhibitory effect of nerve growth factor on cell-free phosphorylation of Nsp100 in PC12h cells. *Cell Struct and Function* 1989 Feb;14(1):87-93.

41. Liu WK, Sze SC, Ho JC, Liu BP, Yu MC. Wheat germ lectin induces G2/M arrest in mouse L929 fibroblasts. *J Cell Biochem.* 2004 Apr 15;91(6):1159-73

42. Yevdokimova NY, Yefimov AS. Effects of wheat germ agglutinin and concanavalin A on the accumulation of glycosaminoglycans in pericellular matrix of human dermal fibroblasts. A comparison with insulin. *Acta Biochim Pol.*2001;48(2):563-72.

43. Sasano H, Rojas M, Silverberg SG. Analysis of lectin binding in benign and malignant thyroid nodules. *Arch Pathol Lab Med.*1989 Feb;113(2):186-9.

44. Lebret M, Rendu F. Further characterization of wheat germ agglutinin interaction with human platelets: exposure of fibrinogen receptors.*Thromb Haemost.*1986 Dec 15;56(3):323-7.

45. Ohmori T, Yatomi Y, Wu Y, Osada M, Satoh K, Ozaki Y. Wheat germ agglutinin-induced platelet activation via platelet endothelial cell adhesion molecule-1: involvement of rapid phospholipase C gamma 2 activation by Src family kinases. *Biochemistry.* 2001 Oct 30;40(43):12992-3001

46. Evolutionary Aspects of Nutrition and Health: Diet, Exercise, Genetics and Chronic Disease. World Review of Nutrition and Dietetics, vol. 84. Edited by A. P. Simopoulos. Basel: Karger. 1999. Pp. 145. Book review: SE Humphries. *Annals of Human Genetics* Volume 63, Issue 4, pages 377–381, July 1999

47. Neolithic Revolution. http://en.wikipedia.org/wiki/Neolithic_Revolution

48. Anil K Gupta. Review article PDF: Origin of agriculture and domestication of plants and animals linked to early Holocene climate amelioration. Dept. of Geology and Geophysics, Indian institute of Technology, Kharagpur 721 302, India.

49. Triticeae glutens www.wikipedia.org (accessed August 2010)

50. Gluten www.wikipedia.org

51. Tamed 11,400 Years Ago, Figs Were Likely First Domesticated Crop. Science daily.

    http://www.sciencedaily.com/releases/2006/06/060602074522.htm

52. Sompayrac Lauren. How The Immune System Works. Blackwell Publishing, 2nd edition, 2003.

53. Ceri H, Falkenberg-Anderson K, Fang R, Costerton JW, howard R and Barnwell JG. Bacteria-lectin interactions in phytohemagglutinin-induced bacterial overgrowth of the small intestine. *Canadian Journal Of microbiology* 34, 1003-8, 1988.

54. Carpender G, Cohen S. Influence of lectins on the binding of 125-1 labelled EGF to human fibroblasts. Biochemical And Biophysical Research Communications 79, pg. 545-52, 1977.

55. JH Ovelgonne, JFJG Koninkxa, A Pusztaib, S bardoczb, W Koka, SWB Ewenc, HGCJM Hendriksa, JE van Dijka. Decreased levels of heat shock proteins in gut epithelial cells after exposure to plant lectins. *Gut.* 2000 May;46(5):679-87.

56. Pusztia A, F Greer and G Grant. Specific uptake of dietary lectins into the systemic circulation of rats, *Biochem Soc. Trans.*, 17: 481-482, 1989.

57.   Pusztai A. Dietary lectins are metabolic signals for the gut and modulate immune and hormonal functions. *Eur. J. Clin. Nutr,* 47: 691-699, 1993.

58.   Vasconcelos IM and JT Oliveira. Antinutritional Properties Of Plant Lectins. *Toxicon,* 44: 385-403, 2004.

59.   Fabian RH, Coulter JD. Transneuronal transport of lectins. *Brain Research* 344, 41-48, 1985.

60.   Wheat germ agglutinin induces NADPH-oxidase activity in human neutrophils by interaction with mobilizable receptors. Infection and Immunity.1999 Jul;67(7):3461-8.

61.   Kidney bean (phaseolus vulgaris) lectin induced lesions in rat small intestine. 2 ultrastructural studies. *The Journal Of Comparitive Pathology* 92, 357-73, 1982.

62.   Zang J, D Li, X Piao and X Tang. Effects Of Soybean Agglutinin On Body Composition And Organ Weights In Rats. *Arch Anim Nutr.,* 60: 245-253, 2006.

63.   Brady PG, AM Vannier and JG Banwell. Identification of dietary lectin, wheat germ agglutinin, in human intestinal contents. *Gastroenterology,* 75: 236., 1978.

64.   Freed DLJ. Dietary lectins and the anti-nutritive effects of gut allergy. In: Protein Transmission Through Living Membranes. Elsevier/North Holland Biomedical Press, pages: 411-422, 1979.

65.   Bulajic M, CuperlovicM, Movsesinjan IM, Borojevil D. Interaction of dietary lectin (phytohemagglutinin) with the mucosa of rat digestive tract. *Immunofluorescence Studies. Periodicum Biologorum,* 38, 331-76, 1986.

66.   Gloria V. Guzyeyeva. Lectin Glycosylation As A Marker of Thin Gut inflammation. *The FASEB Journal.* 2008;22:898.3

67.   Underdown B, Schiff J (1986). "Immunoglobulin A: strategic defense initiative at the mucosal surface". *Annu Rev Immunol* 4: 389–417

68.   Chen K, Xu W, Wilson M, He B, Miller NW, Bengtén E, Edholm ES, Santini PA, Rath P, Chiu A, Cattalini M, Litzman J, B Bussel J, Huang B, Meini A, Riesbeck K, Cunningham-Rundles C, Plebani A, Cerutti A (2009). "Immunoglobulin D enhances immune surveillance by activating antimicrobial, proinflammatory and B cell-stimulating programs in basophils". *Nature Immunology* 10 (8): 889–98.

69.   Geisberger R, Lamers M, Achatz G (2006). "The riddle of the dual expression of IgM and IgD". *Immunology* 118 (4): 429–37.

70.   A. Pusztai. Plant Lectins. Cambridge University Press, 1991.

71.   Jönsson T, Ahrén B, Pacini G, Sundler F, Wierup N, Steen S, Sjöberg T, Ugander M, Frostegård J, Göransson L, Lindeberg S. A Paleolithic diet confers higher

insulin sensitivity, lower C-reactive protein and lower blood pressure than a cereal-based diet in domestic pigs. Nutr Metab (Lond). 2006 Nov 2;3:39.

72. Ludvig M. Sollid. Molecular Basis Of Celiac Disease. Annu. Rev. Immunol, 2000. 18:53-81.

73. Feldman Mark, MD, Friedman Lawrence S, MD, Sleisenger, Marvin H, MD, Gastrointestinal and Liver Disease Pathophysiology/Diagnosis/Management 7th Edition, Volume11, 2002,Saunders

74. Nieuwenhuizen WF, RH Peters, LM Knippels, MC Jansen, and SJ Koppelman. Is Candida Albicans A Trigger In The Onset Of Coeliac Disease? Lancet 361:2152, 2003.

75. Gary B. Huffnagle with Sarah Wernick. The Probiotics Revolution. The Definitive Guide To Safe Natural Health Solutions Using Probiotic And Prebiotic Foods And Supplements, 2007.

Chapter 28

1. Hausch F, Shan L, Santiago NA, Gray GM, Khosla C. Intestinal digestive resistance of immunodominant gliadin peptides. *Am J Physiol Gastrointest Liver Physiol.* 2002;283(4):G996–G1003.

2. Shan L, Qiao SW, Arentz-Hansen H, *et al* (2005). Identification and Analysis of Multivalent Proteolytically Resistant Peptides from Gluten: Implications for Celiac Sprue. *J. Proteome Res.* 4 (5): 1732–41.

3. Evolutionary Aspects of Nutrition and Health: Diet, Exercise, Genetics and Chronic Disease. World Review of Nutrition and Dietetics, vol. 84. Edited by A. P. Simopoulos. Basel: Karger. 1999. Pp. 145. Book review: SE Humphries. *Annals of Human Genetics* Volume 63, Issue 4, pages 377–381, July 1999

4. Neolithic Revolution. http://en.wikipedia.org/wiki/Neolithic_Revolution

5. Anil K Gupta. Review article PDF: Origin of agriculture and domestication of plants and animals linked to early Holocene climate amelioration. Dept. of Geology and Geophysics, Indian institute of Technology, Kharagpur 721 302, India.

6. Tamed 11,400 Years Ago, Figs Were Likely First Domesticated Crop. Science daily. http://www.sciencedaily.com/releases/2006/06/060602074522.htm

Alphabetical Index

A

B

L

M

N

339

Y

Z

CPSIA information can be obtained at www.ICGtesting.com
Printed in the USA
LVOW070744030612

284408LV00004B/4/P

9 781